Asthma

Editors

SUMITA B. KHATRI
SERPIL C. ERZURUM

CLINICS IN CHEST MEDICINE

www.chestmed.theclinics.com

March 2019 • Volume 40 • Number 1

ELSEVIER

1600 John F. Kennedy Boulevard • Suite 1800 • Philadelphia, Pennsylvania, 19103-2899

http://www.theclinics.com

CLINICS IN CHEST MEDICINE Volume 40, Number 1
March 2019 ISSN 0272-5231, ISBN-13: 978-0-323-65536-1

Editor: Colleen Dietzler
Developmental Editor: Casey Potter

Clinics in Chest Medicine (ISSN 0272-5231) is published quarterly by Elsevier Inc., 360 Park Avenue South, New York, NY 10010-1710. Months of issue are March, June, September, and December. Periodicals postage paid at New York, NY and additional mailing offices. Subscription prices are $377.00 per year (domestic individuals), $726.00 per year (domestic institutions), $100.00 per year (domestic students/residents), $423.00 per year (Canadian individuals), $902.00 per year (Canadian institutions), $484.00 per year (international individuals), $902.00 per year (international institutions), and $230.00 per year (international and Canadian students/residents). International air speed delivery is included in all Clinics subscription prices. All prices are subject to change without notice. **POSTMASTER:** Send address changes to Clinics in Chest Medicine, Elsevier Health Sciences Division, Subscription Customer Service, 3251 Riverport Lane, Maryland Heights, MO 63043. **Customer Service: Telephone: 1-800-654-2452** (U.S. and Canada); **1-314-447-8871** (outside U.S. and Canada). **Fax: 1-314-447-8029. E-mail: journalscustomerservice-usa@elsevier.com (for print support); journalsonlinesupport-usa@elsevier.com (for online support).**

Reprints. For copies of 100 or more of articles in this publication, please contact the Commercial Reprints Department, Elsevier Inc., 360 Park Avenue South, New York, NY 10010-1710. Tel.: 212-633-3874; Fax: 212-633-3820; E-mail: reprints@elsevier. com.

Clinics in Chest Medicine is covered in *MEDLINE/PubMed (Index Medicus), Current Contents/Clinical Medicine, EMBASE/ Excerpta Medica, Science Citation Index,* and *ISI/BIOMED.*

Contributors

EDITORS

SUMITA B. KHATRI, MD, MA
Co-Director, Asthma Center, Respiratory
Institute, Research Subject Advocate, Clinical
Research Unit, Associate Professor of
Medicine, Cleveland Clinic Lerner College of
Medicine, Case Western Reserve University
School of Medicine, Cleveland, Ohio, USA

SERPIL C. ERZURUM, MD
Chair, Lerner Research Institute, The Alfred
Lerner Memorial Chair in Innovative Biomedical
Research, Cleveland Clinic, Lerner Research
Institute, Cleveland, Ohio, USA

AUTHORS

RHONDA ALKATIB, MD
Fellow, Allergy and Immunology, Department
of Medicine, University of Arizona, Tucson,
Arizona, USA

MARK A. ARONICA, MD
Staff, Department of Pathobiology, Respiratory
Institute, Cleveland Clinic Lerner College of
Medicine, Case Western Reserve University,
Cleveland, Ohio, USA

KAY BOYCOTT, BA
Asthma UK, London, United Kingdom

STEVEN M. BRUNWASSER, PhD
Research Assistant Professor, Department of
Medicine, Division of Allergy, Pulmonary, and
Critical Care Medicine, Department of
Obstetrics and Gynecology, Vanderbilt
University Medical Center, Nashville,
Tennessee, USA

CARLOS A. CAMARGO Jr, MD, DrPH
Professor of Emergency Medicine,
Massachusetts General Hospital, Harvard
Medical School, Boston, Massachusetts, USA

TARA F. CARR, MD
Associate Professor of Medicine and
Otolaryngology, University of Arizona, Tucson,
Arizona, USA

MARIO CASTRO, MD
Professor of Medicine, Pediatrics and
Radiology, Washington University School of
Medicine, St Louis, Missouri, USA

GEOFFREY CHUPP, MD
Professor of Medicine, Pulmonary and Critical
Care Medicine, Yale School of Medicine, New
Haven, Connecticut, USA

JOSHUA L. DENSON, MD
National Jewish Health, Denver, Colorado,
USA

MAULI DESAI, MD
Assistant Professor of Medicine, Division of
Allergy and Clinical Immunology, Icahn School
of Medicine at Mount Sinai, New York, New
York, USA

NIKITA S. DESAI, MD
Staff Physician, Pulmonary and Critical Care,
Respiratory Institute, Cleveland Clinic,
Cleveland, Ohio, USA

ANNE E. DIXON, MA, BM, BCh
Professor of Medicine, Division of Pulmonary
and Critical Care, University of Vermont,
Burlington, Vermont, USA

JONATHAN M. GAFFIN, MD, MMsc
Division of Respiratory Diseases, Boston
Children's Hospital, Harvard Medical School,
Boston, Massachusetts, USA

BENJAMIN M. GASTON, MD
Children's Lung Foundation Professor of
Pediatrics, Division of Pediatric Pulmonology,
Allergy/Immunology and Sleep Medicine,
University Hospitals Rainbow Babies and
Children's Hospital and Case Western Reserve
University School of Medicine, Cleveland,
Ohio, USA

TINA V. HARTERT, MD, MPH
Professor, Department of Medicine, Division of
Allergy, Pulmonary, and Critical Care Medicine,
Vanderbilt University Medical Center,
Nashville, Tennessee, USA

STEPHEN T. HOLGATE, MD, FMedSci
Clinical and Experimental Sciences, Faculty of
Medicine, University of Southampton, The Sir
Henry Wellcome Research Laboratories,
Southampton General Hospital, Southampton,
United Kingdom

FERNANDO HOLGUIN, MD, MPH
Professor of Medicine, Pediatrics and
Epidemiology, Division of Pulmonary and
Critical Care, University of Colorado, Denver,
Colorado, USA; Allergy & Asthma Clinic,
Aurora, Colorado, USA

OCTAVIAN C. IOACHIMESCU, MD, PhD, MBA
Professor of Medicine, Pulmonary, Critical
Care and Sleep Medicine, Emory University,
Atlanta VA Medical Center, Atlanta, Georgia,
USA

ELLIOT ISRAEL, MD
Division of Pulmonary and Critical Care
Medicine, Department of Medicine, Brigham
and Women's Hospital, Harvard Medical
School, Boston, Massachusetts, USA

NIZAR N. JARJOUR, MD
Professor of Medicine and Radiology, The
Jeffrey Grossman Chair in Medical Leadership,
Allergy, Pulmonary and Critical Care Division
Head, University of Wisconsin-Madison School
of Medicine and Public Health, Madison,
Wisconsin, USA

SUMITA B. KHATRI, MD, MA
Co-Director, Asthma Center, Respiratory
Institute, Research Subject Advocate, Clinical
Research Unit, Associate Professor of
Medicine, Cleveland Clinic Lerner College of
Medicine, Case Western Reserve University
School of Medicine, Cleveland, Ohio, USA

SANDHYA KHURANA, MD
Associate Professor of Medicine, Division of
Pulmonary and Critical Care Medicine,
Co-Director, Mary Parkes Center for Asthma,
Allergy and Pulmonary Care, University of
Rochester Medical Center, Rochester, New
York, USA

CYNTHIA J. KOZIOL-WHITE, PhD
Instructor, Department of Pharmacology,
Robert Wood Johnson Medical School, Rutgers
Institute for Translational Medicine and Science,
Rutgers University, The State University of New
Jersey, New Brunswick, New Jersey, USA

MONICA KRAFT, MD
Professor, Department of Medicine, University
of Arizona, Tucson, Arizona, USA

DAVID M. LANG, MD
Professor of Medicine, Cleveland Clinic Lerner
College of Medicine, Department of Allergy and
Clinical Immunology, Respiratory Institute,
Cleveland Clinic, Cleveland, Ohio, USA

ANNE S. MAINARDI, MD
Fellow in Pulmonary and Critical Care
Medicine, Yale School of Medicine, New
Haven, Connecticut, USA

WENDY C. MOORE, MD
Section on Pulmonary, Critical Care, Allergy
and Immunologic Diseases, Wake Forest
School of Medicine, Winston-Salem, North
Carolina, USA

JOHN OPPENHEIMER, MD
Department of Medicine UMDNJ - Rutgers,
Pulmonary and Allergy Association, Summit,
New Jersey, USA

REYNOLD A. PANETTIERI Jr, MD
Professor, Department of Medicine, Director,
Rutgers Institute for Translational Medicine and
Science, Rutgers University, The State
University of New Jersey, New Brunswick, New
Jersey, USA

R. STOKES PEEBLES Jr, MD
Elizabeth and John Murray Professor of
Medicine, Division of Allergy, Pulmonary and
Critical Care Medicine, Departments of
Medicine, and Pathology, Microbiology, and
Immunology, Vanderbilt University School of
Medicine, VUMC, Nashville, Tennessee, USA

WANDA PHIPATANAKUL, MD, MS
Division of Allergy and Immunology, Boston
Children's Hospital, Harvard Medical School,
Boston, Massachusetts, USA

AMIRA ALI RAMADAN, MD, MSc
Division of Allergy and Immunology, Boston
Children's Hospital, Beth Israel Deaconess
Center, Boston, Massachusetts, USA

KRISTIE R. ROSS, MD, MS
Associate Professor of Pediatrics, Division of
Pediatric Pulmonology, Allergy/Immunology
and Sleep Medicine, University Hospitals
Rainbow Babies and Children's Hospital and
Case Western Reserve University School of
Medicine, Cleveland, Ohio, USA

**MARGARET E. SAMUELS-KALOW, MD,
MPhil, MSHP**
Assistant Professor of Emergency Medicine,
Massachusetts General Hospital, Harvard
Medical School, Boston, Massachusetts, USA

PHILIP E. SILKOFF, MD
Philadelphia, Pennsylvania, USA

PETER J. STERK, MD, PhD
Department of Respiratory Medicine,
Amsterdam UMC, University of Amsterdam,
Amsterdam, The Netherlands

AHILA SUBRAMANIAN, MD, MPH
Respiratory Institute, Cleveland Clinic,
Cleveland Clinic Lerner College of Medicine,
Case Western Reserve University School of
Medicine, Cleveland, Ohio, USA

W. GERALD TEAGUE, MD
Ivy Foundation Distinguished Professor of
Pediatrics, University of Virginia School of
Medicine, Charlottesville, Virginia, USA

SAMANTHA WALKER, PhD
Asthma UK, London, United Kingdom

MICHAEL E. WECHSLER, MD, MMSc
National Jewish Health, Denver, Colorado,
USA

BRIGITTE WEST, BSc
Asthma UK, London, United Kingdom

JOE G. ZEIN, MD, MBA
Assistant Professor of Medicine, Cleveland
Clinic, Cleveland, Ohio, USA

Contents

Asthma is among the most common chronic diseases worldwide and is a significant contributor to the global health burden, highlighting the urgent need for primary prevention. This article outlines several practical and conceptual challenges that accompany primary prevention efforts. It advocates for improved predictive modeling to identify those at high-risk of developing asthma using automated algorithms within electronic medical records systems and explanatory modeling to refine understanding of causal pathways. Understanding the many issues that are likely to affect the success of primary prevention efforts helps the community of individuals invested in asthma prevention organize efforts and maximize their impact.

The SARP, ADEPT, and U-BIOPRED programs are all significant efforts in characterizing asthma and reporting clusters that will assist in designing personalized therapies for asthma, and especially severe asthma. Key aspects of the design of these programs are summarized and major findings are reported in this review.

There are multiple proinflammatory pathways in the pathogenesis of asthma. These include both innate and adaptive inflammation, in addition to inflammatory and physiologic responses mediated by eicosanoids. An important component of the innate allergic immune response is ILC2 activated by interleukin (IL)-33, thymic stromal lymphopoietin, and IL-25 to produce IL-5 and IL-13. In terms of the adaptive T-lymphocyte immunity, CD4+ Th2 and IL-17–producing cells are critical in the inflammatory responses in asthma. Last, eicosanoids involved in asthma pathogenesis include prostaglandin D_2 and the cysteinyl leukotrienes that promote smooth muscle constriction and inflammation that propagate allergic responses.

Airway smooth muscle is the primary cell mediating bronchomotor tone. The milieu created in the asthmatic lung modulates airway smooth muscle contractility and relaxation. Experimental findings suggest intrinsic abnormalities in airway smooth muscle derived from patients with asthma in comparison with airway smooth muscle from those without asthma. These changes to excitation–contraction pathways may underlie airway hyperresponsiveness and increased airway resistance associated with asthma.

> Asthma is a serious global health issue and asthma guidelines recommend a step-wise approach to management with goals to achieve control and minimize future risk. Prior to escalation of pharmacotherapy, steps to confirm accurate diagnosis as well as address comorbidities and triggers are critical to effective asthma management. This article provides readers with a structured approach to evaluation and management of asthma of varying severity.

> Asthma triggers are exogenous or endogenous factors that could worsen asthma acutely to cause an exacerbation, or perpetuate chronic symptoms and airflow limitation. Because it is well known that recent asthma exacerbations and poor symptom control are strong predictors of future disease activity, it is not surprising that the number of (allergic or nonallergic) asthma triggers in the environment correlates with the disease-related quality of life. There is a need to identify and avoid specific triggers as the centerpiece of disease management, especially in those with heightened sensitivity to certain factors.

> The lung and gut microbiome are factors in asthma risk or protection. Relevant elements of the microbiome within both niches include the importance of the early life window for microbiome establishment, the diversity of bacteria, richness of bacteria, and effect of those bacteria on the local epithelium and immune system. Mechanisms of protection include direct anti-inflammatory action or induction of non–type 2 inflammation by certain bacterial colonies. The gut microbiome further impacts asthma risk through the contribution of metabolic products. This article reviews the mechanisms that connect the lung and gut microbiota to asthma development and severity.

> Obesity is a major risk factor for asthma. This association appears related to altered dietary composition and metabolic factors that can directly affect airway reactivity and airway inflammation. This article discusses how specific changes in the western diet and metabolic changes associated with the obese state affect inflammation and airway reactivity and reviews evidence that interventions targeting weight, dietary components, lifestyle, and metabolism might improve outcomes in asthma.

> This article on exposome and asthma focuses on the interaction of patients and their environments in various parts of their growth, development, and stages of life. Indoor and outdoor environments play a role in pathogenesis via levels and duration of exposure, with genetic susceptibility as a crucial factor that alters the initiation and trajectory of common conditions such as asthma. Knowledge of environmental exposures globally and changes that are occurring is necessary to function effectively as medical professionals and health advocates.

Kristie R. Ross, W. Gerald Teague, and Benjamin M. Gaston

Asthma is a heterogeneous developmental disorder influenced by complex interactions between genetic susceptibility and exposures. Wheezing in infancy and early childhood is highly prevalent, with a substantial minority of children progressing to established asthma by school age, most of whom are atopic. Adolescence is a time of remission of symptoms with persistent lung function deficits. The transition to asthma in adulthood is not well understood.

Joe G. Zein, Joshua L. Denson, and Michael E. Wechsler

Asthma is a common disorder that affects genders differently across the life span. Earlier in life, it is more common in boys. At puberty, asthma becomes more common and often more severe in girls and women. The effect of sex hormones on asthma incidence and its severity is difficult to differentiate from other asthma severity risk factors, such as racial background, socioeconomic factors, obesity, atopy, environmental exposure, and, in particular, lung aging. Recognizing gender-associated and age-associated differences is important to understanding the pathobiology of asthma and to providing effective education and personalized care for patients with asthma across the life course.

Amira Ali Ramadan, Jonathan M. Gaffin, Elliot Israel, and Wanda Phipatanakul

Corticosteroids are the most effective treatment for asthma; inhaled corticosteroids (ICSs) are the first-line treatment for children and adults with persistent symptoms. ICSs are associated with significant improvements in lung function. The anti-inflammatory effects of corticosteroids are mediated by both genomic and nongenomic factors. Variation in the response to corticosteroids has been observed. Patient characteristics, biomarkers, and genetic features may be used to predict response to ICSs. The existence of multiple mechanisms underlying glucocorticoid insensitivity raises the possibility that this might indeed reflect different diseases with a common phenotype.

Mauli Desai, John Oppenheimer, and David M. Lang

This review highlights recent data concerning efficacy and safety of biological agents that are currently approved by Food and Drug Administration (FDA), as well as several agents that will likely soon be FDA approved, for management of properly selected patients with severe persistent asthma that is poorly or not well controlled despite "stepped care" management according to best evidence.

Anne S. Mainardi, Mario Castro, and Geoffrey Chupp

Bronchial thermoplasty is an advanced therapy for severe asthma. It is a bronchoscopic procedure in which radiofrequency energy is applied to the airway wall, resulting in decreased airway smooth muscle burden. Human trials have shown that bronchial thermoplasty may reduce asthma exacerbations and improve quality of life in patients with severe uncontrolled asthma. It has been demonstrated to be a safe procedure, with most adverse events being early and mild. More studies are required to understand the precise effects of bronchial thermoplasty on the asthmatic airway and optimal parameters to appropriately select patients for this novel procedure.

The authors examine uses of geographic data to improve asthma care delivery and population health and describe potential practice changes and areas for future research.

Although once considered a single disease entity, asthma is now known to be a complex inflammatory disease engaging a range of causal pathways. The most frequent forms of asthma are identified by sputum/blood eosinophilia and activation of type 2 inflammatory pathways involving interleukins-3, -4, -5, and granulocyte-macrophage colony-stimulating factor. The use of diagnostics that identify T2 engagement linked to the selective use of highly targeted biologics has opened up a new way of managing severe disease. Novel technologies, such as wearables and intelligent inhalers, enable real-time remote monitoring of asthma, creating a unique opportunity for personalized health care.

CLINICS IN CHEST MEDICINE

SERIES OF RELATED INTEREST

Immunology and Allergy Clinics of North America
https://www.immunology.theclinics.com/

THE CLINICS ARE AVAILABLE ONLINE!
Access your subscription at:
www.theclinics.com

Preface
Asthma

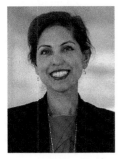 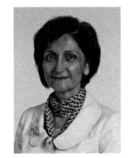

Sumita B. Khatri, MD, MA   Serpil C. Erzurum, MD
Editors

As of late, a palpable feeling of optimism is noted among health care providers caring for patients with asthma. Meanwhile, those individuals who have asthma, including severe asthma, are realizing the potential of advanced therapies that have emerged from translation of fundamental discoveries in the last two decades. The compendium of articles compiled for this issue of *Clinics in Chest Medicine*—Asthma serves as a repository and reference for all clinicians who care for patients with asthma as well as those who want to understand and further explore where the emerging science of asthma is heading.

The authors, who are experts within the field of asthma, provide the current state of asthma care as well as aspirational goals that promise even better care in the future. The possibility for being able to primarily prevent asthma is an exciting start to the issue. Practical considerations for prevention, and novel predictive modeling to identify those at high risk of developing asthma, are presented. The concept of severe asthma phenotypes is subsequently defined through review of the three major cohorts studied in the last 20 years (ie, the Severe Asthma Research Program, Airways Disease Endotyping for Personalized Therapeutics, and the Unbiased BIOmarkers in PREDiction of respiratory disease outcomes). All these studies uncover clusters of types of patients with severe asthma and lay out possibilities for personalizing treatments. Our new understanding of how underlying proinflammatory mechanisms drive asthma is comprehensively summarized. Just as important, the abnormalities that dictate the hypercontractile airway smooth muscle phenotype in asthma are identified. The overarching goals of asthma management are to control symptoms and mitigate future risks of asthma exacerbations, and a structured approach to asthma evaluation and management is provided to ensure accurate diagnosis and to address comorbidities and triggers critical to effective asthma management.

The lifecycle of asthma, based upon age and exposures and gender, is recognized to be a major influence on this disease. To understand the pathways in the pathogenesis of asthma, be it from innate allergic responses, nonallergic inflammatory responses, or the eicosanoid pathways, is essential. In addition to well-known comorbidities that exacerbate asthma, such as obesity, gastroesophageal reflux, obstructive sleep apnea, and chronic rhinitis, the contributions of the microbiome, diet, and metabolism are considered in the factors leading to asthma and more severe asthma. Data on the exposome and asthma highlight how interactions of individuals with their environments over various times of their life play a role in the initiation and trajectory of asthma. There is a life cycle of asthma, from infancy, childhood, adolescence, and adult life, which is modulated by gender, while asthma and its severity vary between genders across the life course. Therefore, one first step to develop personalized asthma care would be to uncover the gender-based differences in asthma outcomes. Corticosteroids remain the most effective treatment for asthma, but there are substantial variations in reponse. Fortunately, we now have several options for beyond stepped care therapy, which are described in articles outlining the use of biologic agents, or novel procedures such as thermoplasty for patients with severe asthma that is poorly controlled. Finally, this issue informs how to deliver care for populations of asthmatics as well as how to deliver care to the individual in a precision manner. Thus, this issue spans from the microscopic to macroscopic, and from intrinsic factors to exposures, all of which we now realize may be modified to prevent, treat, or perhaps cure asthma.

We are grateful to our authors, who worked diligently to provide clear and definitive information for this issue. We hope that readers enjoy the issue and that it will make a difference to the care of individuals with asthma.

Sumita B. Khatri, MD, MA
Asthma Center, Respiratory Institute
Cleveland Clinic
9500 Euclid Avenue, A90
Cleveland, OH 44195, USA

Serpil C. Erzurum, MD
Lerner Research Institute
Cleveland Clinic
9500 Euclid Avenue, NB21
Cleveland, OH 44195, USA

E-mail addresses:
khatris@ccf.org (S.B. Khatri)
erzurus@ccf.org (S.C. Erzurum)

Practical and Conceptual Considerations for the Primary Prevention of Asthma

Steven M. Brunwasser, PhD[a,b], Tina V. Hartert, MD, MPH[a,*]

KEYWORDS

- Asthma • Primary prevention • Prediction models • Explanatory models • Implementation

KEY POINTS

- The primary prevention of asthma is a key priority given its increasing prevalence and large contribution to the global public health burden.
- Clinicians can accelerate and maximize primary prevention efforts by improving identification of high-risk individuals through predictive modeling and understanding of causal disease processes through increasingly precise explanatory modeling.
- Strong collaborations among patients, clinicians, researchers, the public health and health policy community, and stakeholders are needed to address the many challenges of prevention and organize efforts.

INTRODUCTION

Asthma is one of the most common and important noncommunicable diseases worldwide.[1-3] Although there are effective treatments[3] and secondary prevention measures,[4] there is currently no way to prevent asthma, nor a cure.[5] Thus, there is an urgent need for advances in primary prevention. Asthma researchers have identified several modifiable disease processes that are candidate targets for primary prevention[5-8] and several primary prevention strategies have shown promise.[5-7] However, there is insufficient evidence to warrant widespread implementation at this time.[5] In addition, as for other diseases that have both a genetic and environmental component, no single modifiable risk factor will likely prevent disease, meaning that multifaceted approaches are most likely to be effective.[6,9] Advancing primary prevention may be the best way to curb the growing burden of asthma. As such, it should be a central objective for researchers, practitioners, and policymakers.

This article explicates several challenges and considerations that scientists and practitioners face in the pursuit of asthma prevention. Because there have been several recent and extensive reviews of specific candidate targets and interventions,[5-8] we instead focus on broad conceptual issues that must be addressed to maximize prevention efforts.

IMPROVING DELINEATION OF ASTHMA OUTCOMES

There is broad consensus that asthma is an umbrella term that encompasses multiple phenotypes.[5-7,10,11] In some cases, observable differences in disease manifestation seem to emanate from unique etiologic pathways (endotypes).[10,12]

Disclosure Statement: U19AI95227 (National Institutes of Health); K24 AI 77930 (National Institutes of Health); K12 HS022990 (Agency for Healthcare Research and Quality).

a Department of Medicine, Division of Allergy, Pulmonary, and Critical Care Medicine, Vanderbilt University Medical Center, T-1218 Medical Center North, 1161 21st Avenue South, Nashville, TN 37232-2650, USA;
b Department of Obstetrics and Gynecology, Vanderbilt University Medical Center, R-1217 Medical Center North, 1161 21st Avenue South, Nashville, TN 37232-2521, USA
* Corresponding author.
E-mail address: tina.hartert@vumc.org

The fact that asthma, as currently operationalized in clinical and research settings, is an imprecise construct reflecting distinct disease processes complicates prevention efforts considerably. The following sections discuss how advancement toward primary prevention is largely predicated on the ability to improve identification of individuals at high risk for asthma, and understanding of the etiologic processes contributing to asthma. In both of these endeavors, treating asthma as a unitary construct likely impedes progress.[10,13] Fortunately, there has been recent progress toward identifying asthma endotypes from data-driven "omics" research studies[14–17] that could inform increasingly precise prevention efforts.

SELECTING A TARGET POPULATION AND IMPROVING RISK IDENTIFICATION

With limited health care resources and innumerable competing priorities,[18] it is essential to invest prevention resources prudently. Several universal prevention strategies (eg, reducing fossil fuel emissions through political advocacy) are aimed at decreasing exposure to disease processes in entire populations, regardless of risk level. Other low-cost, noninvasive interventions (eg, prenatal providers informing women of the dangers of prenatal cigarette exposure[19]) require little investment, making universal delivery a sound option. However, high-cost and/or invasive prevention strategies should be reserved for those at greatest risk (targeted prevention). Respiratory syncytial virus (RSV) immune-prophylaxis or anti-IgE, both being evaluated for asthma prevention,[20–24] are expensive and require multiple injections for administration.[6,25] This would likely be a poor investment of resources and an unwarranted imposition for families of children with low wheezing or asthma risk. The greatest net benefit will likely come from a combination of universal and targeted prevention approaches, with the former having greater breadth of impact and the latter having greater per-person impact.

Improving Prediction

To optimize targeted primary prevention efforts, the ability to identify those at greatest risk must be improved.[13] This underscores the importance of ongoing efforts to develop and refine clinical prediction tools, and as asthma phenotypes and endotypes and their causal pathways are better understood, developing a precision approach for high-cost or high-intensity prevention efforts.[26,27] Well-calibrated and highly discriminating prediction tools could greatly improve the rate at which precious prevention resources are expended on individuals who would go on to develop asthma and not on those who would not. Existing tools[28,29] improve case identification, but there is considerable room for improvement.[26] In particular, identifying prediction cutpoints that have strong positive and negative likelihood ratios has been challenging.[26]

In many cases, identification of those at risk and prevention interventions (eg, vaccines) are administered in medical settings where there is access to electronic medical record (EMR) platforms. The technological capabilities of many EMR systems provide an opportunity to improve the performance and utility of asthma prediction tools.[30] Automated algorithms for the calculation of risk scores can be embedded within EMRs, allowing for complex calculations without added burden to care providers. A recent study demonstrated the feasibility of integrating an automated version of an established prediction tool within an EMR.[31]

Incorporating prediction tools into EMRs also provides opportunity to evaluate whether the rich data contained within (eg, standard laboratory results) provide incremental predictive value and improve the performance of existing tools. Expanding the set of predictors to include variables that have no known association with asthma, but that are widely available in EMR systems, may help improve predictive accuracy. For example, red cell distribution width has emerged as a powerful and robust predictor of numerous health complications[32,33] even though the mechanism is not always known.[32] A danger in adding many predictors with no theoretic basis is an "overfitted" model that does not perform well in validation samples.[34] However, there are numerous modeling strategies to reduce the degree of overfitting.[34] Beyond that, EMRs constantly accumulate new records, allowing for rigorous and iterative validation and refinement, and elimination of predictors whose predictive utility does not replicate.

From the standpoint of targeted prevention, the most important future direction, as the performance of prediction tools improves, is to conduct rigorous impact evaluations.[34] Prediction tools are most effective if they are developed in conjunction with preventive care models and with clinician input throughout.[35] Researchers could conduct pragmatic randomized controlled trials[36,37] to evaluate whether implementation of prediction tools improves linkage to prevention services and clinical outcomes. These same systems could identify risk factors and targets for prevention (eg, second-hand smoke).

Section Summary

The optimal primary prevention strategy likely involves a combination of low-cost universal interventions and high-cost targeted interventions for those at high risk. The expenditure of targeted prevention resources requires careful consideration and should be informed by well-validated prediction tools. The performance and utility of clinical prediction tools may be advanced considerably by leveraging the technological capabilities of modern EMR systems and the rich data they contain.

SELECTING TARGET DISEASE PROCESSES

Primary prevention efforts targeting asthma will be most successful if they draw on a strong understanding of its etiologic foundations.[5,6] There have been several recent papers reviewing disease processes that hold promise as potential targets for primary prevention of asthma.[3,5–7] Therefore, we focus solely on important conceptual considerations rather than specific disease processes.

Fig. 1 shows a hypothetical model in which there are four disease processes associated with incident asthma. These four disease processes are potential targets for primary prevention and are depicted using circles, with the size of the circles representing the prevalence of the disease processes in the population of interest. There are four potential preventive interventions (depicted as trapezoids), each specifically targeting one of

the four disease processes. Directed arrows emanating from the potential targets to incident asthma represent causal effects of the disease process on the outcome. The unshaded arrows represent the average effect of the target process on the outcome without intervention, with the strength of the effect proportional to the width of the arrow. We also assume that there is a preexisting risk factor (eg, a genetic polymorphism) that is either present (see **Fig. 1**A) or absent (see **Fig. 1**B). The risk factor modifies the strength of some of the associations within the etiologic system.

The goal of the preventive interventions is to reduce risk for the development of asthma by limiting the contribution of the target disease processes. The gray shaded arrows contained within the larger white arrows represent the average effect of the target process after administering the corresponding preventive intervention. Thus, the relative width of the concentric unshaded and shaded arrows represents the magnitude of the effect of the corresponding prevention intervention. If there were no intervention effect at all, the arrow connecting the disease process and incident asthma would be completely shaded. A completely unshaded arrow would indicate that the intervention completely eliminated the effect of the target disease process. We refer to **Fig. 1** to illustrate several of the concepts discussed next.

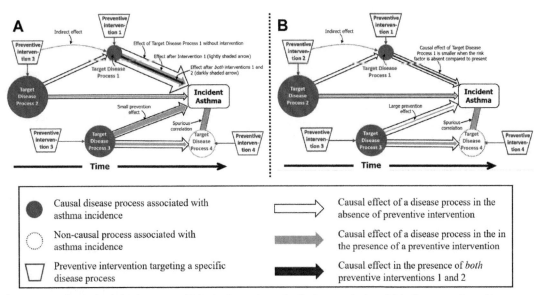

Fig. 1. Hypothetical etiologic system. This depicts a hypothetical scenario in which there are four disease processes (*circles*) associated with asthma incidence. Disease Processes 1 to 3 are causal contributors to asthma, whereas Disease Process 4 is noncausal. The width of the *unshaded arrows* connecting the disease processes and incident asthma represents the effect size in the absence of intervention. The width of the *shaded arrows* represents the effect size when the corresponding interventions (*trapezoids*) are administered. The differences in widths of the *concentric shaded* and *unshaded arrows* represents the magnitude of the intervention effect. The etiologic system is presented when a hypothetical risk factor is present (*A*) and absent (*B*) to show that the effects of specific processes and interventions are moderated by risk.

Evidence of Causality

The most important consideration when selecting a target disease process is whether there is compelling evidence that it is causally associated with asthma development.[38,39] If the target process is not a causal contributor to asthma, then all subsequent considerations in this section are moot. This criterion may be the most difficult to establish in human subjects research given that associations between disease processes and outcomes is often limited to observational rather than experimental designs.[5,39]

Within **Fig. 1**, the association between Disease Process 4 and incident asthma illustrates the pitfall of intervening on a noncausal disease process. Disease Process 4 is linked to asthma incidence by a path without a directional arrow, indicating a noncausal (spurious) correlation. Disease Process 4 and asthma incidence are associated only because they share a common cause (Disease Process 3). Even if Intervention 4 has a strong impact on Disease Process 4, it will have no impact on asthma incidence because Disease Process 4 is not contributing to the outcome. Thus, any investment in Intervention 4 would be wasted.

Distinguishing between processes that are causally related to the outcome and those that are associated but not causal, is difficult in practice. For example, if we were to model the association between maternal prenatal antidepressant use and asthma incidence, the exposure would almost certainly be highly confounded with the severity of maternal prenatal depression. Just as Disease Process 3 induced a spurious correlation between Disease Process 4 and incident asthma in **Fig. 1**, maternal depression could theoretically induce a noncausal association between antidepressant use and child asthma if it is causally related to both. In this hypothetical scenario, efforts to reduce antidepressant medication use would not be expected to reduce asthma risk, and in fact may actually increase exposure to a causal disease process (maternal depression). Thus, misspecification of the causal model could lead to ill-advised prevention efforts.

There have been significant advancements in causal effects modeling in recent years that can improve the plausibility of causal claims from observational data (eg, propensity score methods[40] and instrumental variable analysis[41]). Structural causal modeling can unify many causal frameworks and facilitates the formal explication and evaluation of assumptions necessary for causal inference.[42] Capitalizing on these advances may aid in the identification of disease mechanisms and preclude counterproductive prevention efforts.

Contribution to Disease Burden

It may be possible to maximize primary prevention efforts by targeting the risk factors and disease processes that contribute most to asthma's global disease burden. The contribution will be a function of the magnitude of the disease process's impact on asthma development and its prevalence in the population.[43,44] In **Fig. 1**A, Disease Process 1 clearly has the strongest statistical association (effect size) with asthma incidence. For simplicity, assume for the moment that individuals could be exposed to either Disease Process 1 or Disease Process 3, but not both, and that the two causal disease processes were independent. If one were to reduce Disease Process 1 and Disease Process 3 by an equal amount, those exposed to Disease Process 1 would experience, on average, a greater reduction in asthma risk than those exposed to Disease Process 3. However, Disease Process 3 is twice as prevalent in the population. Far more people could potentially benefit from an intervention ameliorating the effects of Disease Process 3, resulting in a comparable expected impact on the risk for asthma.

Evaluating the potential impact of specific targets is more complicated when the disease processes are dependent. In **Fig. 1**, Disease Process 2 makes a small direct contribution to asthma risk, but it also increases the risk of exposure to Disease Process 1, creating an indirect (mediated) effect.[45] Thus, the potential benefit of targeting Disease Process 2 is a function of its prevalence, its direct effect on asthma risk, and its indirect effect through Disease Process 1. Explanatory models that omit the indirect effect (particularly those that adjust for Disease Process 1 as a confounder) would likely underestimate Disease Process 2's disease contribution.[46] For example, assume that infant RSV contributes to childhood asthma primarily by damaging airway epithelial cells and altering lung development. But RSV may also contribute to asthma indirectly by increasing the probability of infant exposure to antibiotic treatments,[47] altering the microbiome and contributing to type 2 biased immune development.[48] Given this hypothetical scenario, if one developed a statistical model estimating the effect of RSV on incident asthma that controlled for the number of child antibiotic courses rather than modeling it as a mediator, one would likely underestimate the effect of infant RSV exposure.[46]

Effect heterogeneity presents another complexity in estimating the contribution of disease processes to the disease burden. **Fig. 1** presents a scenario in which Disease Process 1 has a large causal effect on incident asthma in the presence of a hypothetical risk factor (see **Fig. 1**A), but only a small effect when the risk factor is absent (see **Fig. 1**B). To make this concrete, assume that the risk factor is a single-nucleotide polymorphism, such as rs117902240,[49] and that Disease Process 1 is childhood dust mite exposure.[50] Assume that the contribution of dust mite exposure to asthma is greater in combination with the polymorphism (a gene × environment interaction).[49] Imagine we developed a statistical regression model of the effect of dust mite exposure on asthma incidence in which we included the genetic risk factor as a binary covariate, but we omitted the gene × dust mite exposure interaction. We may greatly underestimate or overestimate dust mite exposure's causal contribution depending on the arbitrary decision of how to code the genetic risk variable.[51] If the genetic risk variable were coded with the reference value corresponding to the risk being present, we would conclude that RSV makes a strong causal contribution; whereas we would conclude that it has minimal impact if the reference value corresponded to the risk being absent.

Modifiability

All things being equal, asthma risk factors or disease pathways that are easily mutable are preferable prevention targets compared with more intransigent ones. If, for example, a prenatal care provider aimed to prevent asthma by reducing fetal exposure to maternal stress[52] then it would be prudent to target stressors that could feasibly be altered within the pregnancy window (eg, interpersonal conflict with partners[53]) rather than firmly entrenched risk processes (eg, poverty). However, efforts to curb stressors related to entrenched structural processes may ultimately have a greater impact on the disease burden. For example, long-term political advocacy that leads to reduced exposure to air pollution in cities could yield enormous health benefits for asthma and other disease outcomes. Thus, the importance of ease of modifiability is relative to the context (eg, whether there is a critical time window in which to implement the intervention).

Effect on Related Disease Outcomes

Because asthma shares pathophysiologic origins with other chronic diseases,[54,55] it seems imprudent to strive for primary prevention of asthma in isolation. Targeting transdiagnostic disease processes (eg, allergic sensitization, promotion of healthy lung development, obesity) may greatly increase the utility of prevention efforts. **Fig. 2** shows

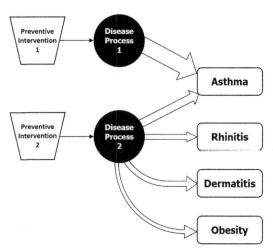

Fig. 2. Disease processes linked to multiple outcomes. This figure depicts a hypothetical scenario in which two equally prevalent disease processes contribute to asthma incidence. Disease Process 1 makes a much stronger contribution to asthma than Disease Process 2, as indicated by the relative width of the *arrow* connecting it to incidence asthma. However, Disease Process 2 also makes small contributions to three related disease outcomes. All things being equal, Disease Process 1 is the preferable disease target and Intervention 1 the preferable intervention if the goal were simply to reduce the burden of asthma. However, targeting Disease Process 2 with Intervention 2 might be preferable if the goal were to reduce the total disease burden across all four conditions. Ultimately, it may be prudent to target transdiagnostic disease processes (Disease Process 2) with preventive interventions rather than asthma-specific processes (Disease Process 1).

an unrealistic scenario in which two disease processes (Disease Process 1 and Disease Process 2) contribute causally to asthma. The effect size for Disease Process 1 is double that of Disease Process 2. However, Disease Process 2 also makes small causal contributions to the risk for rhinitis, dermatitis, and obesity, whereas Disease Process 1 is asthma-specific. Disease Process 2 makes a greater total contribution to the disease outcomes as a whole even though it makes a smaller specific contribution to asthma. Ultimately, it may be best to target asthma disease processes that likely contribute to multiple related conditions and to evaluate the global impact of prevention strategies across these conditions. This could best be achieved through interdisciplinary collaborations among investigators interested in similar disease processes, but different disease outcomes.

Section Summary

The selection of optimal targets for the primary prevention of asthma is challenging because it requires interventionists to weigh numerous factors and potential tradeoffs. Teasing apart these considerations cannot be accomplished by a single clinician or research study. However, the accumulation of research findings could help one make informed judgements about which disease processes are likely to be the most impactful targets. We are not limited to intervening on one, or even a few, targets. But knowing where the greatest potential benefits lie can help set the agenda for asthma prevention efforts. Asthma researchers must continually improve explanatory models, taking care to avoid pitfalls (eg, attributing cause to spurious correlation) that could steer us off course. Researchers should take advantage of modern causal inference methods, and analytical procedures that allow for precise specification and testing of structural models representing hypothesized etiologic pathways.[56]

CONSIDERATIONS FOR SELECTING PREVENTIVE INTERVENTIONS

This section outlines several practical considerations before implementing preventive interventions. The foremost consideration for selecting prevention programs is the degree of evidence of its efficacy. This typically is assessed based on results of randomized trials or meta-analyses. But there are several other important considerations. We address only a few of them, again referring to **Fig. 1** to illustrate key points.

Fig. 1 depicts the degree to which the four hypothetical interventions reduce the impact of the target disease processes. Borrowing an analogy from Pearl and colleagues,[38] one can think of the arrows connecting the causal disease processes (Disease Processes 1–3) to incident asthma as pipes carrying the pathogenic processes. The interventions are thought of as valves whose purpose is to cutoff the pathogenic stream as much as possible. The larger, unshaded arrows reflect the contribution of the disease process to the outcome with no intervention, and the shaded arrows reflect the contribution of the disease processes after implementation of the corresponding preventive intervention. The relative size of the shaded and unshaded arrows, therefore, represents the magnitude of the intervention effect (ie, the degree to which the valve restricts the flow of pathogenic processes).

Heterogeneity in Treatment Effects

In **Fig. 1**, the effect of Intervention 3 is strongly moderated by the presence of the risk factor. When the risk factor is present (see **Fig. 1**A), the contribution of Disease Process 3 (the target disease process) to incident asthma after Intervention

3 is only slightly smaller than it would have been with no intervention (ie, small effect of Intervention 3). When the risk factor is absent, the contribution of Disease Process 3 to incident asthma is much smaller than it would have been without intervention (ie, large effect of Intervention 3). In sum, Intervention 3 seems to be a highly promising intervention that reduces a causal disease process affecting a large portion of the population, but its overall potential to reduce disease burden depends on the prevalence of the risk factor. Identifying moderators of preventive interventions is critical for the long-term success of primary asthma prevention, particularly for high-cost and/or invasive strategies. A statistical model of the effect of Intervention 3 on incident asthma could be highly misleading if the moderator is not accounted for.

Acceptability and Tolerability

Accurate appraisal of preventive intervention effects requires estimation under intention-to-treat.[57] Many preventive interventions have poor uptake.[58] Some preventive interventions are unpleasant to complete (eg, those requiring injections) or time-intensive (multisession behavioral health interventions), and some may carry unwanted side effects (eg, digestive symptoms with probiotic supplementation). To the extent that these factors affect intervention compliance must be factored into the estimation of the intervention effect. Considering **Fig. 1**A, assume that Intervention 1 is an invasive intervention that is often rejected by potential recipients. Our interpretation of Intervention 1's large effect would change considerably depending on whether investigators included or excluded individuals who refused, or did not fully comply with, the intervention. The practical impact of Intervention 1 would be greatly diminished if the compliance rate were 20% compared with 90%. With poor compliance, Intervention 1 would have limited value despite its potential for large preventive effects. Additionally, one could not assume that those who refused the intervention would have shown equal benefit had they received the intervention, so there is a high risk of bias.[57]

Timing

The optimal timing for a primary prevention intervention depends on many factors, but obviously it must be initiated before asthma onset. Because most asthma cases begin in early childhood,[59] primary prevention efforts must begin early. High-risk pregnant women are a logical focus for targeted prevention. There is growing evidence that intrauterine exposures (eg, stress) may play a role in the development of asthma and disease processes linked to asthma.[52,60] Limiting adverse prenatal exposures might alter disease processes before they become entrenched and difficult to modify.[61] Additionally, early intervention efforts may prevent a disease process cascade. For example, prenatal probiotic supplementation for mothers requiring antibiotic treatment could offset the adverse effects on microbial diversity in the maternal gut microbiome. This, in turn, could affect microbial diversity of the fetal microbiome, reduce risk for developing a Th2 immune phenotype, and prevent inflammatory airway responses characteristic of atopic asthma.[62] **Fig. 1** provides a simple example of disease process cascading: Disease Process 2 is the first exposure and it makes a modest direct contribution to asthma incidence, but also a small indirect contribution by reducing exposure to Disease Process 1. By intervening early with Intervention 2, one may affect multiple disease pathways.

Earlier intervention is not always better. It may be counterproductive, for example, to give a high-risk infant a full regimen of RSV immunoprophylaxis during the summer months when RSV is not circulating. In this circumstance, the intervention would presumably be more impactful if administration were delayed until the season when RSV is circulating. Additionally, there are instances when it makes sense to intervene at multiple critical time points.[9] For example, among children at risk for late-onset asthma, there may be early mutable disease processes that serve as a latent diathesis. Later exposures (eg, interpersonal stressors) may activate this latent diathesis, resulting in late-onset asthma. In this scenario, the best prevention strategy might be to intervene early to thwart the development of the early diathesis, and later to ameliorate the exposures that activate the diathesis. In **Fig. 1**A, the directed arrow connecting Disease Process 1 to incident asthma contains two smaller shaded arrows. The lightly shaded arrow represents the contribution of Disease Process 1 to incident asthma if only the Intervention 1 is initiated (effect of Intervention 1 alone). The darker shaded arrow represents the effect of Disease Process 1 if both Intervention 1 and Intervention 2 were used. The curved dotted line emanating from Intervention 2 to Disease Process 1 indicates that there is an indirect effect of Intervention 2 on Disease Process 1 through Intervention 2's effect on Disease Process 2. Intervening early (Intervention 2) and late (Intervention 1) reduces the impact of Disease Process 1 more than implementing Intervention 1 alone.

Transportability

The ultimate utility of a preventive intervention depends in part on whether it retains its potency when transported to new settings, away from the site where it was developed and/or initially tested.[63] Imagine a scenario in which prenatal probiotic supplementation and a prenatal smoking cessation intervention produced identical reductions in asthma incidence in initial efficacy trials (**Fig. 3**). The interventions are then tested for replication at independent sites with independent research teams. The probiotic intervention simply involves providing supplement packs during prenatal care visits. The supplements are obtained easily from local suppliers. The smoking cessation intervention is much more involved, requiring multiple in-person therapy sessions following a detailed structured protocol. It requires highly skilled intervention providers, qualified trainers/supervisors with advanced degrees, dedicated intervention space, and intervention protocol booklets for providers and participants. Assuming all of these components are necessary for the intervention to have an optimal impact, there is a greater risk that the smoking cessation program's intervention effect will attenuate when it is transported.[63] It may also be difficult to replicate the enthusiasm that the initial investigators and their research team had for the intervention. **Fig. 3** depicts a scenario where the intervention effect for probiotic supplementation is better maintained during the transportation from the initial evaluation site to the replication site than the more complex smoking cessation intervention.

Sustainability

In addition to being harder to transport, complex interventions may be more difficult to maintain over time.[64] With our hypothetical smoking cessations intervention, there may be high turnover rates in intervention providers and supervisors in some settings, requiring continued investment in training and potential loss of quality. The extent to which prevention interventions yield insurance reimbursements also affects the ability of many health care settings to continue offering the intervention over time.

Intervention Scope

Some prevention programs are highly focused on a remediating a single disease process.[20] Other intervention programs target multiple disease processes.[9,65] Although the latter approach may increase the probability of an effect on asthma outcomes by hitting multiple putative mediators

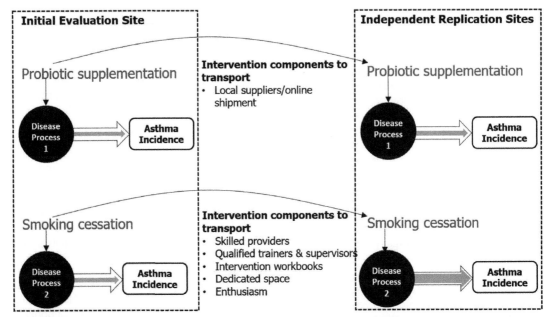

Fig. 3. Intervention transportability. This figure illustrates the concept of intervention transportability. It depicts a hypothetical scenario where two interventions (a prenatal probiotic supplementation and prenatal smoking cessation behavioral intervention) are administered with the goal of preventing asthma. Each intervention targets a specific disease process: Disease Process 1 and Disease Process 2, respectively. The *unshaded arrows* connecting the disease processes to asthma incidence reflect the effect of the disease process without intervention. The *shaded arrows* within the *unshaded arrows* represent the effect of the disease process in the presence of the corresponding intervention. The relative width of the *unshaded* and *shaded arrows* represents the magnitude of the intervention effect. In the initial intervention evaluation sites, the two interventions have equal impact on their targeted disease processes and asthma incidence. When evaluating the intervention in independent sites, there is only minor reduction in the effect of the probiotic intervention, whereas the effect of the smoking cessation intervention diminishes markedly. This may be because the smoking cessation intervention is more complex with multiple essential components that may be difficult to transport effectively to other settings. All things being equal, easily transportable interventions are preferable.

and preventing interactions among them,[66] these interventions are likely to be more costly and difficult to transport and sustain. It can also be challenging to identify which intervention components contributed most to the intervention effect.[5] However, a recent cost-effectiveness study suggests that a multicomponent asthma prevention program, although more costly, may provide greater value than prevention programs targeting only a single disease process.[67]

Return on Investment

Ultimately, whether or not a preventive intervention is broadly disseminated depends on whether it is a prudent investment of resources. Looking at the cost of an intervention is insufficient. High-cost asthma prevention programs may provide a strong return on investment[67] if they obviate high-cost care (eg, hospital stays) or even low-cost care (eg, chronic asthma medications) over a long period of time. It is critical to account not only for financial costs, but also the burden of

living with asthma, a lifelong chronic disease. Financial and nonfinancial burdens can be converted to a standardized scale using concepts like quality-adjusted life year and disability-adjusted life year.[68] Often large investments are made in promising preventive interventions (eg, multiple multi-million-dollar trials) before the issue of costs and return on investment is considered. We recommend making investment evaluation part of the intervention evaluation process from the outset, even if an intervention's economic impact cannot be fully appraised until it progresses to large effectiveness trials.

SUMMARY

The primary prevention of asthma is an important yet challenging endeavor. We addressed only some of the many practical and conceptual challenges for the asthma prevention community. Maximizing prevention efforts requires the consideration of many competing priorities. Selecting optimal disease targets and preventive interventions requires tradeoffs among these competing priorities. However, because of recent advances in defining asthma phenotypes, modeling causal pathways, and developing/implementing interventions, there is tremendous opportunity for progress. As we identify efficacious interventions that can be implemented with reasonable uptake and sustainability among high-risk populations, it will be critical to organize prevention efforts through collaborations among practitioners, researchers, patients, and policymakers.

REFERENCES

1. Asher I, Pearce N. Global burden of asthma among children. Int J Tuberc Lung Dis 2014;18(11):1269–78.
2. Vos T, Barber R, Bell B, et al. Global, regional, and national incidence, prevalence, and years lived with disability for 301 acute and chronic diseases and injuries in 188 countries, 1990–2013: a systematic analysis for the Global Burden of Disease Study 2013. Lancet 2015;386(9995):743–800.
3. Global Initiative for Asthma. Global strategy for asthma management and prevention (2018 update). 2018. Available at: www.ginasthma.org. Accessed April 28, 2018.
4. Kaiser S, Huynh T, Charier L, et al. Preventing exacerbations in preschoolers with recurrent wheeze: a meta-analysis. Pediatrics 2016;137(6). https://doi.org/10.1542/peds.2015-4496.
5. Beasley R, Semprini A, Mitchell E. Risk factors for asthma: is prevention possible? Lancet 2015; 386(9998):1075–85.
6. Jackson D, Hartert T, Martinez F, et al. Asthma: NHLBI workshop on the primary prevention of chronic lung diseases. Ann Am Thorac Soc 2014; 11(Suppl 3):S139–45.
7. Gur M, Hakim F, Bentur L. Better understanding of childhood asthma, towards primary prevention: are we there yet? Consideration of pertinent literature. F1000Res 2017;6:2152.
8. Burbank A, Sood A, Kesic M, et al. Environmental determinants of allergy and asthma in early life. J Allergy Clin Immunol 2017;140(1):1–12.
9. Kuiper S, Maas T, Schayck C, et al. The primary prevention of asthma in children study: design of a multifaceted prevention program. Pediatr Allergy Immunol 2005;16(4):321–31.
10. Skloot G. Asthma phenotypes and endotypes: a personalized approach to treatment. Curr Opin Pulm Med 2016;22(1):3–9.
11. Savenije O, Granell R, Caudri D, et al. Comparison of childhood wheezing phenotypes in 2 birth cohorts: ALSPAC and PIAMA. J Allergy Clin Immunol 2011;127(6):1505–12.e14.
12. Lötvall J, Akdis CA, Bacharier L, et al. Asthma endotypes: a new approach to classification of disease entities within the asthma syndrome. J Allergy Clin Immunol 2011;127(2):355–60.
13. Szefler SJ. Early asthma: stepping closer to primary prevention. J Allergy Clin Immunol 2012;130(2): 308–10.
14. Woodruff P, Modrek B, Choy D, et al. T-helper type 2–driven inflammation defines major subphenotypes of asthma. Am J Respir Crit Care Med 2009;180(5): 388–95.
15. George B, Reif D, Gallagher J, et al. Data-driven asthma endotypes defined from blood biomarker and gene expression data. PLoS One 2015;10(2): e0117445.
16. Turi K, Romick-Rosendale L, Ryckman K, et al. A review of metabolomics approaches and their application in identifying causal pathways of childhood asthma. J Allergy Clin Immunol 2018;141(4): 1191–201.
17. Nair H, Nokes D, Gessner B, et al. Global burden of acute lower respiratory infections due to respiratory syncytial virus in young children: a systematic review and meta-analysis. Lancet 2010;375(9725): 1545–55.
18. Norheim O, Baltussen R, Johri M, et al. Guidance on priority setting in health care (GPS-Health): the inclusion of equity criteria not captured by cost-effectiveness analysis. Cost Eff Resour Alloc 2014;12:18.
19. Silvestri M, Franchi S, Pistorio A, et al. Smoke exposure, wheezing, and asthma development: a systematic review and meta-analysis in unselected birth cohorts. Pediatr Pulmonol 2015;50(4):353–62.
20. Blanken M, Rovers M, Molenaar J, et al. Respiratory syncytial virus and recurrent wheeze in healthy preterm infants. N Engl J Med 2013;368(19):1791–9.
21. Scheltema N, Nibbelke E, Pouw J, et al. Respiratory syncytial virus prevention and asthma in healthy preterm infants: a randomised controlled trial. Lancet Respir Med 2018;6(4):257–64.
22. O'Brien K, Chandran A, Weatherholtz R, et al. Efficacy of motavizumab for the prevention of respiratory syncytial virus disease in healthy Native American infants: a phase 3 randomised double-blind placebo-controlled trial. Lancet Infect Dis 2015;15(12):1398–408.
23. Carroll K, Gebretsadik T, Escobar G, et al. Respiratory syncytial virus immunoprophylaxis in high-risk infants and development of childhood asthma. J Allergy Clin Immunol 2017;139(1):66–71.e3.
24. Mochizuki H, Kusuda S, Okada K, et al. Palivizumab prophylaxis in preterm infants and subsequent recurrent wheezing. Six-year follow-up study. Am J Respir Crit Care Med 2017;196(1):29–38.
25. Thomas G. A cost-benefit analysis of the immunisation of children against respiratory syncytial virus (RSV) using the English Hospital Episode Statistics

(HES) data set. Eur J Health Econ 2018;19(2): 177–87.

26. Smit H, Pinart M, Antó J, et al. Childhood asthma prediction models: a systematic review. Lancet Respir Med 2015;3(12):973–84.

27. Sears M. Predicting asthma outcomes. J Allergy Clin Immunol 2015;136(4):829–36.

28. Castro-Rodríguez J, Holberg C, Wright A, et al. A clinical index to define risk of asthma in young children with recurrent wheezing. Am J Respir Crit Care Med 2000;162(4):1403–6.

29. Schauberger E, Khurana Hershey G, Bernstein D, et al. Predicting asthma development in children using a new personalized asthma risk score. J Allergy Clin Immunol 2018;141(2, Supplement):AB106.

30. Miotto R, Li L, Kidd B, et al. Deep patient: an unsupervised representation to predict the future of patients from the electronic health records. Scientific Rep 2016;6:26094.

31. Kaur H, Sohn S, Wi C-I, et al. Automated chart review utilizing natural language processing algorithm for asthma predictive index. BMC Pulm Med 2018; 18(1):34. https://doi.org/10.1186/s12890-018-0593-9.

32. Patel K, Semba R, Ferrucci L, et al. Red cell distribution width and mortality in older adults: a meta-analysis. J Gerontol A Biol Sci Med Sci 2010;65A(3): 258–65.

33. Wang L, McGregor T, Jones D, et al. Electronic health record-based predictive models for acute kidney injury screening in pediatric inpatients. Pediatr Res 2017;82(3):465–73.

34. Steyerberg E. Clinical prediction models: a practical approach to development, validation, and updating. New York: Springer Science & Business Media; 2009. Available at: https://books.google.com/books?hl=en&lr=&id=kHGK58cLsMIC&oi=fnd&pg=PR2&dq=clinical+prediction+models+a+practical+approach&ots=TNShCYjFhj&sig=8XapmSZMqp4VhEXC-F0jJFujuH8.

35. Reilly B, Evans A. Translating clinical research into clinical practice: impact of using prediction rules to make decisions. Ann Intern Med 2006;144(3):201.

36. Semler M, Wanderer J, Ehrenfeld J, et al. Balanced crystalloids versus saline in the intensive care unit. The SALT randomized trial. Am J Respir Crit Care Med 2017;195(10):1362–72.

37. Feldstein D, Hess R, McGinn T, et al. Design and implementation of electronic health record integrated clinical prediction rules (iCPR): a randomized trial in diverse primary care settings. Implement Sci 2017;12:37.

38. Pearl J, Glymour M, Jewell N. Causal inference in statistics: a primer. Chichester (United Kingdom): John Wiley & Sons; 2016.

39. Hill A. The environment and disease: association or causation? J R Soc Med 2015;108(1):32–7.

40. Austin P, Stuart E. Moving towards best practice when using inverse probability of treatment weighting (IPTW) using the propensity score to estimate causal treatment effects in observational studies. Stat Med 2015;34(28):3661–79.

41. Angrist J, Imbens G, Rubin D. Identification of causal effects using instrumental variables. J Am Stat Assoc 1996;91(434):444–55.

42. Pearl J. Causal inference in statistics: an overview. Stat Surv 2009;3:96–146.

43. Mansournia M, Altman D. Population attributable fraction. BMJ 2018;360:k757.

44. Abreo A, Gebretsadik T, Stone CA Jr, et al. The impact of modifiable risk factor reduction on childhood asthma development. Clin Transl Med 2018; 7(1):15.

45. MacKinnon DP, Fairchild AJ, Fritz MS. Mediation analysis. Annu Rev Psychol 2007;58:593–614.

46. MacKinnon DP, Krull JL, Lockwood CM. Equivalence of the mediation, confounding and suppression effect. Prev Sci 2000;1(4):173–81.

47. Gonzales R, Malone D, Maselli J, et al. Excessive antibiotic use for acute respiratory infections in the United States. Clin Infect Dis 2001;33(6):757–62.

48. Johnson C, Ownby DR. The infant gut bacterial microbiota and risk of pediatric asthma and allergic diseases. Transl Res 2017;179:60–70.

49. Forno E, Sordillo J, Brehm J, et al. Genome-wide interaction study of dust mite allergen on lung function in children with asthma. J Allergy Clin Immunol 2017;140(4):996–1003.e7.

50. Celedón J, Milton D, Ramsey C, et al. Exposure to dust mite allergen and endotoxin in early life and asthma and atopy in childhood. J Allergy Clin Immunol 2007;120(1):144–9.

51. Braumoeller B. Hypothesis testing and multiplicative interaction terms. Int Organ 2004;58(4):807–20.

52. van de Loo K, van Gelder M, Roukema J, et al. Prenatal maternal psychological stress and childhood asthma and wheezing: a meta-analysis. Eur Respir J 2016;47(1):133–46.

53. Spinelli M. Interpersonal psychotherapy for depressed antepartum women: a pilot study. Am J Psychiatry 1997;154(7):1028–30.

54. Weiss ST. Obesity: insight into the origins of asthma. Nat Immunol 2005;6(6):537.

55. Zheng T, Yu J, Oh M, et al. The atopic march: progression from atopic dermatitis to allergic rhinitis and asthma. Allergy Asthma Immunol Res 2011;3(2):67–73.

56. Grace J, Michael A, Han O, et al. On the specification of structural equation models for ecological systems. Ecol Monogr 2010;80(1):67–87.

57. Ranganathan P, Pramesh C, Aggarwal R. Common pitfalls in statistical analysis: intention-to-treat versus per-protocol analysis. Perspect Clin Res 2016;7(3): 144–6.

58. Supplee L, Parekh J, Johnson M. Principles of precision prevention science for improving recruitment and retention of participants. Prev Sci 2018;1–6. https://doi.org/10.1007/s11121-018-0884-7.

59. Yunginger J, Reed C, O'Connell E, et al. A community-based study of the epidemiology of asthma: incidence rates, 1964–1983. Am Rev Respir Dis 1992;146(4):888–94.

60. Slopen N, Loucks E, Appleton A, et al. Early origins of inflammation: an examination of prenatal and childhood social adversity in a prospective cohort study. Psychoneuroendocrinology 2015;51:403–13.

61. Marks G. The allergic paradox: a key to progress in primary prevention of asthma. J Allergy Clin Immunol 2011;128(4):789–90.

62. Lapin B, Piorkowski J, Ownby D, et al. Relationship between prenatal antibiotic use and asthma in at-risk children. Ann Allergy Asthma Immunol 2015; 114(3):203–7.

63. Schoenwald S, Hoagwood K. Effectiveness, transportability, and dissemination of interventions: what matters when? Psychiatr Serv 2001;52(9):1190–7.

64. Johnson K, Hays C, Center H, et al. Building capacity and sustainable prevention innovations: a sustainability planning model. Eval Program Plann 2004;27(2):135–49.

65. Mihrshahi S, Peat J, Marks G, et al. Eighteen-month outcomes of house dust mite avoidance and dietary fatty acid modification in the childhood asthma prevention study (CAPS). J Allergy Clin Immunol 2003; 111(1):162–8.

66. Maas T, Kaper J, Sheikh A, et al. Mono and multifaceted inhalant and/or food allergen reduction interventions for preventing asthma in children at high risk of developing asthma. Cochrane Database of Systematic Reviews 2009, Issue 3. Art. No.: CD006480.

67. Ramos G, Asselt A, Kuiper S, et al. Cost-effectiveness of primary prevention of paediatric asthma: a decision-analytic model. Eur J Health Econ 2014; 15(8):869–83.

68. van Gils PF, Tariq L, Verschuuren M, et al. Cost-effectiveness research on preventive interventions: a survey of the publications in 2008. Eur J Public Health 2011;21(2):260–4.

Three Major Efforts to Phenotype Asthma: Severe Asthma Research Program, Asthma Disease Endotyping for Personalized Therapeutics, and Unbiased Biomarkers for the Prediction of Respiratory Disease Outcome

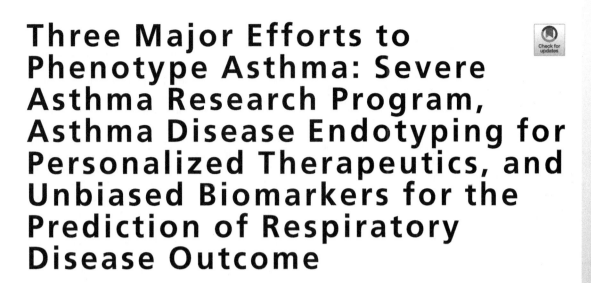

Philip E. Silkoff, MD[a],*, Wendy C. Moore, MD[b],
Peter J. Sterk, MD, PhD[c]

KEYWORDS

• Asthma • Endotypes • Phenotypes • Clustering • Biomarkers

KEY POINTS

• Asthma is increasingly recognized as a syndrome encompassing multiple phenotypes.
• The Asthma Disease Endotyping for Personalized Therapeutics, Severe Asthma Research Program, and Unbiased Biomarkers for the Prediction of Respiratory Disease Outcome programs have enrolled large numbers of asthmatic subjects and healthy controls to better understand this complex syndrome and have used complementary but different approaches.
• Each program has described several clusters that are overlapping in part, but distinct in many aspects, providing novel insights into the processes driving asthma severity.
• The hope is that better understanding of asthma phenotypes/endotypes will enable a personalized approach to asthma management.

Disclosure Statement: P.J. Sterk: The Amsterdam UMC has received a public-private grant by the Innovative Medicines Initiative (IMI) for the U-BIOPRED Study, covered by the European Union (EU) and the European Federation of Pharmaceutical Industries and Associations (EFPIA). P.E. Silkoff: P.E. Silkoff is a full-time employee of Third Pole Inc and declares no conflict of interest regarding the content of this article. W.C. Moore has received funding by the National Heart, Lung and Blood Institute (NHLBI) or the National Institutes of Health (NIH), USA for the SARP program.
[a] 827 North 21st Street, Philadelphia, PA 19130, USA; [b] Department of Internal Medicine, Section on Pulmonary, Critical Care, Allergy and Immunologic Diseases, Wake Forest School of Medicine, Medical Center Boulevard, Winston-Salem, NC 27157, USA; [c] Department of Respiratory Medicine F5-152, Amsterdam UMC, University of Amsterdam, PO Box 22700, 1100 DE Amsterdam, The Netherlands
* Corresponding author.
E-mail address: philsilkoff@gmail.com

Clin Chest Med 40 (2019) 13–28
https://doi.org/10.1016/j.ccm.2018.10.016
0272-5231/19/© 2018 Elsevier Inc. All rights reserved.

INTRODUCTION

Although asthma was once considered to be a uniform disease entity, it is now well established that asthma is a syndrome with multiple phenotypes and endotypes. A distinct functional or pathologic mechanism defines an endotype of a condition, whereas a phenotype is any observable characteristic or trait of a disease, without necessarily implying a mechanism. The usual example given for a phenotype is allergic versus nonallergic asthma where one can observe the associated allergic condition, for example, allergic rhinitis or worsening related to allergen exposure. Defining an endotype for asthma is more challenging unlike other diseases, for example, cystic fibrosis where a definable genetic defect has been linked to dysfunction of the cystic fibrosis transmembrane conductance regulator ion channel. Asthma has genetic underpinnings, but the environment plays a major role with relevant factors, including exposure to viruses, allergens, occupational exposures, and air pollution, as well as behavioral drivers, for example, obesity and exposure to socioeconomic and psychological stressors.

Given the complexity of asthma, alternative approaches to classification have been undertaken in recent years to create subgroups using clustering on clinical, functional, and molecular biological characteristics. Although there have been many efforts in this regard, this article will discuss some background and aspects of 3 major efforts including the Severe Asthma Research Program (SARP), the Unbiased Biomarkers for the Prediction of Respiratory Disease Outcome (U-BIOPRED) program, and the Asthma Disease Endotyping for Personalized Therapeutics (ADEPT) study. These programs used divergent approaches and as might be expected, each provides distinct insights into the enigmatic disease, asthma.

THE SEVERE ASTHMA RESEARCH PROGRAM

In 2000, the American Thoracic Society (ATS) published a workshop summary consensus definition of severe asthma that identified areas of critical need for future research into the disease.[1] In 2001, the National Heart, Lung, and Blood Institute (NHLBI) funded SARP to meet this need. For the first 10 years of funding, SARP (SARP1/2) brought together a consortium of 8 clinical centers composed of 12 universities that collected a cross-sectional cohort of more than 1600 subjects (including 250 children) with mild, moderate, and severe asthma (40% severe).[2] Participants underwent comprehensive clinical characterization including medical history, symptom and quality of life questionnaires, evaluation of atopy (skin prick testing, serum immunoglobulin E [IgE]), extended pulmonary function testing (pre- and postbronchodilator spirometry [after 4–8 puffs of albuterol] and methacholine challenge in those with forced expiratory volume in the first second of expiration [FEV_1] >50% predicted), measurement of exhaled nitric oxide (FeNO) as well as phlebotomy for DNA, inflammatory cellular measures, and collection of serum and plasma specimens. Subsets of participants underwent additional testing including collection of exhaled breath condensate (∼850 subjects)[3]; sputum induction for assessment of inflammatory cells and collection of sputum supernatants (∼450 subjects)[4,5]; and investigative bronchoscopy with collection of bronchoalveolar lavage fluid, bronchial brushings, and biopsies (∼500 subjects).[6] Imaging studies were performed on more than 400 subjects using high-resolution chest computed tomography with imaging at full inspiration and end expiration postbronchodilator.[7]

In 2011, the NHLBI continued their commitment to severe asthma by funding the third iteration of the network (SARP3), a 3-year longitudinal protocol consisting of all the original SARP1/2 clinical sites with the addition of new investigators. The network recruited 715 asthma subjects (527 adult and 188 pediatric) of which 61% had severe asthma compatible with the newly published joint European Respiratory Society (ERS)/ATS refined definition for severe asthma.[8,9] SARP3 adopted the methodology of SARP1/2 applied to longitudinal assessments, with only small changes to incorporate new scientific discoveries in severe asthma and changes in clinical practice, asthma tools, and laboratory methodology in the previous decade. Collection of biospecimens was increased throughout the SARP3 protocol with serum, plasma, and sputum supernatants now processed in greater quantities for full "–omics" analyses.

There are too many findings from analyses of the cross-sectional SARP1/2 cohort to adequately cover the wealth of knowledge that has been attained in this review, but summary statements of findings have been previously published.[10,11] Baseline data from the SARP3 cohort have been analyzed and some published,[9,12,13] but much of the longitudinal analysis is ongoing as subjects continue to participate in annual assessments of their asthma, now in their fourth to fifth year of follow-up. The following is a brief summary of "highlights" from the 18-year network that are closest to affecting clinical care for asthma patients today.

Clinical Phenotypes of Asthma in Severe Asthma Research Program

One of the unique features of the SARP program has been that the cohort includes participants of all ages (both children and adults) and the entire spectrum of asthma severity from mild intermittent to severe persistent asthma.[2,14] The large number of subjects and sheer breadth of the clinical data in SARP makes this cohort ideal for unbiased statistical approaches to identify subgroups of asthma subjects that share clinical characteristics and similar pathobiology to improve disease classification.

An unsupervised cluster analysis was performed in the first 726 subjects ($\geq$12 years of age) of the SARP1/2 cohort using 34 variables that included demographics (current age, age of asthma onset, duration of disease, BMI, gender, self-reported race), extended lung function (pre- and postbronchodilator FEV_1, forced vital capacity (FVC), FEV_1/FVC, % reversibility), atopy assessments (number and type of positive skin prick tests), and extensive questionnaire data (symptoms, exacerbations, comorbidities, medication use).[15] This analysis identified 5 clinical cluster phenotypes (**Fig. 1**)[10] that include the spectrum of childhood-onset allergic asthma (Clusters 1, 2, and 4), adolescent- to early adulthood-onset asthma with poor lung function and chronic airflow obstruction (Cluster 5), and a small group of subjects with very late-onset asthma (>40 years of age) and profound symptoms, but preserved lung function (Cluster 3). Eleven of the original 34 variables were most discriminating in clustering subjects—gender, age of asthma onset and duration of disease, pre- and postbronchodilator lung function variables (FEV_1 and FVC % predicted, FEV1/FVC and % bronchodilator reversibility), frequency of beta-agonist use, and intensity of steroid exposure; 94% of subjects could be correctly assigned to a clinical cluster phenotype using

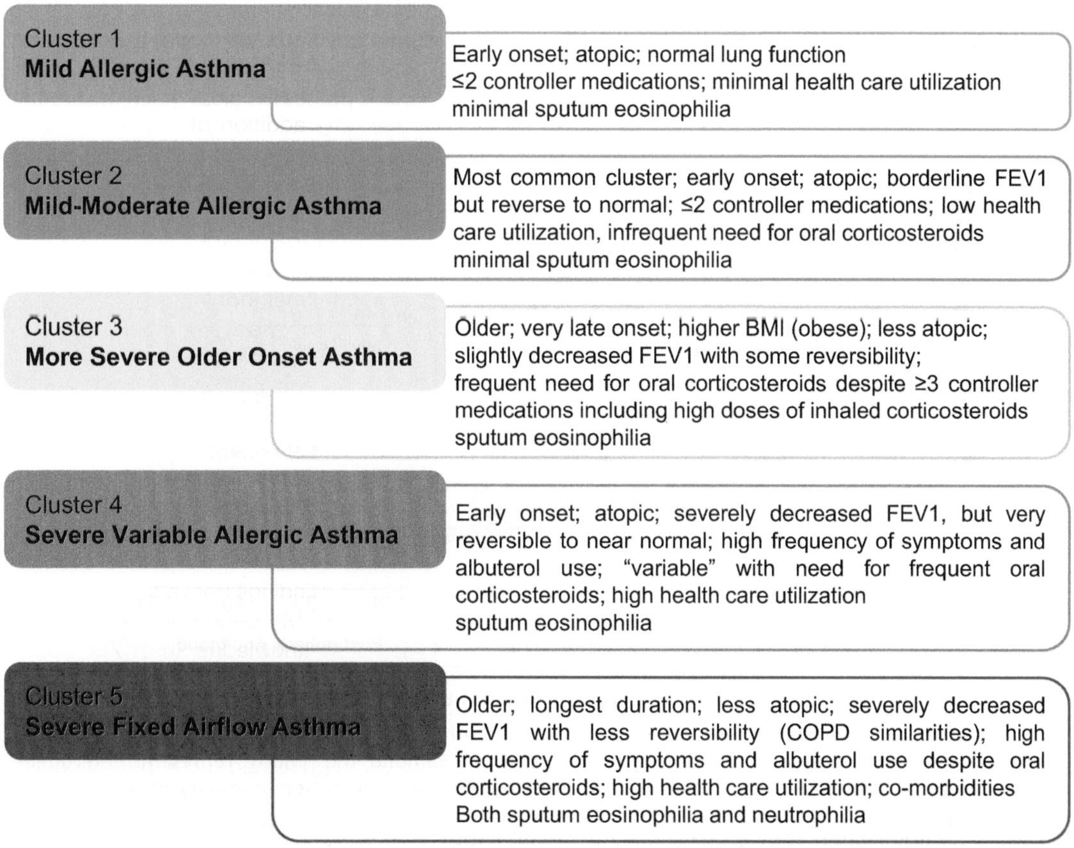

Cluster 1 Mild Allergic Asthma	Early onset; atopic; normal lung function $\leq$2 controller medications; minimal health care utilization minimal sputum eosinophilia
Cluster 2 Mild-Moderate Allergic Asthma	Most common cluster; early onset; atopic; borderline FEV1 but reverse to normal; $\leq$2 controller medications; low health care utilization, infrequent need for oral corticosteroids minimal sputum eosinophilia
Cluster 3 More Severe Older Onset Asthma	Older; very late onset; higher BMI (obese); less atopic; slightly decreased FEV1 with some reversibility; frequent need for oral corticosteroids despite $\geq$3 controller medications including high doses of inhaled corticosteroids sputum eosinophilia
Cluster 4 Severe Variable Allergic Asthma	Early onset; atopic; severely decreased FEV1, but very reversible to near normal; high frequency of symptoms and albuterol use; "variable" with need for frequent oral corticosteroids; high health care utilization sputum eosinophilia
Cluster 5 Severe Fixed Airflow Asthma	Older; longest duration; less atopic; severely decreased FEV1 with less reversibility (COPD similarities); high frequency of symptoms and albuterol use despite oral corticosteroids; high health care utilization; co-morbidities Both sputum eosinophilia and neutrophilia

Fig. 1. The 5 clusters from SARP with the predominant characteristics. (*Reprinted* with permission of the American Thoracic Society. Copyright © 2018 American Thoracic Society. *From* Jarjour NN, Erzurum SC, Bleecker ER, et al. Severe Asthma: Lessons learned from the NHLBI Severe Asthma Research Program. Am J Respir Crit Care Med 2012;185:356-62. PMC3297096. The American Journal of Respiratory and Critical Care Medicine is an official journal of the American Thoracic Society.)

just these 11 clinical characteristics.[15] A separate cluster analysis in the SARP children revealed 4 clusters that were again distinguished by age of onset and duration of disease as well as pre- and postbronchodilator lung function similar to that seen in the adult cohort, especially in the severe asthma clusters (**Fig. 2**).[14,16]

There are important differences in the newer SARP3 cohort at baseline from SARP1/2.[2,9] The enrollment mandate for 60% of the participants to have severe asthma skews the cohort toward more severe disease. The complexity of medication use has increased, and exacerbation rates have decreased likely related to changes in controller medications and asthma management strategies over a decade between the times the 2 cohorts were established. Nonetheless, application of the SARP1/2 eleven variable cluster algorithms to the new SARP3 cohort shows reproducibility of all 5 clinical cluster phenotypes albeit with an expected shift toward the more severe Clusters 3, 4, and 5.[17]

These current cluster phenotypes, reproducible in both SARP1/2 and SARP3 emphasize several important clinical aspects of asthma phenotypes. First, "traditional" early onset allergic asthma exists throughout the disease severity spectrum and even the most severe subjects (pediatric and adult Clusters 4) have the capability to achieve near-normal lung function with bronchodilators despite longer duration of disease. On the other hand, another group of subjects with very low lung function, later-onset disease (adolescent), and less responsiveness to bronchodilators is reminiscent of COPD (adult Cluster 5), with significant comorbidities and presumed high risk for poor clinical outcomes including irreversible lung remodeling. Finally, the identification of a small group with a late-onset, obese asthma phenotype with chronic rhinosinusitis and normal lung function (Cluster 3) was novel in SARP1/2 but represented by a higher proportion of subjects in SARP3 suggesting that this group of subjects may be increasing in prevalence or recognition over time.

Inflammatory Cell Phenotypes in Severe Asthma Research Program

Although the clinical cluster phenotypes are "real world" consistent with what we see in clinic, they lack biomarkers that would inform the underlying important pathobiological mechanisms that

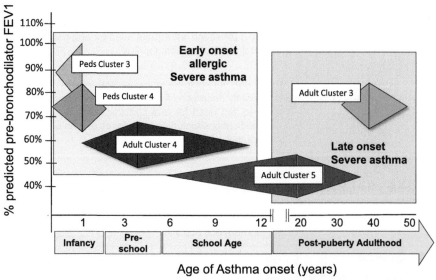

Age of Asthma onset (years)

Fig. 2. The adult and pediatric severe asthma phenotypes identified in the SARP cluster analyses.[15,16] Heterogeneity within each phenotype is indicated by the shape of the diamond; the "width" represents heterogeneity in the age of asthma onset (median *line*, IQR), the "height" symbolizes heterogeneity of lung function within each group (IQR). Note that most of the subjects with severe asthma had abnormal baseline lung function when bronchodilators were appropriately withhold before spirometry, reinforcing the importance of extended lung function testing in the clinic. (*Data from* Moore WC, Meyers DA, Wenzel SE, et al. Identification of asthma phenotypes using cluster analysis in the severe asthma research program. Am J Respir Crit Care Med 2010;181(4):315–23; and Fitzpatrick AM, Teague WG. Severe asthma in children: insights from the National Heart, Lung, and Blood Institute's Severe Asthma Research Program. Pediatr Allergy Immunol Pulmonol 2010;23(2):131–8.)

drive those clinical phenotypes. A major limitation of cluster analysis is that the chosen clustering variables must all be available in all included subjects. Thus, to maximize cohort size in the original cluster analysis, biomarkers were not included. Two additional cluster analyses have been performed on subsets of the SARP1/2 cohort, however, in which inflammatory cells were included.[18,19] Both of these analyses included blood granulocyte counts In their clustering variables but differed in the other clustering variables used.

The first "inflammatory" cluster analysis in SARP1/2 used different statistical methodology, applying a machine learning approach to a dataset containing greater than 100 clinical variable "factors," FeNO, and inflammatory cell counts from blood and bronchoalveolar lavage fluid in 378 subjects, including normal controls.[18] The identified asthma clusters were similar to the original clinical cluster phenotypes, but with the addition of an early onset symptom predominant female cluster that had previously been reported in other cluster analyses,[20] and also recognition of the importance of nasal polyposis in adult-onset disease, a phenotype also reported by others.[21] Importantly, these clusters were predominantly discriminated by clinical variables, not the inflammatory cell counts or biomarkers.

The second "inflammatory" cluster analysis used the same technique as the original clinical cluster analysis but added blood and sputum inflammatory cells to the 11 discriminating clinical variables from the original analysis (demographics, lung function, medication use).[5] In 423 subjects with adequate sputum samples, 4 clusters were identified, which are again reminiscent of the original clinical clusters. Importantly, blood and sputum eosinophilia were present in all groups and were not specific for allergic asthma phenotypes. Sputum neutrophilia, on the other hand, was primarily seen in the 2 more severe sputum clusters, with the most severe subjects manifesting elevations in both granulocytes.[4] Pre-bronchodilator percent predicted FEV_1 and percent sputum neutrophils were the most influential clustering variables by discriminant analysis supporting the role of non-Type 2 (T2-low) inflammatory mechanisms in severe asthma, either alone or in coexistence with T2-high mechanisms. Further –omics analyses in cell-free supernatants in SARP1/2 confirmed elevations in cytokines and chemokines from both the innate immunity (non-T2) and the traditional T2 inflammatory proteins. These findings suggest that in many severe asthma subjects, airway inflammation is complex with mixed non-T2 and T2 pathobiological elements.[4]

Although there is increasing appreciation for the importance of non-T2 inflammatory pathways, nearly all novel immunomodulators currently on the market target T2-high mechanisms. The ability to accurately identify T2-high patients who are good candidates for these treatments is crucial. Unfortunately, although there are positive correlations between the current clinic accessible T2 biomarkers (blood eosinophils, FeNO, and serum IgE), using any of these single biomarkers (or a combination of them) to predict sputum eosinophils (the "gold standard" T2-high biomarker) erroneously classified 25% of SARP1/2 subjects (half inaccurately labeled T2-low, half erroneously labeled T2-high).[22] In the search for a more sensitive T2 biomarker, quantitative polymerase chain reaction of gene expression from RNA isolated from sputum cells collected in SARP3 (n = 269) defined a "Type 2 Gene Mean (T2GM)" consisting of an average of gene expression measurements of the typical T2-high interleukin 4 (IL-4, IL-5, and IL-13).[23] Slightly more than half (55%) of the severe asthma subjects had "high" T2GM signatures. This means, however, that 45% of severe asthma subjects failed to show T2-high inflammation when defined by the T2GM furthering the observation that non-T2 (or T2-low) mechanisms may be predominant in many patients.

In conclusion, the SARP has comprehensively characterized close to 2400 subjects with asthma over the 18 years of funding. Phenotypes identified in SARP by cluster analysis are an evidenced-based approach to disease severity classification that aims to divide patients by extended clinical characteristics, lung function testing, and pathobiological mechanisms (biomarkers), rather than the treatment-oriented stepwise guidelines approach. The spectrum of allergic asthma phenotypes from mild to severe is in line with the concept of traditional atopic asthma. However, the finding of later-onset (non-childhood) phenotypes with marked comorbidities,[24–26] high health care utilization, and evidence for non-T2 with or without persistent steroid refractory T2-high biomarkers identifies a group of "nontraditional" patients in critical need.

In SARP1/2, investigations into pathobiological mechanisms have spanned many tissue compartments (airway samples, sputum, blood, and urine) and many biological pathways with diverse mechanistic studies[24,27–33] and genetics.[11,34–36] The newer SARP3 cohort provides cross-sectional data at baseline that will allow validation and expansion of the findings from SARP1/2. The longitudinal data collected in SARP3 will allow investigation into the stability of these clinical and pathobiological findings over time, analyses that are already in progress. Whether the pattern and trajectory of cluster phenotypes or mediators can predict adverse outcomes being assessed in annual follow-up in SARP3 (lung function decline, exacerbation risk) is the pivotal question.

THE ASTHMA DISEASE ENDOTYPING FOR PERSONALIZED THERAPEUTICS STUDY

The ADEPT study had a primary objective to characterize the clinical, physiologic, and molecular profiles of healthy nonsmoking subjects and nonsmoking subjects with mild, moderate, and severe asthma to facilitate directed drug discovery. ADEPT was a program funded by the pulmonary division of Janssen R&D. There was no formal hypothesis.

The ADEPT study was first reported in 2015[37] summarizing the study design and baseline parameters across cohorts. In brief, the study included screening, baseline visits, and follow-up visits at 3, 6, and 12 months, to allow assessment of stability of biomarkers over time. The study enrolled 157 adult nonsmoking mild/moderate and severe asthma subjects who underwent physical examination, completed the asthma control 7-item questionnaire (ACQ7) and the asthma quality of life questionnaire (AQLQ), with blood sampled for routine chemistry and hematology and specific IgE. Pulmonary function included pre- and postbronchodilator spirometry and airway hyperresponsiveness using methacholine. Biomarkers included exhaled nitric oxide (FENO), induced sputum in all subjects, bronchoscopy with endobronchial biopsy and brushing in a subset, and serum and whole blood biomarkers. Thirty healthy nonsmoking control subjects underwent all the procedures except those relevant to asthma, including induced sputum and bronchoscopy, during screening and baseline visits only.

Mild asthma was defined as a prebronchodilator (pre-BD) FEV_1 greater than or equal to 80% predicted and use of short-acting bronchodilators alone (ie, nonsteroid-treated). Moderate asthmatics had pre-BD FEV_1 between 60% and greater than 80% predicted, on low-medium doses of inhaled corticosteroids (ICS) alone or in combination with any other controller medication aside oral corticosteroids (OCS), whereas severe asthmatics had pre-BD FEV_1 from 50%

to less than 80% predicted and were on high-dose ICS with any other controller permitted including OCS. Of note, subjects with recent exacerbations or who were significantly uncontrolled were excluded. All asthmatics were required to show bronchodilator reversibility (BDR) or a provocative concentration resulting in a decline of FEV_1 of 20% (PC20) for methacholine less than 16 mg/ml or a FEV_1/FVC ratio less than 0.7 tested sequentially during screening.

Because of concerns for morbidity associated with bronchoscopy, the ADEPT population did not include the most refractory asthmatic subjects, smoking asthmatics (and those with >10 pack year history), or subjects with morbid obesity, and only one subject was on chronic OCS. In addition, ADEPT did not include pediatric asthma and non-Caucasian representation was small.

Age, asthma duration, and BMI increased with asthma severity, whereas those undergoing bronchoscopies were approximately 10 years younger than those who did not (**Fig. 3**, **Tables 1** and **2**).[37]

The major contributions of the ADEPT study to date are (1) evaluation of ways to define Type-2 high inflammation, (2) assessment of the longitudinal stability of asthma characteristics, and (3) defining asthma clusters that will all be summarized here.

Defining Type 2 Inflammation

Recently, classifying asthma as Type-2 or T-helper 2 (Th2) lymphocyte–driven asthma, characterized by elaboration of Type-2 cytokines, IL-4, IL-5, and IL-13 by CD4+Th2 cells has gained prominence. Evaluation of IL-13–driven gene expression in airway samples can identify Type-2-high asthmatics who have high expression of Type-2 cytokines in airway biopsies. Type-2 asthmatics also have enhanced airway hyperresponsiveness, elevated serum IgE, blood and airway eosinophilia, subepithelial fibrosis, and airway mucin gene expression.[38] Importantly, lung function improves after ICS only in Type-2-high asthma. The emergence of therapeutics that target Type-2-high asthmatics, for example, monoclonal antibodies targeting IL-13, IL-4, IL-5, and TSLP, has created a need to define the Type-2 high subset in clinical practice.

The ADEPT study revisited ways to define Type-2 status.[39] First, ADEPT evaluated IL-13–driven gene expression in several human cell lines and then defined Type-2 status based on gene expression for CCL26 (the highest differentially

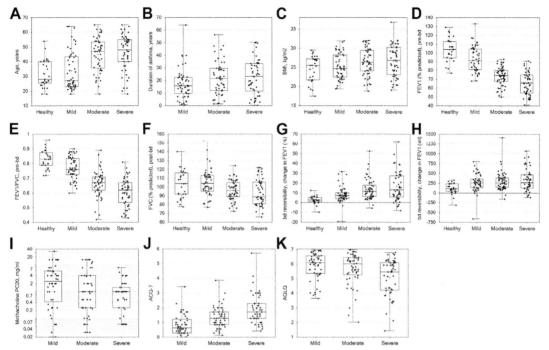

Fig. 3. Reproduced from Silkoff and colleagues (see Fig. 2). Demographic and clinical characteristics. The values for the indicated variables (y-axis) are shown for healthy control and asthma severity groups (x-axis). Data presented as symbols representing individual subjects and summarized by box (interquartile range and median) and whiskers (range), with "+" indicating mean. (*From* Silkoff PE, Strambu I, Laviolette M, et al. Asthma characteristics and biomarkers from the airways disease endotyping for personalized therapeutics (ADEPT) longitudinal profiling study. Respir Res 2015;16:142; with permission.)

expressed gene), periostin (as previously reported[40]), and an IL-13 multigene in vitro signature (IVS) in a subset from ADEPT of 25 healthy subjects, 28 mild, 29 moderate, and 26 severe asthmatic subjects. As bronchoscopy is not practical for screening patients for Type-2 status, ADEPT evaluated the diagnostic capability of clinically accessible biomarkers namely FENO, and blood eosinophil count (bEOS) but also assessed serum CCL26 and CCL17 (TARC), which could be used in the clinical arena in the future.

Mucosal expression of CCL26, periostin, and the IL-13 IVS were all effective in segregating subjects into Type-2-high and low groups, but CCL26 was optimal in the ADEPT dataset. All mucosal CCL26-Type-2-high subjects had FENO values greater than 35 ppb and bEOS counts greater than 300 cells/mm³ and demonstrated sputum eosinophilia. Looking at different combinations of clinical biomarkers in moderate-severe asthma, the combination of a FENO value ≥35 ppb OR a bEOS≥300 AND sCCL17 high status was optimal with a 93% sensitivity, 85% specificity, and receiver operator characteristic (ROC) value of

0.89 for the identification of Type-2-high CCL26 inflammation.

Potential issues with defining Type-2 status by bronchial mucosal expression include the impact of ICS. In the ADEPT subset, the proportion of mucosal CCL26-Type-2-high subjects decreased from mild steroid-nontreated asthmatics (16/28) to moderate-severe asthmatics (13/55) probably due to response to ICS. Another issue is that the expression of Type-2 inflammation in the bronchial mucosa may be heterogeneous leading to sampling error.

In summary, defining Type-2 status by mucosal CCL26 expression is novel. This expression allowed the evaluation of the diagnostic capability of "clinically accessible" biomarkers, FENO and bEOS, as well as the novel use of serum CCl26 and CCL17, which if available could have a role in clinical diagnosis and selection of therapeutics.

Longitudinal Stability of Asthma Characteristics

ADEPT addressed the stability of asthma characteristics in the cohort of 51 mild, moderate and

Table 1
Asthma disease characteristics by cohort at baseline visit (screening or baseline for PC20)

Cohorts	Healthy	Mild	Moderate	Severe	P-Value[c]
N	30	52	55	51	—
Pre-BD FEV1 (L)	3.98 (0.81)[a]	3.35 (0.81)	2.39 (0.62)	2.10 (0.71)	<.0001
Pre-BD FEV1 (% predicted normal)	103.3 (13.4)	92.7 (14.3)	73.6 (10.4)	65.4 (12.7)	<.0001
Post-BD FEV1 (L)	4.10 (0.84)	3.61 (0.87)	2.67 (0.66)	2.43 (0.81)	<.0001
Post-BD FEV1 (% predicted normal)	106.2 (13.7)	101.4 (14.0)	82.7 (10.2)	75.7 (15.4)	<.0001
Pre-BD FEV/FVC ratio	0.83 (0.06)	0.77 (0.08)	0.66 (0.09)	0.61 (0.09)	<.0001
Post-BD FVC (% predicted normal)	103.8 (15.9)	105.0 (15.5)	96.4 (11.4)	94.0 (15.1)	.0004
BDR (%)	2.9 (4.1)	8.5 (8.3)	15.2 (10.3)	18.3 (14.5)	.0016
BDR (mL)	114.8 (140.6)	265.1 (231.7)	335.2 (234.3)	355.7 (270.6)	.45
PC20 methacholine (mg/mL)	NA	1.68 (+10.85/−0.26)[b]	0.93 (+6.49/−0.13)[b]	0.63 (+2.62/−0.15)[b]	.034
ACQ7	NA	0.84 (0.69)	1.33 (0.71)	1.92 (1.01)	<.0001
Controlled ACQ <0.75 (N, %)	NA	29 (56%)	10 (18%)	4 (8%)	—
Partially controlled ACQ 0.75–1.5 (N, %)	NA	13 (25%)	24 (44%)	16 (31%)	<.0001
Uncontrolled ACQ ≥1.5 (N, %)	NA	10 (19%)	21 (38%)	31 (61%)	—
AQLQ	NA	5.86 (0.93)	5.68 (1.11)	5.09 (1.28)	.0016

[a] Mean (standard deviation) reported by cohort, unless otherwise indicated.
[b] Geometric mean (asymmetric standard deviation).
[c] P-value (ANOVA F-test, or Fisher's exact test when N, % reported) for differences across severity cohorts, excluding healthy control cohort (based on log-transformed data when geometric means reported).
   Data from Silkoff PE, Strambu I, Laviolette M, et al. Asthma characteristics and biomarkers from the Airways Disease Endotyping for Personalized Therapeutics (ADEPT) longitudinal profiling study. Respir Res 2015;16:142.

severe asthmatics as defined over 12 months.[41] Repeated assessments were made for patient questionnaires (ACQ, AQLQ), spirometry, bronchodilator reversibility, FENO, and induced sputum biomarkers.

There were no significant changes in group mean data over the 12 months of the study. However, individual data demonstrated significant variability. The FEV_1/FVC ratio was highly reproducible (intraclass correlation [ICC] 0.88) but pre-BD FEV_1 and FVC were only moderately reproducible (ICC 0.60–0.72 and 0.62–0.79, respectively) reflecting asthma variability. Of note, bronchodilator reversibility to albuterol was poorly reproducible (ICC 0.39–0.45), with the nonreversible phenotype much more stable compared with

the reversible phenotype. The ACQ7 had moderate reproducibility for the combined asthma cohorts (ICC = 0.76), but the uncontrolled asthma phenotype (ACQ7 >1.5) was highly variable in mild and moderate asthma but stable in severe asthma 1.5 at baseline (with 87% concordance at third month). The FENO-low phenotype (FENO <35 ppb) was more stable than the FENO-high phenotype (FENO ≥35 ppb). Induced sputum inflammatory phenotypes were markedly variable for 3 sputum samples taken over 6 months.

The data reflect the inherent variability in asthma and could be related to seasonal exposures including viral infections but has implications for clinical trials that require BDR for enrollment. The same subject could on this basis qualify for a

Table 2
Clinical biomarkers and sputum differential counts by cohort at screening/baseline visits

Cohorts	Healthy	Mild	Moderate	Severe	P-Value[c]
n (blood/sputum)	30/20	52/32	55/38	51/40	—
FENO (ppb)[a]	NA	32.9 (+64.2/−16.9)	29.1 (+61.0/−13.9)	28.8 (+64.7/−12.9)	NA/.59
bEOS, cells/μL[a]	112 (+218/−57)	178 (+347/−91)	197 (+435/−89)	210 (+452/−97)	.0018/.54
bNEU, 1000 cells/μL[a]	3.47 (+4.96/−2.42)	3.59 (+4.72/−2.74)	3.64 (+4.92/−2.69)	3.94 (+5.89/−2.63)	.35/.32
Serum IgE, RFU[a]	1.0 (+2.1/−0.7)	8.3 (+25.3/−6.2)	9.8 (+26.7/−7.2)	12.1 (+31.0/−8.7)	<.0001/.35
Sputum eosinophils, % of WBC[a]	0.38 (+0.78/−0.25)	1.12 (+5.38/−0.93)	3.12 (+13.62/−2.54)	2.70 (+12.27/−2.21)	<.0001/.033
Sputum lymphocytes, % of WBC[b]	1.16 (1.05)	1.29 (1.42)	0.98 (1.19)	0.94 (1.25)	.64/.48
Sputum macrophages, % of WBC[b]	44.57 (19.42)	50.20 (31.17)	32.10 (21.45)	43.04 (26.46)	.031/.019
Sputum neutrophils, % of WBC[b]	53.57 (20.06)	43.88 (30.90)	56.99 (26.13)	48.10 (25.52)	.19/.13

[a] Geometric mean (asymmetric standard deviation) reported by cohort.
[b] Mean (standard deviation) reported by cohort.
[c] P-value (ANOVA F-test) for differences across severity cohorts, inclucing/excluding healthy control cohort (based on log-transformed data when geometric means reported); NA = not applicable (not measured in healthy cohort).
Data from Silkoff PE, Strambu I, Laviolette M, et al. Asthma characteristics and biomarkers from the Airways Disease Endotyping for Personalized Therapeutics (ADEPT) longitudinal profiling study. Respir Res 2015;16:142.

specific clinical trial on one occasion but not on another. The variability in the high FENO phenotype also could have implications for the use of this biomarker to select patients for Type-2 therapies. In addition, the variability in the inflammatory phenotype based on induced sputum should drive caution in relying on a single induction to define the phenotype of asthma. Repeated measures over time may be necessary to truly understand the fluctuations in the phenotype of airway inflammation over time.

Clustering on the Asthma Disease Endotyping for Personalized Therapeutics Cohort

One aim of establishing the ADEPT dataset was to evaluate ways to define distinct subsets that could require different therapeutic approaches. SARP and U-BIOPRED have also evaluated clustering on their datasets.

ADEPT used fuzzy partition-around-medoid (PAM) clustering on 156 asthma subjects.[42,43] This methodology is tolerant to outliers, missing data, and independently suggests the optimal number of clusters. The PAM method assigns probabilities for each subject belonging to a cluster. The clustering was performed on 9 variables that are widely available: pre-BD FEV_1 and FVC expressed as % predicted, FEV_1/FVC ratio, BDR, airway hyperresponsiveness (AHR) expressed as log-transformed provocative concentration of methacholine resulting in 20% decline in FEV_1 (PC20), ACQ-7, AQLQ, log-transformed FENO, and bEOS expressed as absolute counts per μL. Of note, the clustering was intentionally based on the current status of the disease and did not include demographic details, for example, age or gender, BMI etc., nor historical aspects, for example, age of onset, thus differing from prior efforts in this area.

The PAM methodology determined that 4 clusters was the ideal number.[42,43] These four clusters (**Table 3**) are as follows: A1: predominantly (93%) nonsteroid-treated well-controlled mild asthma, normal lung function, early age-of-onset, no BDR, and low AHR; the degree of airway inflammation was low; A2: predominantly moderate asthmatics with marked AHR and marked degree of eosinophilic inflammation (highest FENO and sputum eosinophilia); A3 (the largest cluster): fixed obstruction with noneosinophilic inflammation (normal FENO, neutrophilic inflammation); and A4: severe asthma with marked BDR, the poorest asthma control, and a mixed inflammatory phenotype. The cluster phenotypes were robust to perturbation. A full description of the clusters can be found in the publication, which is open access.[43] Notable, the 4 ADEPT clusters correspond to phenotypes that are commonly seen in clinical practice. The repeated visits of ADEPT subjects over 12 months allowed examination of the stability of the ADEPT clusters. In general, there was remarkable stability of the ADEPT clusters with only a minority of subjects changing their original cluster assignment.

Independent validation

Importantly and uniquely, validation of the 4 ADEPT clusters was subsequently obtained using a subset of the U-BIOPRED data that contained subjects who most closely corresponded to the ADEPT inclusion criteria, for example, excluding smokers and those on OCS (82 of 397 participants). When applying the same PAM clustering methodology as ADEPT, the U-BIOPRED subset (US) optimally partitioned to 4 clusters, US1, 2, 3, and 4, which demonstrated remarkable similarity to the ADEPT clusters. ADEPT is the first study to identify robust stable clinically relevant

Table 3
The 4 clusters in ADEPT derived using PAM clustering methodology

N = 158	Pre-BD FEV$_1$% Predicted	ACQ7	PC20	FeNO Ppb/Geo.mean	N; Proportion Mild/Moderate/ Severe %
A1: *mild* controlled asthma	103.5 ± 11.8	0.5 ± 0.5	2.8 + 11.3/−2.2	35.2 + 28.1/−15.6	28;93/7/0
A2: *Hyperreactive eosinophilic*	77.4 ± 10.2	1.1 ± 0.5	0.3 + 1.4/−0.3	43.8 + 36.7/−20.0	44;16/52/32
A3: *Fixed obstruction noneosinophilic*	76.5 ± 9.8	1.2 ± 0.5	2.2 + 7.0/−1.7	16.4 + 9.7/−6.1	49;27/43/31
A4: *Severe uncontrolled asthma* with mixed inflammatory phenotype	66.8 ± 11.5	2.6 ± 0.9	0.6 + 2.8/−0.5	37.7 + 47.8/−21.1	35;11/26/63

phenotypes of asthma using data from 2 independent cohorts.

In summary, ADEPT evaluated a range of severity of asthma against healthy controls over a 12-month period. This dataset has provided valuable insights into ways to determine type2 status, the longitudinal stability of asthma outcome measures, and inflammatory phenotypes and identified 4 clusters that reproduce well in an independent cohort.

UNBIASED BIOMARKERS FOR THE PREDICTION OF RESPIRATORY DISEASE OUTCOME

In 2008, the European Union (EU) and the European Federation of Pharmaceutical Industries and Associations (EFPIA) joined forces to establish the Innovative Medicines Initiative (IMI) as part of a major public-private collaboration (Joint Undertaking) in Europe. The objective of IMI was, and is, to not only speed up but also change the paradigms for the development, testing, and implementation of new medicines in areas with major medical needs. The program has resulted in unprecedented funding, collaborations, and assets that have become the backbone of biomedical progress in Europe.

Novel Collaborations

The IMI calls are driven by EFPIA members, whereas the academics and other research institutes write and submit the grants. The EU coordinates the peer review and EFPIA members can join the approved grants for matching funding with the EU. One of the first calls was "Understanding severe asthma," aimed to provide a step-change in the treatment of patients with severe asthma by a renewed focus on the complexity of its underlying mechanisms. The U-BIOPRED project received funding for its objective to phenotype patients with severe asthma by integrating clinical and high-throughput biological disease markers in a systems medicine approach.[44] The structure of the project was and still is extremely successful, allowing basic and clinical scientists from academia, pharmaceutical industry, small-medium enterprises, and charities to really join forces in a precompetitive setting.[45]

A major step-change of this project was the true participation and control by individual patients and their organizations at all levels of the project.[46,47] In retrospect, the project could not have been successful without patient participation! Another major accomplishment at the time of setting up U-BIOPRED was that the SARP generously shared their Standard Operating Procedures (SOPs) in order to allow future comparison of data that have been derived from similar sampling and measurement procedures between projects. Subsequently, U-BIOPRED has provided its SOPs to several other new consortia around the world, so that harmonization between consortia is becoming the standard. In fact, it can be questioned whether new projects without such methodological streamlining should still be funded. The Research Agency of the ERS is now heavily promoting such fine tuning of big projects in respiratory research as an indispensable aspect of quality and impact. Taken together, U-BIOPRED is an exponent of a new attitude in collaborative biomedical research, which has become sustained in the U-BIOPRED Alliance ensuring continuity toward new projects and collaborations in its postfunding period.

The Clinical Approach

The first issue required for adequately phenotyping patients with severe asthma is distinguishing truly severe asthma from difficult-to-treat asthma. The latter group represents patients whose asthma is hard to control because of other reasons than the disease itself, such as environmental exposures and treatment adherence. U-BIOPRED has provided a stepwise decision tree in order to delineate the patients with genuinely severe asthma amongst those who are difficult to treat.[48] The resulting decision tree has had immediate applicability, not only for pinpointing the prevalence of severe asthma (3%–4% of the asthmatics)[49] but also for improving clinical care.

Inevitably, the pediatric[50] and adult[51] cohorts of U-BIOPRED are representative of a European sample. The pediatric cohorts include severe preschool wheeze, mild-moderate preschool wheeze, severe school-age asthma, and mild-moderate school-age asthma,[50] whereas the adult cohorts comprise nonsmoking severe asthma, smoking severe asthma, mild-moderate asthma, and healthy controls.[51] When performing an unbiased cluster analysis on the clinically available patient characteristics, 4 clinical phenotypes could be discriminated based on distinguishing characteristics such as age of onset, gender, severity of airflow limitation, frequency of exacerbations, circulating eosinophil counts, and oral steroid dose.[52] This resembles and extends previous cluster analyses in severe asthma.[15,20] In those adult patients consenting for bronchial biopsies, the severity of mucosal airway inflammation does not seem to be a distinguishing characteristic of severe asthma.[53] This suggests that simply the numbers of inflammatory cells in the bronchial wall is not associated with the severity of asthma.

Biological complexity

Apparently, severe asthma exhibits far from simple pathophysiology underlying its heterogeneous clinical presentation. The complex biology of severe asthma requires the identification of the various cellular and biological networks. Even though single biomarkers (eg, sputum eosinophils and exhaled nitric oxide) are gradually being introduced in the management of severe asthma (based on the latest meta-analyses),[54] the U-BIOPRED study has postulated that composite biomarker fingerprints will provide more comprehensive pathobiological information of these diseases and their underlying molecular phenotypes. Indeed, there is increasing evidence that complex biology can be better captured by pattern recognition, based, for example, on machine learning, than by unraveling multiple individual molecular pathways.[55] It should be emphasized that this leads to molecular phenotypes, rather than so-called "endotypes." The latter term should be used very carefully because it requires solid establishment of causative molecular pathways (almost always pending). The term "endotypes" is not used and is unknown outside the respiratory field.

These high-throughput "omics" technologies based on unbiased systems biology approaches, including transcriptomics, proteomics, lipidomics, and metabolomics, are being used by U-BIOPRED for biomarker discovery in severe asthma.[56] The leading principle here is to strictly obey the recent guidelines on the quality and validation of omics analysis in clinical medicine.[57]

The first unbiased biomarkers for the prediction of respiratory disease outcome molecular fingerprints

U-BIOPRED sampled blood, urine, nasal lavage, sputum, and bronchial brushes and biopsies for comprehensive 'omics' analysis. Even though gene expression profiles in blood,[58] sputum, and bronchial brushes and biopsies differ between clinical and inflammatory subgroups (eosinophilic, neutrophilic, Th2, non-Th2, IL-1 receptor),[59–61] these comprise previously unknown and complementary information leading to newly discovered severe asthma phenotypes. For instance, unbiased transcriptomic analysis in sputum from patients with moderate and severe asthma identified 3 distinct transcriptome-associated clusters, one being Th2-high and eosinophilic, whereas the other 2 were Th2-low and either associated with inflammasome or metabolic/mitochondrial pathways.[59] Hence, this revealed previously undiscovered molecular phenotypes that are currently input for the development of targeted interventions. Not unexpectedly, such fingerprints

diverge between nonsmoking and smoking severe asthmatics, highlighting the need for taking lifestyle and environmental factors into account.[62]

Gene expression does not track between sample locations (blood, sputum, biopsies),[63] which indicates that severe asthma phenotypes may require local as well systemic sampling. It remains to be established whether relatively noninvasive signatures as provided from blood, sputum, nasal lavage, urine, or exhaled air can still largely cover the major severe asthma phenotypes by themselves. Supervised analysis of transcriptomic fingerprints is demonstrating differences between adult- and childhood-onset asthma[63] and between patients with and without fixed airflow limitation.[64] This suggests that these clinical entities are associated with partially divergent molecular mechanisms. The differential gene expression between clinical, severe asthma categories (eg, childhood- vs adult-onset) varies between sample sites (sputum, bronchial brushes, and nasal brushes)[63] as shown in **Fig. 4**. This indicates that the phenotypic molecular signatures depend on local cellular environments, which is to be expected.

These data from U-BIOPRED indicate that there are multiple bioclinical phenotypes of severe asthma that are linked to distinct molecular mechanisms. A major observation is that patients with severe asthma with or without sputum eosinophilia apparently exhibit distinct subnodes of sputum proteomic signatures.[65] Further analysis is providing the driving proteins for such separate proteomic clusters and in combination with a transcriptome analysis from the same cells in sputum allows projection into pathway analysis and in a connectivity map for potential drug target identification. This comes close to the core objective of U-BIOPRED, namely to identify novel bioclinical phenotypes of (severe) asthma by unsupervised discovery.

Noninvasive methods may be able to capture molecular phenotypes of severe asthma, as seems from analysis of exhaled air from the U-BIOPRED severe asthma cohorts by cross-reactive sensor technology (electronic nose: eNose).[66] eNose provides metabolomic fingerprints, based on comprehensive and composite signatures of exhaled volatile organic compounds. The data show eNose-driven clusters of severe asthma patients that differ with regard to systemic eosinophilic and neutrophilic inflammation.[67] When considering the first prospective follow-up data, the individual eNose signatures of the patients are changing over time in association with changes in eosinophilic inflammation[67], suggesting that molecular fingerprints can monitor the longitudinal course and dynamics of severe asthma phenotypes. These findings may have broader implications,

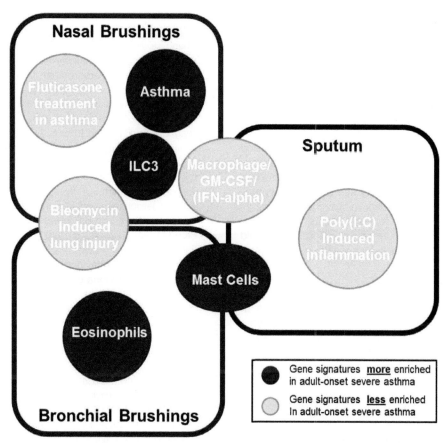

Fig. 4. Differential gene expression at various sample sites (sputum, bronchial brushes, and nasal brushes) between patients with adult-onset versus childhood-onset severe asthma as measured by gene-set variation analysis. Some gene-sets are more enriched in adult-onset asthma (*blue*), whereas other gene-sets are less enriched (*gray*). (*From* Hekking PP, Loza MJ, Pavlidis S, et al. Pathway discovery using transcriptomic profiles in adult-onset severe asthma. J Allergy Clin Immunol 2018;141(4):1280; with permission.)

because it seems that inflammatory profiles can also be identified by eNose amongst a collective cohort of patients with asthma, COPD, or their overlap independent of their clinical diagnosis.[68]

Multiomics: the severe asthma handprints
The most recent efforts of U-BIOPRED are focusing on multiscale analysis, linking various "omics" fingerprints by similarity network fusion.[69] This attempts to combine the information derived from multiple fingerprints (eg, transcriptomics, proteomics, and metabolomics), thereby called handprints. To that end, U-BIOPRED has developed its multiomics toolbox, which is a stepwise format for ensuring the quality and validation of this type of analysis.[70] External validation of those handprints is currently being done by using data from the ADEPT and Asthma Bridge datasets. Recent evidence indicates that the sample size required for the identification of phenotypes by such multiomics analyses with sufficient statistical

power is actually decreasing with increasing number of omics platforms.[71] This is good news and may intuitively be right: the more we have measured from a particular patient, the easier she/he can be distinguished from others. This observation will undoubtedly promote the discovery of new (severe) asthma phenotypes. Linking those to rapid and noninvasive diagnostic procedures will facilitate implementation of data-driven management of the disease.

In Summary, U-BIOPRED has delivered its cohorts and its clinical phenotypes. The first unbiased molecular fingerprints obtained by various omics technologies in samples from the airways, blood, urine, and exhaled air have been established. This has led to discovery of new (severe) asthma phenotypes that were previously unknown and is now helping to abolish 2 major roadblocks in severe asthma. First, finding new targets for therapy: not only those drugs that provide clinical control or those that suppress exacerbations (as is the target by the currently available biologics) but also those drugs that can accomplish true disease modification by efficacy against the development of severe asthma and against its prognostic deterioration. This requires linking the observed fingerprints and handprints to detailed, existing knowledge on molecular pathways in health and disease. Recently, the AsthmaMap has been developed for that very purpose.[72] Second, the newly discovered phenotypes will allow tailoring existing and novel drugs to the right individual patient. To that end, the U-BIOPRED fingerprints and handprints should be assessed at baseline in prospective therapeutic trials, in order to analyze their predictive capacity for responders and nonresponders. This is currently ongoing and should be expanded as widely as possible.

ACKNOWLEDGEMENT

PJS expresses his gratitude to the patients of U-BIOPRED and all the partners and collaborators in the U-BIOPRED Study Group (http://www.europeanlung.org/projects-and-research/projects/u-biopred/home)

REFERENCES

1. Proceedings of the ATS workshop on refractory asthma: current understanding, recommendations, and unanswered questions. American Thoracic Society. Am J Respir Crit Care Med 2000;162(6): 2341–51.
2. Moore WC, Bleecker ER, Curran-Everett D, et al. Characterization of the severe asthma phenotype by the National Heart, Lung, and Blood Institute's Severe Asthma Research Program. J Allergy Clin Immunol 2007;119(2):405–13.
3. Liu L, Teague WG, Erzurum S, et al. Determinants of exhaled breath condensate pH in a large population with asthma. Chest 2011;139(2):328–36.
4. Hastie AT, Moore WC, Meyers DA, et al. Analyses of asthma severity phenotypes and inflammatory proteins in subjects stratified by sputum granulocytes. J Allergy Clin Immunol 2010;125(5): 1028–36.e13.
5. Moore WC, Hastie AT, Li X, et al. Sputum neutrophil counts are associated with more severe asthma phenotypes using cluster analysis. J Allergy Clin Immunol 2014;133(6):1557–63.e5.
6. Moore WC, Evans MD, Bleecker ER, et al. Safety of investigative bronchoscopy in the Severe Asthma Research Program. J Allergy Clin Immunol 2011; 128(2):328–36.e3.
7. Choi S, Hoffman EA, Wenzel SE, et al. Quantitative computed tomographic imaging-based clustering differentiates asthmatic subgroups with distinctive clinical phenotypes. J Allergy Clin Immunol 2017; 140(3):690–700.e8.
8. Chung KF, Wenzel S, European Respiratory Society/American Thoracic Society Severe Asthma International Guidelines Task Force. From the authors: International European Respiratory Society/American Thoracic Society guidelines on severe asthma. Eur Respir J 2014;44(5):1378–9.
9. Teague WG, Phillips BR, Fahy JV, et al. Baseline Features of the Severe Asthma Research Program (SARP III) Cohort: differences with age. J Allergy Clin Immunol Pract 2018;6(2):545–54.e4.
10. Jarjour NN, Erzurum SC, Bleecker ER, et al. Severe asthma: lessons learned from the National Heart, Lung, and Blood Institute Severe Asthma Research Program. Am J Respir Crit Care Med 2012;185(4): 356–62.
11. Wenzel SE, Busse WW. Severe asthma: lessons from the Severe Asthma Research Program. J Allergy Clin Immunol 2007;119(1):14–21 [quiz: 22–3].
12. Denlinger LC, Phillips BR, Ramratnam S, et al. Inflammatory and comorbid features of patients with severe asthma and frequent exacerbations. Am J Respir Crit Care Med 2017;195(3):302–13.
13. Phipatanakul W, Mauger DT, Sorkness RL, et al. Effects of age and disease severity on systemic corticosteroid responses in asthma. Am J Respir Crit Care Med 2017;195(11):1439–48.
14. Fitzpatrick AM, Teague WG, Meyers DA, et al. Heterogeneity of severe asthma in childhood: confirmation by cluster analysis of children in the National Institutes of Health/National Heart, Lung, and Blood Institute Severe Asthma Research Program. J Allergy Clin Immunol 2011;127(2):382–9. e1-13.
15. Moore WC, Meyers DA, Wenzel SE, et al. Identification of asthma phenotypes using cluster analysis in the Severe Asthma Research Program. Am J Respir Crit Care Med 2010;181(4):315–23.
16. Fitzpatrick AM, Teague WG. Severe asthma in children: insights from the national heart, lung, and blood institute's severe asthma research program. Pediatr Allergy Immunol Pulmonol 2010;23(2):131–8.
17. Moore WCLX, Li H, Castro M, et al, for the NHLBI Severe Asthma Research Program. Clinical cluster phenotypes from the Severe Asthma Research Program (SARP1/2): reproducibility in SARP 3 and the importance of baseline lung function in disease stability and progression. Am J Respir Crit Care Med 2016;193.
18. Wu W, Bleecker E, Moore W, et al. Unsupervised phenotyping of Severe Asthma Research Program participants using expanded lung data. J Allergy Clin Immunol 2014;133(5):1280–8.
19. Moore WCHA, Li X, Li H, et al. Sputum neutrophil counts are associated with more severe asthma phenotypes using cluster analysis. J Allergy Clin Immunol 2013;133(6):1557–663.e5.

20. Haldar P, Pavord ID, Shaw DE, et al. Cluster analysis and clinical asthma phenotypes. Am J Respir Crit Care Med 2008;178(3):218–24.

21. Amelink M, de Groot JC, de Nijs SB, et al. Severe adult-onset asthma: a distinct phenotype. J Allergy Clin Immunol 2013;132(2):336–41.

22. Hastie A, Moore WC, Li H, et al. Biomarker surrogates do not accurately predict sputum eosinophil and neutrophil percentages in asthmatic subjects. J Allergy Clin Immunol 2013;132(1):72–80.

23. Peters MC, Kerr S, Dunican EM, et al. Refractory airway type 2 inflammation in a large subgroup of asthmatic patients treated with inhaled corticosteroids. J Allergy Clin Immunol 2018. [Epub ahead of print].

24. Holguin F, Bleecker ER, Busse WW, et al. Obesity and asthma: an association modified by age of asthma onset. J Allergy Clin Immunol 2011;127(6): 1486–93.e2.

25. Luyster FS, Strollo PJ Jr, Holguin F, et al. Association between insomnia and asthma burden in the severe asthma research program (SARP) III. Chest 2016; 150(6):1242–50.

26. Zein JG, Dweik RA, Comhair SA, et al. Asthma is more severe in older adults. PLoS One 2015;10(7): e0133490.

27. Dweik RA, Sorkness RL, Wenzel S, et al. Use of exhaled nitric oxide measurement to identify a reactive, at-risk phenotype among patients with asthma. Am J Respir Crit Care Med 2010;181(10): 1033–41.

28. Comhair SA, Ricci KS, Arroliga M, et al. Correlation of systemic superoxide dismutase deficiency to airflow obstruction in asthma. Am J Respir Crit Care Med 2005;172(3):306–13.

29. Lara A, Khatri SB, Wang Z, et al. Alterations of the arginine metabolome in asthma. Am J Respir Crit Care Med 2008;178(7):673–81.

30. Planaguma A, Kazani S, Marigowda G, et al. Airway lipoxin A4 generation and lipoxin A4 receptor expression are decreased in severe asthma. Am J Respir Crit Care Med 2008;178(6):574–82.

31. Ricklefs I, Barkas I, Duvall MG, et al. ALX receptor ligands define a biochemical endotype for severe asthma. JCI Insight 2018;3(6) [pii:120932].

32. Wenzel SE, Balzar S, Ampleford E, et al. IL4R alpha mutations are associated with asthma exacerbations and mast cell/IgE expression. Am J Respir Crit Care Med 2007;175(6):570–6.

33. Comhair SA, Gaston BM, Ricci KS, et al. Detrimental effects of environmental tobacco smoke in relation to asthma severity. PLoS One 2011;6(5):e18574.

34. Li X, Hawkins GA, Ampleford EJ, et al. Genome-wide association study identifies TH1 pathway genes associated with lung function in asthmatic patients. J Allergy Clin Immunol 2013;132(2): 313–20.e15.

35. Hawkins GA, Robinson MB, Hastie AT, et al. The IL6R variation Asp(358)Ala is a potential modifier of lung function in subjects with asthma. J Allergy Clin Immunol 2012;130(2):510–5.e1.

36. Li X, Ampleford EJ, Howard TD, et al. Genome-wide association studies of asthma indicate opposite immunopathogenesis direction from auto-immune diseases. J Allergy Clin Immunol 2012; 130(4):861–8.e7.

37. Silkoff PE, Strambu I, Laviolette M, et al. Asthma characteristics and biomarkers from the Airways Disease Endotyping for Personalized Therapeutics (ADEPT) longitudinal profiling study. Respir Res 2015;16:142.

38. Woodruff PG, Modrek B, Choy DF, et al. T-helper type 2-driven inflammation defines major subphenotypes of asthma. Am J Respir Crit Care Med 2009; 180(5):388–95.

39. Silkoff PE, Laviolette M, Singh D, et al. Identification of airway mucosal type 2 inflammation by using clinical biomarkers in asthmatic patients. J Allergy Clin Immunol 2017;140(3):710–9.

40. Jia G, Erickson RW, Choy DF, et al. Periostin is a systemic biomarker of eosinophilic airway inflammation in asthmatic patients. J Allergy Clin Immunol 2012; 130(3):647–54.e10.

41. Silkoff PE, Laviolette M, Singh D, et al. Longitudinal stability of asthma characteristics and biomarkers from the Airways Disease Endotyping for Personalized Therapeutics (ADEPT) study. Respir Res 2016;17:43.

42. Loza MJ, Adcock I, Auffray C, et al. Longitudinally stable, clinically defined clusters of patients with asthma independently identified in the ADEPT and U-BIOPRED asthma studies. Ann Am Thorac Soc 2016;13(Suppl 1):S102–3.

43. Loza MJ, Djukanovic R, Chung KF, et al. Validated and longitudinally stable asthma phenotypes based on cluster analysis of the ADEPT study. Respir Res 2016;17(1):165.

44. Auffray C, Adcock IM, Chung KF, et al. An integrative systems biology approach to understanding pulmonary diseases. Chest 2010;137(6):1410–6.

45. Riley JH, Erpenbeck VJ, Matthews JG, et al. U-BIOPRED: evaluation of the value of a public-private partnership to industry. Drug Discov Today 2018; 23(9):1622–34.

46. Supple D, Roberts A, Hudson V, et al. From tokenism to meaningful engagement: best practices in patient involvement in an EU project. Res Involv Engagem 2015;1:5.

47. European Lung Foundation: A short guide to successful patient involvement in EU funded research. Lessons learnt from the U-BIOPRED project. Available at: http://www.europeanlung.org/assets/files/publications/ubiobookletpip.pdf.

48. Bel EH, Sousa A, Fleming L, et al. Diagnosis and definition of severe refractory asthma: an

international consensus statement from the Innovative Medicine Initiative (IMI). Thorax 2011;66(10): 910–7.

49. Hekking PP, Wener RR, Amelink M, et al. The prevalence of severe refractory asthma. J Allergy Clin Immunol 2015;135(4):896–902.

50. Fleming L, Murray C, Bansal AT, et al. The burden of severe asthma in childhood and adolescence: results from the paediatric U-BIOPRED cohorts. Eur Respir J 2015;46(5):1322–33.

51. Shaw DE, Sousa AR, Fowler SJ, et al. Clinical and inflammatory characteristics of the European U-BIOPRED adult severe asthma cohort. Eur Respir J 2015;46(5):1308–21.

52. Lefaudeux D, De Meulder B, Loza MJ, et al. U-BIOPRED clinical adult asthma clusters linked to a subset of sputum omics. J Allergy Clin Immunol 2017; 139(6):1797–807.

53. Wilson SJ, Ward JA, Sousa AR, et al. Severe asthma exists despite suppressed tissue inflammation: findings of the U-BIOPRED study. Eur Respir J 2016; 48(5):1307–19.

54. Petsky HL, Li A, Chang AB. Tailored interventions based on sputum eosinophils versus clinical symptoms for asthma in children and adults. Cochrane Database Syst Rev 2017;(8):CD005603.

55. Yu XT, Wang L, Zeng T. Revisit of machine learning supported biological and biomedical studies. Methods Mol Biol 2018;1754:183–204.

56. Wheelock CE, Goss VM, Balgoma D, et al. Application of 'omics technologies to biomarker discovery in inflammatory lung diseases. Eur Respir J 2013; 42(3):802–25.

57. McShane LM, Cavenagh MM, Lively TG, et al. Criteria for the use of omics-based predictors in clinical trials: explanation and elaboration. BMC Med 2013;11:220.

58. Bigler J, Boedigheimer M, Schofield JPR, et al. A severe asthma disease signature from gene expression profiling of peripheral blood from U-BIOPRED cohorts. Am J Respir Crit Care Med 2017; 195(10):1311–20.

59. Kuo CS, Pavlidis S, Loza M, et al. A transcriptome-driven analysis of epithelial brushings and bronchial biopsies to define asthma phenotypes in U-BIOPRED. Am J Respir Crit Care Med 2017;195(4): 443–55.

60. Kuo CS, Pavlidis S, Loza M, et al. T-helper cell type 2 (Th2) and non-Th2 molecular phenotypes of asthma using sputum transcriptomics in U-BIOPRED. Eur Respir J 2017;49(2) [pii:1602135].

61. Rossios C, Pavlidis S, Hoda U, et al. Sputum transcriptomics reveal upregulation of IL-1 receptor family members in patients with severe asthma. J Allergy Clin Immunol 2018;141(2):560–70.

62. Takahashi K, Pavlidis S, Ng Kee Kwong F, et al. Sputum proteomics and airway cell transcripts of current and ex-smokers with severe asthma in U-BIOPRED: an exploratory analysis. Eur Respir J 2018;51(5) [pii:1702173].

63. Hekking PP, Loza MJ, Pavlidis S, et al. Pathway discovery using transcriptomic profiles in adult-onset severe asthma. J Allergy Clin Immunol 2018; 141(4):1280–90.

64. Hekking PP, Loza MJ, Pavlidis S, et al. Transcriptomic gene signatures associated with persistent airflow limitation in patients with severe asthma. Eur Respir J 2017;50(3) [pii:1602298].

65. Burg D, Schofield JPR, Brandsma J, et al. Large-scale label-free quantitative mapping of the sputum proteome. J Proteome Res 2018;17(6):2072–91.

66. Boots AW, Bos LD, van der Schee MP, et al. Exhaled molecular fingerprinting in diagnosis and monitoring: validating volatile promises. Trends Mol Med 2015;21(10):633–44.

67. Brinkman P, Wagener AH, Hekking PP, et al. Identification and prospective stability of eNose derived inflammatory phenotypes in severe asthma. J Allergy Clin Immunol 2018. [Epub ahead of print].

68. de Vries R, Dagelet YWF, Spoor P, et al. Clinical and inflammatory phenotyping by breathomics in chronic airway diseases irrespective of the diagnostic label. Eur Respir J 2018;51(1) [pii: 1701817].

69. Wang B, Mezlini AM, Demir F, et al. Similarity network fusion for aggregating data types on a genomic scale. Nat Methods 2014;11(3):333–7.

70. De Meulder B, Lefaudeux D, Bansal AT, et al. A computational framework for complex disease stratification from multiple large-scale datasets. BMC Syst Biol 2018;12(1):60.

71. Li CX, Wheelock CE, Skold CM, et al. Integration of multi-omics datasets enables molecular classification of COPD. Eur Respir J 2018;51(5) [pii:1701930].

72. Mazein A, Knowles RG, Adcock IM, et al. Asthma-Map: an expert-driven computational representation of disease mechanisms. Clin Exp Allergy 2018; 48(8):916–8.

Proinflammatory Pathways in the Pathogenesis of Asthma

R. Stokes Peebles Jr, MD[a,b,*], Mark A. Aronica, MD[c]

KEYWORDS

- Asthma • Innate • Adaptive • Prostaglandin leukotriene

KEY POINTS

- An important component of the innate allergic immune response is ILC2 activated by interleukin (IL)-33, thymic stromal lymphopoietin, and IL-25 to produce IL-5 and IL-13.
- CD4+ Th2 cells are an important component of the adaptive allergic immune response and produce IL-4, IL-5, and IL-13 in response to specific antigenic stimulation.
- CD4+ Th17 cells produce IL-17A and IL-17F that in turn induce the production of cytokines and chemokines that promote the chemotaxis and survival of neutrophils in the airway and lung.
- Eicosanoids involved in asthma pathogenesis include PGD_2 and the cysteinyl leukotrienes that promote smooth muscle constriction and inflammation that propagate allergic responses.

The most recent Guidelines for the Diagnosis and Management of Asthma from the National Asthma Education and Prevention Program define the disease as follows: "Asthma is a chronic inflammatory disorder of the airways in which many cells and cellular elements play a role: in particular, mast cells, eosinophils, neutrophils (especially in sudden-onset, fatal exacerbations, occupational asthma, and patients who smoke), T lymphocytes, macrophages, and epithelial cells."[1]

The idea of asthma as a disease of inflammation has gone in and out of style over the years. Aretaeus the Cappadocian (120–180 AD) described asthma as an inflammation of the lungs, although his understanding of inflammation was vastly different than it is today. Henry Hyde Salter (1823–1871) was the first to describe eosinophils in the sputum of asthmatic individuals; this was closely followed by the description of Charcot-Leyden crystals. During the dawn of modern medicine Sir William Osler published in his textbook of medicine "all authors agree that there is, (in asthma) a strong neurotic element." It was not until his colleague Robert Cooke took over as editor in 1932 that the text was changed, "In all its types asthma is fundamentally the expression of an allergic reaction." In the early 1960s, asthma was thought to be a disease of the smooth muscle. In the 1980s, human data returned the focus of asthma to inflammation. The discovery and classification of Th1 and Th2 cells in mice by Mosmann and colleagues in 1986,[2] laid the foundation for the

The authors do not have a relationship with a commercial company that has a direct financial interest in subject matter or materials discussed in the article.

Funded by: National Institute of Allergy and Infectious Diseases (NIAID). Grant number(s): R01 AI 111820; R01 AI 124456; R01 AI 145265; U19 AI 095227.

[a] Division of Allergy, Pulmonary and Critical Care Medicine, Department of Medicine, Vanderbilt University School of Medicine, VUMC, T-1218 MCN, 1161 21st Avenue South, Nashville, TN 37232-2650, USA; [b] Department of Pathology, Microbiology, and Immunology, Vanderbilt University School of Medicine, VUMC, T-1218 MCN, 1161 21st Avenue South, Nashville, TN 37232-2650, USA; [c] Department of Pathobiology, Respiratory Institute, Cleveland Clinic Lerner College of Medicine, CWRU, 9500 Euclid Avenue, NB2-85, Cleveland, OH 44195, USA

* Corresponding author. Division of Allergy, Pulmonary and Critical Care Medicine, Vanderbilt University School of Medicine, VUMC, T-1218 MCN, 1161 21st Avenue South, Nashville, TN 37232-2650.

E-mail address: stokes.peebles@vanderbilt.edu

classification of asthma as a predominately "Th2 disease." The discoveries over the subsequent 30 years have shown us that a simple classification of asthma is no longer feasible. Furthermore, the contribution of the importance of research using mice in the discovery of the elements of the allergic inflammatory response cannot be overstated. Many of the cytokines that we now know are critical to the allergic response in humans were first described in mice, initially by discovering their presence in allergic inflammatory response, then by antagonizing those cytokines to determine their specific effect on allergic inflammation, in addition to their contribution on the physiology and pathology of the asthma phenotype.

The link between asthma and inflammation is clear; what has been less clear but has been coming into focus is the heterogeneity and impact of the various inflammatory pathways and the role they play in the currently described asthma phenotypes. Therefore, in this article, we define the known proinflammatory pathways involved in allergic airway inflammation in both mice and humans, and briefly describe therapies that antagonize these pathways and their effectiveness in human asthma. We also identify elements of these pathways for which there are not currently available therapies, but that could be a future target for asthma treatment.

For the past 50 years, the adaptive immune response has been considered the linchpin of allergic inflammation. Although innate immune cells, such as mast cells, eosinophils, and basophils, were known to have a central role in allergic inflammation, they were dependent on products produced by B and T lymphocytes to be activated. This adaptive immunity-centric view of the allergic world changed with the first reports of group 2 innate lymphoid cells (ILC2) in 2010.[3–5] With the discovery of ILC2, there was a paradigm shift in that innate cells were recognized to have the ability to produce allergic proinflammatory mediators without the need or assistance of adaptive T-cell and B-cell products. In this review, we start by detailing the mediators involved in activation of the recently discovered innate immunity-mediated ILC2-centric pathway. Next, we focus on specific aspects of the adaptive immune response that do not overlap with the ILC2 response. Finally, we review lipid mediators in the prostaglandin and leukotriene pathways that regulate allergic inflammatory responses.

INNATE IMMUNITY-MEDIATED ALLERGIC RESPONSE
Group 2 Innate Lymphoid Cells

ILC2 is an innate lymphoid subset that is present in tissues in which the host interacts with the environment to direct immune responses against pathogens, especially helminths (**Fig. 1**). These tissues in which ILC2 are embedded are predominantly mucosal surfaces of the respiratory and gastrointestinal tracts, in addition to the skin. ILC2 are lineage-negative (Lin⁻) in that they do not express markers for T cells, B cells, dendritic cells, macrophages, or granulocytes.[6] ILC2 have many features of lymphocytes, but lack rearranged antigen receptors, and instead of responding to specific antigens, these cells are activated by soluble mediators that include interleukin (IL)-33, IL-25, and thymic stromal lymphopoietin (TSLP). IL-33, IL-25, and TSLP are all expressed by epithelial cells in response to proteases.[6] In vivo experiments reveal that lung ILC2 have a critical role in rapid inflammation in response to protease exposure.[6] Proteases are important constituents of many allergens, such as Alternaria and dust mites (see **Fig. 1**).[7] The inflammatory response created by helminth infections has many features of allergic inflammation, as is discussed later, and is related to the high protease activities of these organisms.[7] Proteases disrupt mucosal integrity by digesting cell adhesion molecules and also act on protease-activated receptors to activate epithelial cells.[6] ILC2 produce a cytokine profile that is very similar to CD4+ Th2 cells, such as IL-4, IL-5, IL-9, and IL-13; however, the amount of these cytokines is much greater than is produced by Th2 cells. ILC2 indirectly activated by allergens infiltrate the lung and are a major innate source of IL-13.[8] There is very strong evidence suggesting ILC2 may be critical in the genesis and propagation of allergic responses.[9–11] Therefore, we first focus on the cytokines that activate ILC2, before turning our attention to those made by ILC2.

Interleukin-33

IL-33 is predominantly expressed by tissue cell types, including epithelial cells, fibroblasts, and endothelial cells, whereas its expression may be induced in immune cells such as mast cells and dendritic cells.[12] IL-33 expression is immediately upregulated in the lung from the first day of life and this is closely followed by a wave of IL-13–producing ILC2. The arrival of lung ILC2 coincides with the appearance of alveolar macrophages and their early polarization to an IL-13–dependent anti-inflammatory M2 phenotype.[13] In mice, IL-33 is predominantly expressed in the lung by alveolar type II pneumocytes, whereas human lung IL-33 is expressed by bronchial epithelial cells. IL-33 has 2 major domains, an N-terminal nuclear domain and an IL-1-like domain, and these domains connect

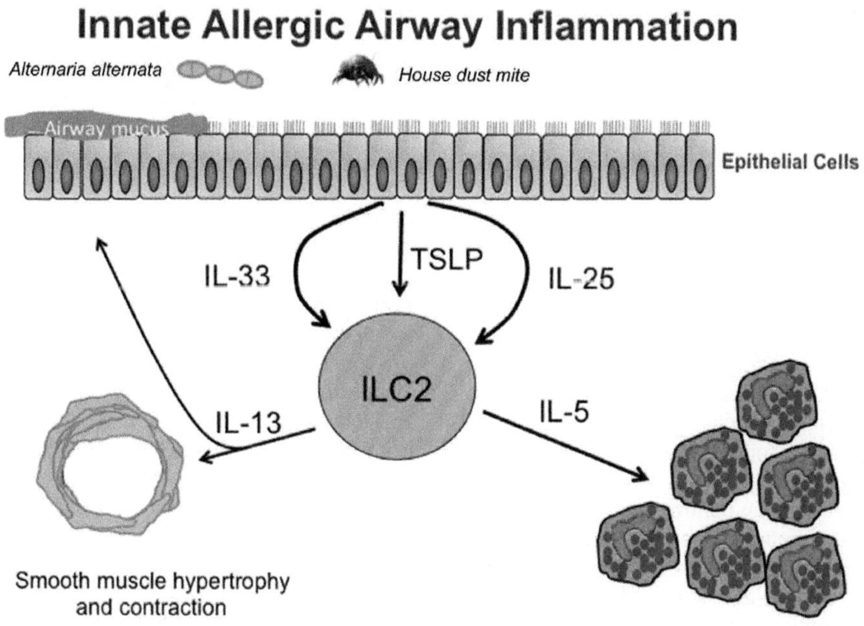

Innate Allergic Airway Inflammation

Fig. 1. Pathway of innate allergic inflammation.

by a central domain. The N-terminal domain is essential for nuclear translocation and chromatin association of IL-33.[12] The IL-1–like domain is key to the binding to the IL-33 receptor ST2. Alternative splicing of ST2 produces 2 different isoforms: a long, transmembrane signaling form of the receptor named ST2L, and a soluble form that lacks transmembrane and intracellular domains called sST2. sST2 is currently believed to be solely a decoy receptor that blocks IL-33 signaling. IL-1R accessory protein is a coreceptor for IL-33 signaling. ST2 is primarily expressed by immune cells, including ILC2, CD4+ T cells, CD8+ T cells, follicular T cells, regulatory T cells (Tregs), mast cells, macrophages, eosinophils, dendritic cells (DCs), basophils, natural killer (NK) cells, and NKT cells. By binding to ST2, IL-33 stimulates receptor-bearing cells to produce and secrete cytokines and growth factors that promote local and systemic immunity. Multiple genome-wide association studies revealed that IL-33 and ST2 are significantly associated with asthma.[14–16] Not only does IL-33 have an important role in Th2-type cytokine production by ILC2 in the innate allergic immune response, but IL-33 also induces antigen-specific IL-5+ CD4+ T cells and promotes allergen-induced inflammation independent of IL-4.[17]

IL-33 is rapidly released into the airway following allergen exposure and elevated levels in bronchoalveolar lavage (BAL) fluid occur within 1 hour.[12] The current concept is that IL-33 exits the cell that produces it by 2 mechanisms: passive release and active secretion.[18] Passive release of full length IL-33 from the nucleus occurs when the cell is damaged and undergoes necrosis, and in this situation, IL-33 is considered as a damage-associated molecular pattern that activates the immune response as a result of cellular injury. Active secretion of IL-33 occurs when cells encounter factors that either cause cellular stress or minor repairable injury. For instance, in normal bronchial airway epithelial cells (NHBE), allergens such as *Alternaria* or cockroach induced the translocation of IL-33 from the nucleus to the cytoplasm, followed by extracellular release of the cytokine without apparent cell death.[19] The signaling pathways that are responsible for active IL-33 secretion are not known; however, several elements have been described. Fungal allergen-induced IL-33 release from NHBE cells involved extracellular accumulation of ATP, autocrine, and paracrine P2 purinergic receptor activation, and resultant increase in intracellular Ca^{2+}.[20] Recently, activation of NADPH oxidase dual oxidase 1 resulting from the engagement of P2 purinergic receptors was identified as a mechanism for IL-33 release by airway epithelial cells stimulated with *Alternaria* or house dust mite.[21]

Airway exposure of naïve mice to a clinically relevant ubiquitous fungal allergen, *Alternaria alternata*, increases BAL levels of IL-33, followed by IL-5 and IL-13 production and airway eosinophilia without T or B cells.[22] This innate type 2 response to the allergen is nearly abolished in mice deficient in ST2, and ILC2 in the lungs are required and sufficient to mediate the response.[22] Airway exposure of naïve mice to IL-33 results in a rapid production of IL-5 and IL-13 that occurs in less than 12 hours, in addition to marked airway eosinophilia independent of adaptive immunity.[22]

Comparison of IL-25 and IL-33 pathway knockout (KO) mice demonstrates that IL-33 signaling plays a more important in vivo role in airways hyperresponsiveness than IL-25.[23] In addition, methacholine-induced airway contraction ex vivo increases after treatment with IL-33, but not IL-25. This is dependent on expression of ST2 and type 2 cytokines. Confocal studies with IL-13 reporter mice reveal that IL-33 potently induces expansion of IL-13–producing ILC2, correlating with airway contraction. This predominance of IL-33 activity is supported in vivo, as IL-33 is more rapidly expressed and released in comparison with IL-25. These data reveal that IL-33 plays a critical role in the rapid induction of airway contraction by stimulating the prompt expansion of IL-13–producing ILC2.

Not only does IL-33 stimulate ILC2, but it also promotes the pro-allergic inflammatory properties of CD4 T cells. In a murine model of asthma, ST2 KO mice had attenuated airway inflammation and IL-5 production.[17] Conversely, IL-33 administration induced IL-5–producing T cells and exacerbated allergen-induced airway inflammation in wild-type (WT), as well as in IL-4 KO mice. IL-33 is also a chemoattractant for human Th2 cells, but not Th1 cells.[24] IL-33, in the presence of antigen, polarized murine and human naïve CD4+ T cells into a population of T cells that produced mainly IL-5, but not IL-4.

Although IL-33 has been comprehensively studied in mouse models of allergic airway inflammation, very few studies have examined its expression in human asthma. ST2L expression was examined in endobronchial brushings and biopsies in patients stratified by asthma severity, as well as by Th2-like biomarkers.[25] ST2L expression was significantly increased in severe asthma and significantly associated with multiple indicators of Th2-like inflammation, including blood eosinophils, exhaled nitric oxide, and both epithelial CLCA1 and eotaxin-3 messenger RNA (mRNA) expression. Multiple single nucleotide polymorphisms in *IL1RL1* were found in relation to dichotomous expression of both ST2L and sST2. sST2 expression was associated with interferon (IFN)-γ expression in BAL, while inducing its expression in vitro in primary human epithelial cells. In another study, the BAL concentrations of IL-33, TSLP, IL-4, IL-5, IL-13, and IL-12p70, but not IL-25, IL-2,

or IFN-γ, were significantly elevated in asthmatic individuals compared with controls.[25] The concentrations of IL-33 and TSLP, but not IL-25, significantly correlated inversely with lung function as measured by forced expiratory volume in 1 second (FEV$_1$), independently of corticosteroid therapy. These data support a role for IL-33 in the pathogenesis of asthma characterized by persistent airway inflammation and impaired lung function, despite intensive corticosteroid therapy, spotlighting them as potential molecular targets for asthma therapy. Currently, there are no IL-33 antagonists that are currently approved by the Food and Drug Administration (FDA); however, there is a major effort by several pharmaceutical companies to develop such molecules, given that IL-33 is upstream of Th2 development and ILC2 activation.[26] One candidate therapeutic, AMG-282, is an anti-ST2 antibody and is currently in phase I clinical trials for mild allergic asthma and chronic rhinosinusitis (NCT01928368 and NCT02170337). A second candidate therapeutic, ANB020, is being evaluated in phase II trials for the treatment of peanut allergy (NCT02920021).

Thymic Stromal Lymphopoietin

TSLP is a member of the IL-2 cytokine family and is expressed during allergic inflammation by epithelial cells, keratinocytes, and stromal cells.[27] The initial prevailing paradigm was that TSLP produced by epithelial cells as a result of exposure to allergen increased DC expression of OX40L to drive Th2 differentiation when antigen was presented by DCs to naïve T cells, initiating an allergic inflammatory response.[28] Therefore, determining the mechanisms that regulate TSLP expression and receptor function have been an area of intense investigation over the past decade. However, as TSLP research has progressed, this initial paradigm has become more complex, although the key element that TSLP drives Th2 differentiation and is an important regulator of Th2 responses is widely accepted.[27] The TSLP receptor (TSLPR) is a heterodimer consisting of a unique TSLPR subunit and the IL-7Rα chain. TSLPR is expressed by a host of hematopoietic cells, including T cells, B cells, NK cells, monocytes, basophils, eosinophils, and DCs, as well as by epithelial cells, which are not hematopoietic in origin.[27] In TSLP signaling, TSLPR subunit associated JAK2 interacts with IL-7Rα-associated JAK1 to induce STAT5 and STAT1 phosphorylation in CD4 T cells. TSLP has also been shown to act directly on T cells. TSLP, in the presence of CD4 T-cell activation through T-cell receptor stimulation, promoted the proliferation and differentiation of Th2 cells via induction of *Il4* gene transcription. IL-4 also upregulated the expression of TSLPR on CD4 Th2 cells compared with Th1 and Th17 cells, thus amplifying Th2 responses. The increase in cell surface CD4 T-cell TSLPR expression was associated with TSLP's capability to augment the proliferation and survival of activated Th2 cells. B cells express TSLPR and TSLP promotes B-cell lymphopoiesis. Innate immune cells also express TSLPR, and NKT cells, mast cells, and eosinophils all increase cytokine production in response to TSLP stimulation.[27]

Mouse models of asthma reveal an important role of TSLP in allergic inflammatory responses. TSLP expression was increased in the lungs of mice with allergen-induced asthma, whereas TSLP receptor KO mice had considerably reduced disease.[28] Lung-specific expression of a *Tslp* transgene, induced airway inflammation and hyperreactivity characterized by Th2 cytokines and increased immunoglobulin (Ig)E. The lungs of *Tslp*-transgenic mice had massive infiltration of leukocytes, goblet cell hyperplasia, and subepithelial fibrosis. TSLP treatment of bone marrow–derived DCs resulted in their production of the Th2 cell-attracting chemokine (C-C motif) ligand 17 CCL17. In a very recent report, TSLP induced the development of pathogenic Th2 cells, which produce increased amounts of the IL-5 and IL-13, while promoting allergic disorders, including asthma.[29] TSLP signaling in mouse CD4 T cells initiated transcriptional changes associated with Th2 cell programming. IL-4 signaling amplified and stabilized the genomic response of T cells to TSLP, which increased the frequency of T cells producing IL-4, IL-5, and IL-13. In addition, TSLP- and IL-4–programmed Th2 cells developed a pathogenic phenotype and produced significantly increased amounts of IL-5 and IL-13 and other proinflammatory cytokines than did Th2 cells stimulated with IL-4 alone. TSLP-mediated Th2 cell induction involved distinct molecular pathways, including activation of the transcription factor STAT5 through the kinase JAK2 and repression of the transcription factor BCL6. In human CD4 T cells, TSLP and IL-4 promoted the generation of Th2 cells that produced greater amounts of IL-5 and IL-13.[29] In this report, asthmatic children showed enhancement of such T-cell responses in peripheral blood compared with healthy controls.

There is evidence that TSLP may mediate corticosteroid-resistant inflammation in the lung, both in mice and in humans. TSLP synthesized during airway inflammation induced ILC2 corticosteroid resistance in vitro and in vivo, by controlling phosphorylation of STAT5 and expression of Bcl-xL in mouse ILC2 cells.[30] Blockade of TSLP with a neutralizing antibody or blocking the

TSLP/STAT5 signaling pathway with low-molecular-weight STAT5 inhibitors, such as pimozide, restored corticosteroid sensitivity. Dexamethasone inhibited chemoattractant receptor-homologous molecule expressed on Th2 lymphocytes (CRTH2) and Th2 cytokine expression by human blood ILC2 stimulated with IL-25 and IL-33.[31] However, it did not do so when ILC2 were stimulated with IL-7 and TSLP, 2 ligands of IL-7Rα. Unlike blood ILC2, BAL fluid ILC2 from asthmatic patients were resistant to dexamethasone. BAL fluid from asthmatic patients had increased TSLP but not IL-7 levels, and BAL fluid TSLP levels significantly correlated with steroid resistance of ILC2.[31]

As opposed to IL-33, there are published clinical trials targeting TSLP in asthma. In a double-blind, placebo-controlled study, 31 patients with mild allergic asthma were treated with 3 monthly doses an anti-TSLP antibody (tezepelumab) or placebo intravenously and allergen challenges were conducted on days 42 and 84.[32] Tezepelumab attenuated allergen-induced early and late asthmatic responses and significantly decreased blood and sputum eosinophils before and after the allergen challenge, while it also reduced the fraction of exhaled nitric oxide. A more recent phase 2 study of tezepelumab (See Mauli Desai and colleagues', "Immunomodulators and Biologics: Beyond Stepped-Care Therapy", in this issue) showed a significantly reduced the rate of asthma exacerbations regardless of blood eosinophil counts at enrollment.[33] These 2 studies provide proof of concept in humans that TSLP has an important role in the pathogenesis of human asthma.

Interleukin-25

IL-25 is expressed by both airway epithelial cells and hematopoietic cells involved in allergic responses, such as Th2 cells, mast cells, basophils, and eosinophils.[34,35] Similar to IL-33, IL-25 is stored in epithelial cells and released when the cell is exposed to protease-containing antigens, such as house dust mite.[36] IL-25 is a member of the IL-17 family and is also known as IL-17E. The IL-25 receptor is a heterodimer of IL-17RA and IL-17RB and signaling results in activation of NF-kB, leading to the expression and release of Th2 cytokines, including IL-4, IL-5, and IL-13.[37,38] The IL-25 heterodimeric receptor complex is expressed on antigen-presenting cells (APCs), airway smooth muscle, airway epithelial cells, fibroblasts, eosinophils, invariant NKT cells, and ILC2.[39] IL-25 activates ILC2 to produce IL-5 and IL-13, but IL-33 is a much more potent and rapid stimulator of ILC2 than IL-25.[6] Mouse models of allergic inflammation reveal that IL-25 inhibition results in significant decreases in BAL fluid concentrations of IL-5 and IL-13, serum IgE, pulmonary eosinophilia, and abrogated airways responsiveness.[40,41] IL-25 also had a critical role in recruitment of endothelial progenitor cells to the lung and subsequent neovascularization in an allergen challenge model, suggesting a direct role for IL-25 during angiogenesis in vivo. Interestingly, neutralization of IL-25 abrogated the secretion of IL-33 and TSLP, indicating a possible therapeutic strategy for inhibiting all 3 of these cytokines.[41]

Human studies support a possible role of IL-25 in asthma pathogenesis. In steroid-naïve patients with asthma, who are stratified based on IL-25 mRNA levels in airway brushings, those with greater IL-25 mRNA levels had a greater allergic phenotype based on allergen skin test positivity and serum IgE levels compared with the IL-25 low subjects or healthy controls.[42] Additionally, the subjects with asthma with greater IL-25 mRNA also had greater methacholine responsiveness and evidence of eosinophil activation compared with the IL-25 mRNA low or control subjects. In another study, higher plasma levels of IL-25 and eosinophil receptor expression of IL-17RB were present in patients with allergic asthma compared with healthy controls.[43] In vitro studies revealed that IL-25 augmented methacholine-induced smooth muscle contractility in bronchial rings of subjects with asthma compared with healthy controls.[44]

Examination of the in vivo role of IL-25 in human asthma is incomplete, as there has only been one intervention study.[45] In this trial, a monoclonal antibody targeting IL-17RA, brodalumab, was used in 300 subjects with moderate to severe asthma and there was no therapeutic benefit. However, the IL-17RA subunit is not only a component of the IL-25 receptor, but is also a shared subunit with the IL-17A and IL-17F receptors. In addition, the subjects in this trial were not phenotyped based on characteristics of IL-25, IL-17A, or IL-17F inflammation. It is interesting that a post hoc analysis revealed a trend toward improvement with brodalumab treatment in subjects with greater bronchodilator reversibility. Additional data targeting subjects with an IL-25 high phenotype is needed to develop a more complete picture as to the role of IL-25 in asthma pathogenesis.

Interleukin-5

Before being given the name IL-5, this protein had been known as either T-cell–replacing factor (TRF) or eosinophil differentiation factor (EDF).[46] As EDF, IL-5 stimulated the production of functional eosinophils in liquid bone marrow cultures and was reported to be specific for the eosinophil lineage in hematopoietic differentiation.[47,48] As TRF, IL-5 was a potent inducer of IL-2 receptor expression and synergized with IL-2 in the induction of the terminal differentiation of B cells into immunoglobulin-secreting cells.[49] These points are important to remember when considering therapies that target IL-5, as they not only affect eosinophils, but will also impact T and B function. IL-5 signals through a receptor composed of an IL-5–specific α chain and the common β-subunit that maintains the survival and functions of eosinophils and B cells.[50] In transgenic mice that overexpress IL-5, there is a significant increase in eosinophils and B cells.[51]

Animal models of allergic airway inflammation reveal an important role of IL-5 in pulmonary eosinophilia and airways responsiveness. One-time IL-5 challenge of guinea pig airways induced a dose-dependent significant increase in the number of eosinophils, neutrophils, and epithelial cells in BAL fluid 24 hours after administration, and this cell recruitment was inhibited by corticosteroids and ketotifen.[52] In a guinea pig model of acute allergic inflammation induced by ovalbumin sensitization and challenge, anti–IL-5 antibody treatment significantly reduced BAL eosinophils 4 hours after allergen challenge.[53] In a guinea pig model of chronic ovalbumin challenge, anti–IL-5 treatment not only significantly reduced BAL eosinophilia, but also histamine-induced airway reactivity, whereas the number of airway neutrophils was not affected.[54] Anti–IL-5 treatment also decreased ovalbumin-induced airway responsiveness in mice.[55] Genetic deficiency of IL-5 receptor α subunit reduced allergen-induced BAL eosinophils and airways responsiveness to acetylcholine compared with WT animals, whereas there was no difference in BAL IL-5 levels or serum antigen-specific IgE.[56] The importance of IL-5 in driving airway eosinophilia is further supported by studies revealing that IL-5 overexpression in airway epithelial cells of mice resulted in a dramatic accumulation of peribronchial eosinophilia, bronchial-associated lymphoid tissue, goblet cell hyperplasia, focal collagen deposition, and airways responsiveness to methacholine compared with nontransgenic mice.[57] The importance of eosinophils in IL-5–associated pathology is evident in studies using mice that can generate IL-5, but that have a genetic deletion of eosinophils (PHIL mice). Allergen challenge of PHIL mice revealed that eosinophils were required for pulmonary mucus accumulation and the airway responsiveness associated with asthma.[58] Allergen-sensitized and challenged PHIL mice had reduced airway levels of Th2 cytokines relative to WT mice and this correlated with a reduced ability to recruit effector T cells to the lung.[59] In contrast, the combined transfer of antigen-specific T cells and eosinophils into PHIL mice restored the number of effector T cells, airway Th2 immune responses, and asthma-like histopathologic changes. In this model, eosinophils induced the expression of the Th2 chemokines TARC (thymus and activation-regulated *chemokine*)/CCL17 and MDC (macrophage-derived chemokine)/CCL22 in the lung after allergen challenge, and neutralization of these chemokines inhibited the recruitment of effector T cells. These results suggest that pulmonary eosinophils are required for the localized recruitment of effector T cells.[59]

These animal studies strongly suggested an important role for IL-5 in human asthma. This was supported by data showing that IL-5 was increased in the serum and bronchial biopsies of patients with asthma.[60,61] Further, increased serum IL-5 and blood eosinophils were associated with a decrease in FEV_1 during the late-phase reactions.[62] In addition, inhaled IL-5 led to airways responsiveness and sputum eosinophilia in subjects with asthma.[63] Although the first trial using an IL-5 neutralizing antibody, SCH55700, failed to show benefit despite it resulting in a significant reduction in blood eosinophils,[64] subsequent studies targeting therapy to the eosinophilic asthma phenotype has supported and confirmed the important role of IL-5 in this subset of asthma (See Mauli Desai and colleagues', "Immunomodulators and Biologics: Beyond Stepped-Care Therapy", in this issue.)

Interleukin-13

IL-13 was first described as a cytokine produced by activated human T lymphocytes that had similar properties to IL-4 in suppressing lipopoly saccharide-induced IL-6, IL-1β, tumor necrosis factor (TNF)-α, and IL-8 from human peripheral blood mononuclear cells.[65] Mapping of the *Il13* gene revealed that it was closely linked to the *Il4* gene on human chromosome 5q 23 to 31.[65] The similar biologic effects of IL-4 and IL-13 stem from the fact that they share a common receptor element, IL-4 receptor α (IL-4Rα). The IL-13 receptor complex, also known as the IL-4 type 2, is composed of the IL-4Rα and IL-13 receptor α1 (IL-13Rα1). The primary IL-4 receptor is composed of the IL-4Rα and the common γ chain (γc). Signaling through IL-4Rα leads to activation and phosphorylation of the transcription factor signal transducer and activator of transcription 6 (STAT6), which when phosphorylated forms a homodimer that can translocate to the nucleus and bind to the GATA-3 promoter, leading to GATA-3 transcription.[66,67] The IL-13R is expressed on airway smooth muscle cells, endothelial cells, fibroblasts, bronchial epithelial cells, and most leukocytes, including eosinophils, basophils, mast cells, and B lymphocytes.[68–72] It is not expressed on Th1 or Th2 CD4 cells, but is expressed on CD4 Th17 cells.[73–75] The interaction between IL-17A and IL-13 is very complex. IL-17A enhances IL-13 activity by upregulating IL-13–induced STAT6 activation, whereas IL-13 inhibits IL-17A intracellular signaling.[76]

Mouse studies reveal an important role of IL-13 in driving the pathognomonic physiologic changes seen in human asthma. In vivo neutralization of IL-13, either by antibody or soluble IL-13R, inhibited allergen challenge driven airway responsiveness and mucus metaplasia, but did not affect airway eosinophils, lymphocytes, or serum antigen-specific IgE concentrations.[77,78] Airway challenge with recombinant IL-13 resulted in induction of airway responsiveness, mucus metaplasia, eosinophilia, and serum IgE.[77,78] Administration of either IL-13 or IL-4 resulted in an asthma-like phenotype to mice lacking adaptive immune cells by an IL-4Rα chain-dependent pathway. Thus, the IL-13 and IL-4 pathways may explain the genetic associations of asthma with both the human 5q31 locus and the IL-4 receptor.[77]

IL-13 has several functional properties that amplify allergic responses. IL-13 and IL-4 selectively induced vascular cell adhesion molecule-1 (VCAM-1) expression in human endothelial cells, suggesting a role in eosinophil tissue accumulation as the VCAM-1 ligand, VLA-4, is expressed on eosinophils.[79] IL-13 is a B-cell–stimulating factor and acts at different stages of the B-cell maturation pathway as it enhances the expression of CD23/FcεRII and major histocompatibility complex (MHC) II on resting B cells and stimulates B-cell proliferation.[80] In human B cells, IL-13 induces germ-line IgE heavy-chain gene transcription, in a similar fashion to the effect of IL-4 on IgE isotype switching.[81]

IL-13 has been identified in biologic fluids and tissues of patients with asthma, supporting a role for this cytokine in disease pathogenesis. In patients with asthma and rhinitis, there was a significant enhancement of both IL-13 transcripts and secreted proteins in the allergen-challenged BAL compared with the saline-challenged controls, whereas the expression of IL-13 transcripts was not detected in the BAL of healthy subjects challenged with the same dose of allergen. The cellular source of IL-13 mRNA was identified in the mononuclear cell fraction of the allergen-challenged BAL.[82] In a model of endobronchial allergen challenge in humans, there was a highly significant increase in the numbers of eosinophils and both IL-4 and IL-13 after 18 hours in the allergen-exposed segment. In contrast to IL-4, the concentration of IL-13 strongly correlated with the eosinophil numbers found 18 hours after allergen challenge.[83] IL-13 may be involved in asthma pathogenesis irrespective of the patient's allergic status. Biopsy specimens from subjects with asthma, whether the subjects were atopic or nonatopic, had statistically equivalent quantities of IL-13 mRNA, and these quantities were significantly elevated compared with those in specimens from both the atopic and nonatopic control subjects.[84] The quantities of IL-13 mRNA reflected the numbers of activated eosinophils per unit area of submucosa in the biopsy specimens as determined by immunohistochemistry and were statistically equivalent in the atopic and nonatopic subjects with asthma and significantly elevated as compared with those in both the atopic and nonatopic control subjects without asthma. However, there was no correlation between the quantities of IL-13 mRNA and disease severity.[84] There is also evidence that IL-13 may contribute to impaired glucocorticoid responsiveness during inflammatory illnesses by decreasing glucocorticoid receptor-binding affinity.[85]

Although the presence of IL-13 in BAL or lung tissue is present in patients with asthma, and therefore is associated with disease pathogenesis, recent intervention studies strongly suggest that IL-13 has an important role in disease. A key issue is to phenotype patients to determine which of those subjects may be more responsive to IL-13 antagonists and therefore have a more favorable outcome. Using microarray and polymerase chain reaction analyses of airway epithelial brushings from patients with mild-to-moderate asthma and healthy control subjects, serum periostin, the product of the IL-13-inducible gene POSTN was identified as increased in Th2-high asthma.[86] Serum periostin was then used as a biomarker in a randomized, double-blind, placebo-controlled trial of the anti–IL-13 antibody lebrikizumab in patients who were inadequately controlled despite inhaled glucocorticoid therapy. At the conclusion of the 12-week trial, there was a significant increase in the mean FEV_1 in the lebrikizumab group than in the placebo group.[87] Among patients in the high-periostin subgroup, the increase from baseline FEV_1 was a statistically significant 8.2% points higher in the lebrikizumab group than in the placebo group. However, in the low-periostin subgroup, the increase from baseline FEV_1 was not different in the lebrikizumab group than in the placebo group. This trial suggested that patients with asthma who had evidence of IL-13–mediated pathobiology of asthma responded to an IL-13 antagonist to a greater degree than those who did not. Recent randomized trials of lebrikizumab have produced mixed results. In the replicate, randomized, double-blind, placebo-controlled trials LUTE and VERSE, treatment with lebrikizumab reduced the rate of asthma exacerbations, with an effect that was more pronounced in the periostin-high patients (60% reduction) than in the periostin-low patients (5% reduction) compared with placebo.[88] Lung function was also improved following lebrikizumab treatment, with the greatest increase in FEV_1 in periostin-high patients. However, in replicate phase 3 studies (LAVOLTA I and LAVOLTA II) of patients with uncontrolled asthma despite inhaled corticosteroids and at least 1 second controller medication, lebrikizumab did not consistently show significant reduction in asthma exacerbations in biomarker-high patients.[89] In the most recent trial of lebrikizumab in adult patients with mild-to-moderate asthma, lebrikizumab did not significantly improve FEV_1 in patients with mild-to-moderate asthma at a dose expected to inhibit the IL-13 pathway.[90]

There have been other strategies to inhibit the IL-13R signaling pathway, most focused on blocking IL-4Rα or GATA3, that have included soluble IL-4Rα, an agent that prevents assembly of the IL-4Rα with either the γc or IL-13Rα1, or antibodies against IL-4Rα. A phase I dose-ranging study of a soluble IL-4Rα in patients with moderate asthma maintained FEV_1, asthma symptom scores, and β2-agonist rescue use compared with placebo despite withdrawal of inhaled corticosteroids.[91] In a follow-up randomized trial of subjects who had asthma exacerbations when inhaled corticosteroids were withdrawn, the soluble IL-4Rα prevented decline in FEV_1 and worsening asthma symptom scores compared with placebo, yet there was no difference in withdrawal from the study based on asthma exacerbations.[92] Another strategy to prevent IL-4Rα signaling was pitrakinra, a human recombinant protein that prevents assembly of the IL-4Rα with either γc or IL-13Rα1. In 2 independent randomized, double-blind, placebo-controlled, parallel group phase 2a clinical trials, patients with atopic asthma were treated with pitrakinra or placebo by either subcutaneous injection or nebulization twice daily. Inhaled allergen challenge was performed before and after 4 weeks of treatment.[93] There was no difference in maximum percentage decrease in FEV_1 between pitrakinra and placebo when the agents were given subcutaneously, but pitrakinra decreased asthma-related adverse events and decreased β2-agonist rescue events compared with placebo. Pitrakinra nebulization significantly increased FEV_1 compared with placebo, but there were too few asthma-related adverse events to assess the effect of pitrakinra on adverse events.

Monoclonal antibodies against IL-4Rα have also been used to determine the effect of this signaling cascade on asthma pathogenesis. In a randomized controlled, phase 2 study of AMG 317, a fully human monoclonal antibody to IL-4Rα, in patients with moderate to severe asthma, the intervention did not demonstrate clinical efficacy across the overall group of patients.[94] However, treatment with dupilumab, a fully human monoclonal antibody to IL-4Rα was associated with fewer asthma exacerbations when long-acting β-agonists and inhaled glucocorticoids were withdrawn in patients with persistent, moderate to severe asthma and elevated eosinophil levels.[95] Dupilumab also improved lung function and reduced levels of Th2-associated inflammatory markers. More recently, dupilumab increased lung function and reduced severe exacerbations in patients with uncontrolled persistent asthma, irrespective of baseline eosinophil count.[96] These results suggest that blocking IL-13 by itself may not be sufficient in reducing Th2 inflammation, and that the combination of blocking IL-4 and IL-13 signaling through the IL-4Rα may be a more robust strategy to inhibit this pathway. These studies also reveal that there is a drug-specific effect, as AMG 317 was not effective whereas studies with dupilumab have shown it to be efficacious. The U.S. Food and Drug Administration has approved dupilumab as an add-on maintenance therapy in patients with moderate-to-severe asthma aged 12 years and older with an eosinophilic phenotype or with oral corticosteroid-dependent asthma.

Signaling through IL-4Rα activates STAT6, which can then translocate to the nucleus to activate GATA3 transcription. SB010, a DNA enzyme that cleaves and inactivates GATA3 messenger RNA, was examined in patients with allergic asthma and sputum eosinophilia and who had biphasic early-phase and late-phase reactions to inhaled allergen challenge.[97] The GATA3 antagonist significantly reduced both the early-phase and the late-phase reactions compared with placebo, attenuated allergen-induced sputum eosinophilia, decreased serum IL-5 levels, and decreased sputum tryptase levels, while having no impact on the levels of fractional exhaled nitric oxide or methacholine-induced airway responsiveness.

To date, clinical trials modulating the IL-13 pathway alone or the combined IL-13/IL-4 pathways have not revealed serious safety concerns, such as increased risk for infections, malignancy, or cardiovascular events.[98] It will be interesting to follow additional methods developed to antagonize the IL-13 signaling to further define the role of this pathway in asthma pathobiology.

ADAPTIVE IMMUNITY-MEDIATED ALLERGIC RESPONSE

Immune recognition of common environmental antigens is initially regulated by specialized APCs, such as DCs, macrophages, B lymphocytes, and several other cell types.[48,49] The dendritic cell is the most potent activator of naïve T cells.[50] Antigens processed by APCs through the endocytic pathway are presented as 8 to 10 amino acid epitopes in MHC class II molecules to CD4+ T lymphocytes. CD4 T lymphocytes are generally divided into classes that are characterized by the cytokine array produced by the cell.[54] Th1 cells are important in the immune response to intracellular pathogens, such as viruses and mycobacteria and produce IFN-γ, lymphotoxin, and IL-2.[55] Th2 cells, as well as mast cells and basophils, produce IL-4, an important factor for B lymphocytes to switch antibody production to the IgE isotype.[55] Th2 cells additionally make a variety of other proallergic inflammatory cytokines, such as IL-5, IL-9, IL-10 and IL-13. As previously mentioned, IL-5 is an important eosinophil regulatory factor and IL-13 is believed to be a central mediator in airway hyperreactivity.[55,56] Eosinophilic inflammation is one of the hallmarks of the allergic inflammatory response in the airway.[57] The allergic response to an inhaled antigen is characterized by antigen-specific IgE production by B lymphocytes, whereupon IgE can bind to IgE receptors on tissue mast cells and peripheral blood basophils. When these antigen-specific IgE molecules bound to mast cells and basophils are cross-linked by the specific antigen on antigenic reexposure, the mast cells and basophils undergo a degranulation process. With degranulation, preformed mediators within the mast cell and basophil, such as histamine and tryptase, are released, and other mediators, such as certain prostaglandins and leukotrienes are generated through the metabolism of arachidonic acid from the cell membrane, as will be detailed in a subsequent section.[57] Although there are many mediators responsible for the full expression of the adaptive allergic response, IL-4 is one of the most important in the adaptive allergic response pathway given its effect on polarizing naïve CD4 lymphocytes to the Th2 pathway and its role in B lymphocyte IgE class switching (**Fig. 2**). Th17 cells are discussed in this section given their importance in neutrophilic inflammation and a review of Tregs is beyond the scope of this article.

Interleukin-4

IL-4 was originally known as B-cell growth factor, and then B-cell stimulatory factor-1, as it

Mechanisms of allergen-specific immunotherapy: multiple suppressor factors at work in immune tolerance to allergens

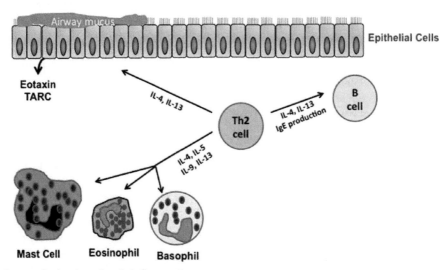

Fig. 2. Pathway of adaptive allergic inflammation.

augmented the proliferative response of B cells to anti-IgM.[99] In 1986, IL-4 was identified as a potent switch factor for B-cell IgE synthesis.[100] *Il4* maps to the human chromosome 5q31 and is 12 kB from the *Il13* gene.[101] IL-4 predominantly signals through the type I IL-4 receptor that is composed of the IL-4Rα and γc. In lymphoid cells, IL-4Rα associated with JAK1 and γc with JAK3. IL-4 and IL-13 are unique in that they are the only ligands that caused STAT6 phosphorylation.[102] IL-4 signaling through the type I IL-4 receptor acts relatively early for naïve CD4 T cells to acquire IL-4–producing capacity and develop into Th2 cells.[103] CD4 Th2 cells are capable of producing IL-4, IL-5 and IL-13, and are critical for the humoral immune response against extracellular pathogens and in the induction of allergic diseases, including asthma. Although STAT6 is downstream of IL-4R signaling, enhanced STAT5 signaling also induced Th2 differentiation independent of IL-4 signaling, and although it did not upregulate GATA-3 expression, it did require the presence of GATA-3 for its action. Therefore, there is a critical role for GATA-3 in Th2 cell differentiation (both IL-4 dependent and IL-4 independent) and in inhibiting Th1 differentiation.[104] In addition to CD4 Th2 cells, other cells that produce IL-4 induce NKT cells, basophils, mast cells, and eosinophils.[105–110] ILC2 can be induced to produce IL-4 in response to cysteinyl leukotrienes.[111]

In addition to IL-4 promoting IgE isotype switching and polarization of naïve T cells into Th2 cells,

IL-4 also induced expression of VCAM-1, which directed the migration of T cells, monocytes, basophils, and particularly eosinophils to sites of allergic inflammation.[112,113] IL-4 also induced mucin gene expression, resulting in increased airway mucus.[114]

Allergen challenge studies in mice revealed the importance of IL-4 in the development of the asthma phenotype. Allergen-sensitized and challenged C57BL/6 mice resulted in substantially fewer eosinophils in BAL and much less peribronchial inflammation in IL-4 KO mice compared with WT mice.[115] These results suggested that IL-4 is a central mediator of allergic airway inflammation, regulating antigen-induced eosinophil recruitment into the airways by a T-cell–dependent mechanism.[115] The relationship between IL-4, IL-5, and airway eosinophils was further defined when CD4 T cells, and not CD8 T cells, were necessary to induce eosinophilic inflammation.[116] Finally, antibody neutralization of IL-4 during the period of systemic immunization abrogated airway responsiveness, but had little effect on the influx of eosinophils.[117] Administration of anti–IL-4 only during the period of the aerosol challenge did not affect the subsequent airway response to acetylcholine. Administration of anti–IL-5 antibodies at levels that suppressed eosinophils to less than 1% of recruited cells had no effect on the subsequent airway responses. These results revealed that IL-4 generated during the period of lymphocyte priming with antigen was critical in generating airway responsiveness to inhaled antigen, whereas no role for IL-5 or eosinophils in airway responsiveness could be demonstrated.[117]

Many investigators found IL-4 present in biologic fluids and cells from patients with asthma, supporting a role for this cytokine in the pathogenesis of allergic airway inflammation. In subjects with mild atopic asthma, mRNA expression of IL-4, IL-5, granulocyte-macrophage colony-stimulating factor (GM-CSF), and IL-2 was greater in BAL cells compared with healthy control subjects, whereas there was no difference between the 2 groups in mRNA expression of IFN-γ in BAL cells as assessed by simultaneous in situ hybridization and immunofluorescence.[118] This study revealed that atopic asthma was associated with a pattern compatible with predominant activation of the Th2-like T-cell population.[118] Others found a distinction in IL-4 expression based on whether the patient had allergic or nonallergic asthma. In one study, increased levels of IL-4 and IL-5 characterized allergic asthmatic individuals, and this elevated IL-4 contributed to the increased IgE levels found in these allergic subjects. In contrast, nonallergic asthmatic individuals had elevated levels of IL-2 and IL-5, with IL-2 contributing to T-cell activation. In both types of asthma, the close correlation of IL-5 levels with eosinophilia suggests that IL-5 is responsible for the characteristic eosinophilia of asthma. Thus, there was evidence of distinct T-cell activation resulting in different spectra of cytokines in allergic and nonallergic asthma.[119] Corticosteroids reduced the number of IL-4–expressing cells and eosinophils in BAL fluid, while increasing the number of IFN-γ–expressing cells.[120] Finally, whole lung allergen challenge increased the number of activated CD4 T cells expressing IL-4 and IL-5 24 hours after the challenge, whereas there was no evidence of activation of CD8 T cells.[121] At the 24-hour post-challenge time point, there was a significant increase in the number of eosinophils that correlated with the maximal late fall in FEV_1. These results revealed that cytokines produced by activated Th2-type CD4 T cells in the airway contributed to late asthmatic responses by mechanisms that included eosinophil accumulation.[121]

Although antagonists targeting IL-4R signaling have been used to determine the contribution of this pathway in asthma pathogenesis, as was reviewed in the IL-13 section, specific IL-4 antagonists have not been approved by the FDA for asthma therapy.

Interleukin-17

IL-17A and IL-17F have been strongly implicated in the neutrophilic inflammation that occurs in a subset of patients with asthma.[122] IL-17A and IL-17F regulate neutrophilic influx into tissues by inducing airway epithelial cell and stromal cell production of cytokines, such as granulocyte colony-stimulating factor (G-CSF), GM-CSF, and IL-6, in addition to chemokines such as chemokine (C-X-C motif) ligand 8 (CXCL8), CXCL6, and CXCL1, that promote neutrophil chemotaxis and survival (**Fig. 3**).[123] Thus, IL-17A and IL-17F do not directly cause neutrophil chemotaxis, but act indirectly by promoting the release of pro-neutrophilic mediators.[124] A number of cell types, including CD4 Th17 cells, γδ T cells, NKT cells, NK cells, ILC3, and mast cells express IL-17A and IL-17F.[125,126] Although some investigators report that neutrophils express IL-17A and IL-17F, others do not.[127] IL-17A and IL-17F share a common receptor complex, IL-17RA and IL-17RC, and is likely the predominant reason for the common biological function of these 2 cytokines.[128] In terms of importance to asthma pathogenesis, the IL-17 receptor is expressed on airway smooth muscle cells, epithelial cells, fibroblasts, macrophages, and endothelial cells. CD4 Th17 cells are a major source of IL-17A and IL-17F. Based on our current understanding, there are 3 different combinations of cytokines that differentiate naïve CD4 T cells into Th17 cells. These include IL-6 and transforming growth factor (TGF)-β, with additive potentiating effects of IL-1β and TNF; IL-21 and TGF-β; and IL-6, IL-1β, and IL-23.[129–131] Key transcription factors activated in the Th17 differentiation process include STAT3 and RORC2.[130]

Animal models investigating the impact of Th17 cytokines suggest an important role in asthma pathogenesis. IL-17RA KO mice that are unable to respond to IL-17A or IL-17F had decreased ovalbumin-induced allergic airway inflammation compared with WT mice.[132] IL-17A protein expression synergized with IL-13 present during allergic airway inflammation to increase airways responsiveness in a complement C5a-dependent manner.[133] Th17 cells mediated steroid-resistant airway inflammation and airway responsiveness in mice.[134] These results suggest that IL-17A increases Th2-mediated airway responsiveness and airway inflammation. However, it is important to note that other groups have reported that IL-17A had an anti-inflammatory role in allergic airway inflammation. For instance, instillation of recombinant mouse IL-17A during ovalbumin challenge decreased airways hyperresponsiveness, eosinophil infiltration into the airways, and expression of CCL5, CCL11, and CCL17.[132] Further, neutralization of IL-17A during allergic airway inflammation increased airway responsiveness and eosinophil infiltration into the airways.[135]

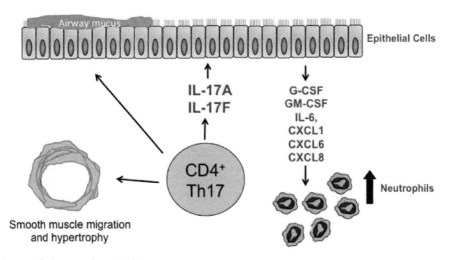

IL-17A Mediated Airway Pathology

Fig. 3. Pathway of Th17-mediated inflammatory responses.

Most studies investigating the presence of IL-17A in asthma support that this cytokine was increased in the airway cells and BAL fluid. IL-17A was increased in the airways of asthma subjects and induced human bronchial fibroblasts to produce proinflammatory cytokines.[136] There was increased expression of airway cells expressing IL-17A and IL-17F in patients with mild-moderate asthma compared with healthy controls.[137] Further, there was increased IL-17 mRNA in the sputum of subjects with mild and moderate/severe asthma compared with healthy controls and this was associated with an increase of the percentage of neutrophils to total granulocytes.[138] In vitro studies support a role for IL-17A in asthma pathogenesis. IL-17 enhanced production of eotaxin, an important chemokine in eosinophil migration, by primary airway smooth muscle cells.[139] IL-17A also increased proliferation of human primary tracheal epithelial cells.[140] IL-17A induced MUC5AC and MUC5B mucins in primary human tracheobronchial epithelial cells.[141,142] IL-17A, IL-17F, and IL-22 are associated with increased airway smooth muscle proliferation and migration.[143,144]

Although there are abundant data from in vivo mouse experiments, human airway surveys, and in vitro studies using human cells, as mentioned earlier, the lone human asthma clinical trial examining IL-17 antagonism with brodalumab did not show clinical improvement.[45] Recently, the FDA issued a black box warning after 6 patients treated with brodalumab across 4 clinical trials committed suicide[145]; therefore, there will likely be no further clinical asthma trials for this drug. However, further exploration of the IL-17 pathway antagonism is warranted in appropriately phenotyped patients who have a Th17 signature with neutrophilic inflammation given the association of neutrophilic inflammation with severe disease.

EICOSANOID PATHWAY

Eicosanoids are 20 carbon chain lipids formed from the metabolism of arachidonic acid that have potent activities in a number of biologic properties. In terms of allergic disease, the 2 pathways that most promote allergic inflammation are PGD_2 and the cysteinyl leukotrienes (LTs), formed from the cyclooxygenase (COX) and leukotriene pathways, respectively. As shown in **Fig. 4**, arachidonic acid is formed by the cytosolic phospholipase A_2 cleavage of membrane phospholipids. There are 2 COX enzymes. COX-1 is largely constitutively expressed, whereas COX-2 may be induced by inflammatory stimuli, such as lipopolysaccharide, IL-1, or TNF. Both COX-1 and COX-2 metabolize arachidonic acid into an unstable intermediate, PGH_2, and then tissue-specific enzymes and isomerase synthesize the 5 primary PGs, which are PGD_2, PGE_2, $PGF_{2\alpha}$, PGI_2, and thromboxane A_2 (TXA_2). LTs are generated when the 5-lipoxygenase (5-LO) pathway metabolizes arachidonic acid.[146] The released arachidonic acid binds to 5-LO activating protein for presentation to 5-LO for oxygenation and the production of LTA_4.[147] LTA_4 can be metabolized by LTA_4 hydrolase into LTB_4, or can be

Arachidonic Acid Metabolism

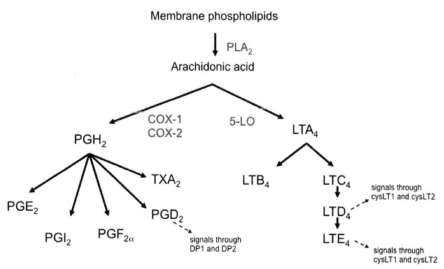

Fig. 4. Metabolism of arachidonic acid through the COX and 5-LO pathways.

metabolized by LTC_4 synthase (LTC_4S) to LTC_4, which can then sequentially be metabolized to LTD_4 and finally LTE_4. LTC_4, LTD_4, and LTE_4 are known as the cysteinyl LT because of the presence of cysteine in their structure.

Prostaglandin D_2

PGD_2 is the major mast cell–derived prostanoid and is released in nanogram quantities in these cells in response to IgE-mediated activation.[148] Eosinophils also synthesize PGD_2.[149] The prostanoids signal through distinct 7-transmembrane, G-protein–coupled receptors. The receptors through which PGD_2 signals are termed D-prostanoid $(DP)_1$ and DP_2 (see **Fig. 4**).[148] DP_1 is expressed on mucus-secreting goblet cells in the nasal and colonic mucosa, nasal serous glands, vascular endothelium, Th2 cells, DCs, basophils, and eosinophils. DP_1 stimulation activates adenylate cyclase, resulting in increased intracellular cyclic AMP (cAMP) and protein kinase A activity. DP_2 is also known as CRTH2, and is expressed on eosinophils, basophils, and the T-cell subsets CD4 Th2 and CD8 Tc2 cells. PGD_2 induces chemotaxis in each of these immune cells in a DP_2-dependent manner. DP_2 is preferentially expressed by T cells expressing IL-4 and IL-13 compared with T cells expressing IFN-γ in the BAL fluid of subjects with asthma.[150] DP_2 signaling in eosinophils augments their release from bone marrow, increases their respiratory burst, stimulates the chemotactic response to other chemokines, such as eotaxin,

and primes them for degranulation. Further, DP_2 signaling upregulated microvascular permeability, reduction of goblet cells, and constricted coronary arteries. In contrast to DP_1 signaling, activation of DP_2 reduced intracellular cAMP.[148] Therefore, PGD_2 signaling through DP_2, by suppressing cAMP, would be predicted to facilitate allergic inflammation through its effect on chemotaxis and mediator release by effector cells. PGD_2 stimulated human peripheral blood ILC2 to secrete large amounts of IL-13 to the same level produced in response to IL-25 and IL-33, whereas the addition of IL-25 and IL-33 to PGD_2 synergistically increased IL-13 expression by ILC2.[151] In these experiments, PGD_2 increased IL-13 production by ILC2 mainly through activation of DP_2.[151] Others similarly reported that PGD_2 enhanced human ILC2 function.[152] DP_2 signaling enhanced ILC2 migration and production of Th2-like cytokines by ILC2. PGD_2 activation through DP_2 increased ILC2 expression of the IL-33 and IL-25 receptor subunits, ST2 and IL-17RA, respectively.[152] Cysteinyl LT, particularly LTE_4, enhances the activation of ILC2 by PGD_2.[153] LTE_4 increased Type 2 cytokine production stimulated by PGD_2, IL-25, IL-33, and TSLP, in addition to IL-2–induced increases in IL-33 and IL-25 receptor expression on ILC2.

Inhalation challenge of allergic subjects with asthma with allergens to which the subjects were sensitized augmented PGD_2 in BAL.[154] PGD_2 levels in BAL were increased in patients with severe asthma, even at baseline in the absence of allergen challenge.[155] Asthma exacerbations, poor asthma control, and markers of Th2 inflammation were associated with higher PGD_2 levels, hematopoietic PGD synthase, and DP2.[155] PGD_2 was also increased in the nasal lavage from subjects with allergic rhinitis,[156] in tears from persons experiencing allergic conjunctivitis,[157] and in the fluid obtained from experimentally produced skin blisters in patients with late-phase reactions of the skin.[158]

There are several published trials of DP_2 antagonists in humans with asthma and other allergic diseases. OC000459 significantly improved quality of life and nighttime symptom score and reduced geometric mean sputum eosinophil count compared with pretreatment baseline, but not placebo.[159] This DP_2 antagonist has also shown some efficacy in adult patients with corticosteroid-dependent or corticosteroid-refractory eosinophilic esophagitis.[160]

The DP_2 antagonist BI 671800 significantly improved nasal symptom scores, decreased nasal eosinophils, and reduced nasal IL-4 and eotaxin levels in a dose-related manner in patients with seasonal allergic rhinitis.[161] BI 671800 was also examined in patients with asthma in 2 separate trials.[162] In the first trial, BI 671800 significantly increased FEV_1 greater than the change in FEV_1 seen with placebo; however, there was no significant change in asthma control questionnaire (ACQ). In the second trial, BI 671800 significantly increased FEV_1 compared with placebo and significantly increased the mean ACQ score at a high dose, although this increase was not deemed to be clinically significant.[162] In a more recent phase IIa, 12-week, BI 6718000 treatment did not result in a statistically significant or clinically meaningful difference in the ACQ scores compared with placebo.[163] The oral DP_2 antagonist fevipiprant was examined in patients with mild-to-moderate uncontrolled allergic asthma.[164] Although there was no benefit with fevipiprant in the entire study population, a subgroup analysis revealed that patients with an FEV_1 less than 70% predicted at baseline had a significant improvement in trough FEV_1 and ACQ7 score compared with placebo. In another study, fevipiprant-treated patients had a decrease in the mean sputum eosinophil percentage, and this was significantly greater than the change in sputum eosinophils in the placebo-treated patients.[165] The DP_2 antagonist AZD1981 was examined in adults with asthma and the treatment had no significant effect on morning peak expiratory flow. In another study of patients with uncontrolled asthma despite inhaled corticosteroid therapy, AZD1981 significantly increased ACQ-5 scores, but there was no dose-response relationship.[166]

Additional studies will be important to confirm the clinical usefulness of DP_2 antagonism in asthma, but these trials suggest that PGD_2 is involved in asthma pathogenesis.

Cysteinyl Leukotrienes

The major cellular sources of cysteinyl LTs are eosinophils, basophils, mast cells, and macrophages, each of which express LTC_4S. LTC_4S expression is sharply upregulated in human mast cells by IL-4-STAT6–dependent transcription, potentially reflecting a mechanism for upregulating cysteinyl LT production in allergic inflammation.[167] Both LTB_4 and LTC_4 are exported by specific respective transporter proteins, members of the multidrug resistance proteins (MRPs). MRP1 is a specific transmembrane protein that transports LTC_4 to the extracellular space. There are 3 cysteinyl LT receptors: cysLT1, cysLT2, and cysLT3. CysLT1 is expressed on airway smooth muscle cells, eosinophils, B cells, mast cells, monocytes, and macrophages.[168,169] Signaling through cysLT1 induced bronchoconstriction, mucus secretion, and airway edema. Therapeutic cysLT1 antagonists include montelukast, pranlukast, and zafirlukast. CysLT1 expression is upregulated at the transcriptional level by type 2 cytokines, including IL-4 and IL-13, providing an explanation for increased cysLT1 expression in subjects with allergic diseases. CysLT2 is expressed on lung macrophages, airway smooth muscle, peripheral blood leukocytes, mast cells, and brain tissue.[170] In mice, cysLT2 is expressed in the lung on bronchial smooth muscle, alveolar macrophages, conventional dendritic cells, and eosinophils.[171] A cysLT2 antagonist inhibited multiple antigen challenge-induced increases in eosinophils and mononuclear cells into the lung.[171] Currently, there are no selective cysLT2 inhibitors in clinical use, thus the function of cysLT2 is based on animal studies. Studies in cysLT2 KO mice suggest that signaling through cysLT2 promotes vascular permeability, inflammation, and tissue fibrosis, but not bronchoconstriction. CysLT3 was recently discovered and was previously known as GPR99. The predominant ligand for cysLT3 is LTE_4 and there are no known human cysLT3 antagonists. Animal studies using cysLT3 KO mice revealed that these mice had a dose-dependent loss of LTE_4-mediated vascular permeability, but not to LTC_4 or LTD_4, suggesting a preference of cysLT3 for LTE_4 even when $CysLT_1$ is present.[172] CysLT3 was detected on lung and nasal epithelial cells in mice.[173] Following either *Alternaria alternata* or LTE_4 airway challenge in mice, cysLT3 KO mice were protected against profound epithelial cell mucin release and swelling. CysLT3 KO mice have decreased baseline numbers of goblet cells, suggesting a function of this receptor in regulating epithelial cell homoeostasis.[173]

There have been 2 productive therapeutic strategies to antagonize LTs. The first is to decrease the production of the LTs by inhibiting their synthesis through 5-LO. The second strategy is to reduce LT binding on target tissues via LT receptor antagonists. Inhibiting 5-LO synthesis would have the combined benefit of reducing production of both LTB_4 and the cysteinyl LTs. Theoretically, 5-LO inhibition would blunt cysteinyl LT-induced bronchoconstriction and vascular permeability, as well as LTB_4-mediated neutrophil and eosinophil chemotaxis. Zileuton is the only 5-LO inhibitor approved for the treatment of asthma.[174] Unfortunately, zileuton has therapeutic shortcomings that have limited its widespread acceptance for asthma treatment. These include a short half-life and the potential for liver toxicity. Thus, 5-LO inhibitor use requires multiple daily doses and liver function testing. An extended-release form of zileuton is available that may be prescribed twice daily as opposed to 4 times a day; however, the total daily dose is the same.

CysLT1 antagonists include montelukast, pranlukast, and zafirlukast. Most of the clinical trials examining the therapeutic effect of LTs in asthma and allergic diseases have been in this class of medications and confirmed that cysteinyl LTs contributed a major portion of the bronchospasm that resulted from allergen challenge. Administration of the cysLT1 antagonist zafirlukast before allergen challenge inhibited immediate-phase bronchospasm by approximately 80% and reduced the late phase by 50%.[175,176] CysLT1 antagonists and 5-LO inhibitors blunted the influx of airway inflammatory cells after segmental allergen challenge.[177,178] Exercise-induced bronchospasm is consistently blunted by both cysLT1 antagonists and 5-LO inhibitors by approximately 30% to 60%.[179–182]

Approximately 10% of adults with asthma will have asthma symptoms and reduction in pulmonary function after ingesting aspirin or other nonsteroidal anti-inflammatory drugs, and this is termed aspirin-exacerbated respiratory disease (AERD).[183] The exact mechanisms causing this adverse response are not fully defined; however, there is increased expression of LTC_4 synthase and cysLT2 by mast cells and eosinophils in patients with AERD. It is unknown whether the increase in LTC_4 synthase expression is an underlying mechanism leading to AERD. Treatment with both cysLT1 antagonists and 5-LO inhibitors reduced AERD pulmonary function abnormalities and symptoms, strongly suggesting that cysLTs are involved in AERD pathogenesis. Several studies revealed that there is almost 100% inhibition of aspirin-induced bronchospasm by LT antagonists.[184–186] 5-LO inhibition decreased aspirin-induced urinary LTE_4 and mast cell–produced tryptase in nasal secretions.[185,187] These results substantiate that LT antagonists impact mast cells and their activation, but the importance of LT generation as a result of mast cell activation in this setting needs further definition.

SUMMARY

Discovery of proinflammatory pathways involved in asthma pathogenesis is far from complete. Just when it seems that we know all there to know is about asthma inflammation, a major paradigm shift occurs that teaches us that we still have a lot to learn. The 2 most recent examples of this include the discovery of the Th17 cells in the early 2000s and the recognition of ILC2 earlier this decade. Continued close observation and investigation will lead the field to future discoveries of molecules and cells that are increased in patients with asthma. These targets will be able to be antagonized quickly in both mice and people because of advancements in molecular biology and pharmacology, providing the opportunity to directly test their involvement in the asthma phenotype, with the goal of improving patient care of people with this disease.

REFERENCES

1. National Heart Lung and Blood Institute. Guidelines for the diagnosis and management of asthma (EPR-3). 2007.
2. Mosmann TR, Cherwinski H, Bond MW, et al. Two types of murine helper T cell clone. I. Definition according to profiles of lymphokine activities and secreted proteins. J Immunol 1986;136(7):2348–57.
3. Durbin JE, Johnson TR, Durbin RK, et al. The role of IFN in respiratory syncytial virus pathogenesis. J Immunol 2002;168(6):2944–52.
4. Neill DR, Wong SH, Bellosi A, et al. Nuocytes represent a new innate effector leukocyte that mediates type-2 immunity. Nature 2010;464(7293):1367–70.
5. Price AE, Liang HE, Sullivan BM, et al. Systemically dispersed innate IL-13-expressing cells in type 2 immunity. Proc Natl Acad Sci U S A 2010; 107(25):11489–94.
6. Halim TY, Krauss RH, Sun AC, et al. Lung natural helper cells are a critical source of Th2 cell-type

cytokines in protease allergen-induced airway inflammation. Immunity 2012;36(3):451–63.

7. Phillips C, Coward WR, Pritchard DI, et al. Basophils express a type 2 cytokine profile on exposure to proteases from helminths and house dust mites. J Leukoc Biol 2003;73(1):165–71.

8. Barlow JL, Bellosi A, Hardman CS, et al. Innate IL-13-producing nuocytes arise during allergic lung inflammation and contribute to airways hyperreactivity. J Allergy Clin Immunol 2012;129(1):191–8.

9. Doherty TA, Khorram N, Chang JE, et al. STAT6 regulates natural helper cell proliferation during lung inflammation initiated by *Alternaria*. Am J Physiol Lung Cell Mol Physiol 2012;303(7): L577–88.

10. Drake LY, Iijima K, Bartemes K, et al. Group 2 innate lymphoid cells promote an early antibody response to a respiratory antigen in mice. J Immunol 2016;197(4):1335–42.

11. McKenzie AN. Type-2 innate lymphoid cells in asthma and allergy. Ann Am Thorac Soc 2014; 11(Suppl 5):S263–70.

12. Liew FY, Girard JP, Turnquist HR. Interleukin-33 in health and disease. Nat Rev Immunol 2016; 16(11):676–89.

13. Saluzzo S, Gorki AD, Rana BMJ, et al. First-breath-induced type 2 pathways shape the lung immune environment. Cell Rep 2017;18(8):1893–905.

14. Moffatt MF, Gut IG, Demenais F, et al. A large-scale, consortium-based genomewide association study of asthma. N Engl J Med 2010;363(13): 1211–21.

15. Savenije OE, Mahachie John JM, Granell R, et al. Association of IL33-IL-1 receptor-like 1 (IL1RL1) pathway polymorphisms with wheezing phenotypes and asthma in childhood. J Allergy Clin Immunol 2014;134(1):170–7.

16. Torgerson DG, Ampleford EJ, Chiu GY, et al. Meta-analysis of genome-wide association studies of asthma in ethnically diverse North American populations. Nat Genet 2011;43(9):887–92.

17. Kurowska-Stolarska M, Kewin P, Murphy G, et al. IL-33 induces antigen-specific IL-5+ T cells and promotes allergic-induced airway inflammation independent of IL-4. J Immunol 2008;181(7): 4780–90.

18. Morita H, Nakae S, Saito H, et al. IL-33 in clinical practice: size matters? J Allergy Clin Immunol 2017;140(2):381–3.

19. Drake LY, Kita H. IL-33: biological properties, functions, and roles in airway disease. Immunol Rev 2017;278(1):173–84.

20. Kouzaki H, Iijima K, Kobayashi T, et al. The danger signal, extracellular ATP, is a sensor for an airborne allergen and triggers IL-33 release and innate Th2-type responses. J Immunol 2011; 186(7):4375–87.

21. Hristova M, Habibovic A, Veith C, et al. Airway epithelial dual oxidase 1 mediates allergen-induced IL-33 secretion and activation of type 2 immune responses. J Allergy Clin Immunol 2016; 137(5):1545–56.e11.

22. Bartemes KR, Iijima K, Kobayashi T, et al. IL-33-responsive lineage- CD25+ CD44(hi) lymphoid cells mediate innate type 2 immunity and allergic inflammation in the lungs. J Immunol 2012;188(3): 1503–13.

23. Barlow JL, Peel S, Fox J, et al. IL-33 is more potent than IL-25 in provoking IL-13-producing nuocytes (type 2 innate lymphoid cells) and airway contraction. J Allergy Clin Immunol 2013;132(4):933–41.

24. Komai-Koma M, Xu D, Li Y, et al. IL-33 is a chemo-attractant for human Th2 cells. Eur J Immunol 2007; 37(10):2779–86.

25. Traister RS, Uvalle CE, Hawkins GA, et al. Phenotypic and genotypic association of epithelial IL1RL1 to human TH2-like asthma. J Allergy Clin Immunol 2015;135(1):92–9.

26. Borish L. The immunology of asthma: asthma phenotypes and their implications for personalized treatment. Ann Allergy Asthma Immunol 2016; 117(2):108–14.

27. Roan F, Bell BD, Stoklasek TA, et al. The multiple facets of thymic stromal lymphopoietin (TSLP) during allergic inflammation and beyond. J Leukoc Biol 2012;91(6):877–86.

28. Zhou B, Comeau MR, De ST, et al. Thymic stromal lymphopoietin as a key initiator of allergic airway inflammation in mice. Nat Immunol 2005;6(10): 1047–53.

29. Rochman Y, Dienger-Stambaugh K, Richgels PK, et al. TSLP signaling in CD4+ T cells programs a pathogenic T helper 2 cell state. Sci Signal 2018; 11(521) [pii:eaam8858].

30. Kabata H, Moro K, Fukunaga K, et al. Thymic stromal lymphopoietin induces corticosteroid resistance in natural helper cells during airway inflammation. Nat Commun 2013;4:2675.

31. Liu S, Verma M, Michalec L, et al. Steroid resistance of airway type 2 innate lymphoid cells from patients with severe asthma: the role of thymic stromal lymphopoietin. J Allergy Clin Immunol 2018; 141(1):257–68.

32. Gauvreau GM, O'Byrne PM, Boulet LP, et al. Effects of an anti-TSLP antibody on allergen-induced asthmatic responses. N Engl J Med 2014;370(22): 2102–10.

33. Corren J, Parnes JR, Wang L, et al. Tezepelumab in adults with uncontrolled asthma. N Engl J Med 2017;377(10):936–46.

34. Andreakos E, Papadopoulos NG. IL-25: the missing link between allergy, viral infection, and asthma? Sci Transl Med 2014;6(256): 256fs238.

35. Corrigan CJ, Wang W, Meng Q, et al. T-helper cell type 2 (Th2) memory T cell-potentiating cytokine IL-25 has the potential to promote angiogenesis in asthma. Proc Natl Acad Sci U S A 2011;108(4): 1579–84.

36. Kouzaki H, Tojima I, Kita H, et al. Transcription of interleukin-25 and extracellular release of the protein is regulated by allergen proteases in airway epithelial cells. Am J Respir Cell Mol Biol 2013; 49(5):741–50.

37. Rickel EA, Siegel LA, Yoon BR, et al. Identification of functional roles for both IL-17RB and IL-17RA in mediating IL-25-induced activities. J Immunol 2008;181(6):4299–310.

38. Su J, Chen T, Ji XY, et al. IL-25 downregulates Th1/Th17 immune response in an IL-10-dependent manner in inflammatory bowel disease. Inflamm Bowel Dis 2013;19(4):720–8.

39. Chang SH, Dong C. Signaling of interleukin-17 family cytokines in immunity and inflammation. Cell Signal 2011;23(7):1069–75.

40. Ballantyne SJ, Barlow JL, Jolin HE, et al. Blocking IL-25 prevents airway hyperresponsiveness in allergic asthma. J Allergy Clin Immunol 2007; 120(6):1324–31.

41. Gregory LG, Jones CP, Walker SA, et al. IL-25 drives remodelling in allergic airways disease induced by house dust mite. Thorax 2013;68(1): 82–90.

42. Cheng D, Xue Z, Yi L, et al. Epithelial interleukin-25 is a key mediator in Th2-high, corticosteroid-responsive asthma. Am J Respir Crit Care Med 2014;190(6):639–48.

43. Tang W, Smith SG, Beaudin S, et al. IL-25 and IL-25 receptor expression on eosinophils from subjects with allergic asthma. Int Arch Allergy Immunol 2014;163(1):5–10.

44. Willis CR, Siegel L, Leith A, et al. IL-17RA signaling in airway inflammation and bronchial hyperreactivity in allergic asthma. Am J Respir Cell Mol Biol 2015;53(6):810–21.

45. Busse WW, Holgate S, Kerwin E, et al. Randomized, double-blind, placebo-controlled study of brodalumab, a human anti-IL-17 receptor monoclonal antibody, in moderate to severe asthma. Am J Respir Crit Care Med 2013;188(11): 1294–302.

46. Loughnan MS, Takatsu K, Harada N, et al. T-cell-replacing factor (interleukin 5) induces expression of interleukin 2 receptors on murine splenic B cells. Proc Natl Acad Sci U S A 1987;84(15):5399–403.

47. Sanderson CJ, O'Garra A, Warren DJ, et al. Eosinophil differentiation factor also has B-cell growth factor activity: proposed name interleukin 4. Proc Natl Acad Sci U S A 1986;83(2):437–40.

48. Sanderson CJ, Warren DJ, Strath M. Identification of a lymphokine that stimulates eosinophil differentiation in vitro. Its relationship to interleukin 3, and functional properties of eosinophils produced in cultures. J Exp Med 1985;162(1):60–74.

49. Azuma C, Tanabe T, Konishi M, et al. Cloning of cDNA for human T-cell replacing factor (interleukin-5) and comparison with the murine homologue. Nucleic Acids Res 1986;14(22):9149–58.

50. Takatsu K. Interleukin-5 and IL-5 receptor in health and diseases. Proc Jpn Acad Ser B Phys Biol Sci 2011;87(8):463–85.

51. Tominaga A, Takaki S, Koyama N, et al. Transgenic mice expressing a B cell growth and differentiation factor gene (interleukin 5) develop eosinophilia and autoantibody production. J Exp Med 1991;173(2): 429–37.

52. Iwama T, Nagai H, Suda H, et al. Effect of murine recombinant interleukin-5 on the cell population in Guinea-pig airways. Br J Pharmacol 1992;105(1): 19–22.

53. Chand N, Harrison JE, Rooney S, et al. Anti-IL-5 monoclonal antibody inhibits allergic late phase bronchial eosinophilia in Guinea pigs: a therapeutic approach. Eur J Pharmacol 1992;211(1):121–3.

54. Van Oosterhout AJ, Ladenius AR, Savelkoul HF, et al. Effect of anti-IL-5 and IL-5 on airway hyperreactivity and eosinophils in Guinea pigs. Am Rev Respir Dis 1993;147(3):548–52.

55. Nakajima H, Iwamoto I, Tomoe S, et al. CD4+ T-lymphocytes and interleukin-5 mediate antigen-induced eosinophil infiltration into the mouse trachea. Am Rev Respir Dis 1992;146(2):374–7.

56. Tanaka H, Kawada N, Yamada T, et al. Allergen-induced airway inflammation and bronchial responsiveness in interleukin-5 receptor alpha chain-deficient mice. Clin Exp Allergy 2000;30(6):874–81.

57. Lee JJ, McGarry MP, Farmer SC, et al. Interleukin-5 expression in the lung epithelium of transgenic mice leads to pulmonary changes pathognomonic of asthma. J Exp Med 1997;185(12):2143–56.

58. Lee JJ, Dimina D, Macias MP, et al. Defining a link with asthma in mice congenitally deficient in eosinophils. Science 2004;305(5691):1773–6.

59. Jacobsen EA, Ochkur SI, Pero RS, et al. Allergic pulmonary inflammation in mice is dependent on eosinophil-induced recruitment of effector T cells. J Exp Med 2008;205(3):699–710.

60. Corrigan CJ, Haczku A, Gemou-Engesaeth V, et al. CD4 T-lymphocyte activation in asthma is accompanied by increased serum concentrations of interleukin-5. Effect of glucocorticoid therapy. Am Rev Respir Dis 1993;147(3):540–7.

61. Humbert M, Corrigan CJ, Kimmitt P, et al. Relationship between IL-4 and IL-5 mRNA expression and disease severity in atopic asthma. Am J Respir Crit Care Med 1997;156(3 Pt 1):704–8.

62. van der Veen MJ, Van Neerven RJ, De Jong EC, et al. The late asthmatic response is associated

with baseline allergen-specific proliferative responsiveness of peripheral T lymphocytes in vitro and serum interleukin-5. Clin Exp Allergy 1999;29(2): 217–27.

63. Shi HZ, Xiao CQ, Zhong D, et al. Effect of inhaled interleukin-5 on airway hyperreactivity and eosinophilia in asthmatics. Am J Respir Crit Care Med 1998;157(1):204–9.

64. Leckie MJ, Jenkins GR, Khan J, et al. Sputum T lymphocytes in asthma, COPD and healthy subjects have the phenotype of activated intraepithelial T cells (CD69+ CD103+). Thorax 2003;58(1): 23–9.

65. Minty A, Chalon P, Derocq JM, et al. Interleukin-13 is a new human lymphokine regulating inflammatory and immune responses. Nature 1993; 362(6417):248–50.

66. Ho IC, Vorhees P, Marin N, et al. Human GATA-3: a lineage-restricted transcription factor that regulates the expression of the T cell receptor alpha gene. EMBO J 1991;10(5):1187–92.

67. Palmer-Crocker RL, Hughes CC, Pober JS. IL-4 and IL-13 activate the JAK2 tyrosine kinase and Stat6 in cultured human vascular endothelial cells through a common pathway that does not involve the gamma c chain. J Clin Invest 1996;98(3):604–9.

68. Kaur D, Hollins F, Woodman L, et al. Mast cells express IL-13R alpha 1: IL-13 promotes human lung mast cell proliferation and Fc epsilon RI expression. Allergy 2006;61(9):1047–53.

69. Laporte JC, Moore PE, Baraldo S, et al. Direct effects of interleukin-13 on signaling pathways for physiological responses in cultured human airway smooth muscle cells. Am J Respir Crit Care Med 2001;164(1):141–8.

70. Lordan JL, Bucchieri F, Richter A, et al. Cooperative effects of Th2 cytokines and allergen on normal and asthmatic bronchial epithelial cells. J Immunol 2002;169(1):407–14.

71. Murata T, Husain SR, Mohri H, et al. Two different IL-13 receptor chains are expressed in normal human skin fibroblasts, and IL-4 and IL-13 mediate signal transduction through a common pathway. Int Immunol 1998;10(8):1103–10.

72. Wang IM, Lin H, Goldman SJ, et al. STAT-1 is activated by IL-4 and IL-13 in multiple cell types. Mol Immunol 2004;41(9):873–84.

73. Newcomb DC, Boswell MG, Huckabee MM, et al. IL-13 regulates Th17 secretion of IL-17A in an IL-10-dependent manner. J Immunol 2012;188(3): 1027–35.

74. Newcomb DC, Boswell MG, Zhou W, et al. Human Th17 cells express a functional IL-13 receptor and IL-13 attenuates IL-17A production. J Allergy Clin Immunol 2011;127(4):1006–13.e1-4.

75. Wilson MS, Ramalingam TR, Rivollier A, et al. Colitis and intestinal inflammation in IL10-/- mice results from IL-13Ralpha2-mediated attenuation of IL-13 activity. Gastroenterology 2011;140(1): 254–64.

76. Hall SL, Baker T, Lajoie S, et al. IL-17A enhances IL-13 activity by enhancing IL-13-induced signal transducer and activator of transcription 6 activation. J Allergy Clin Immunol 2017;139(2):462–71. e4.

77. Grunig G, Warnock M, Wakil AE, et al. Requirement for IL-13 independently of IL-4 in experimental asthma [see comments]. Science 1998;282(5397): 2261–3.

78. Wills-Karp M, Luyimbazi J, Xu X, et al. Interleukin-13: central mediator of allergic asthma. Science 1998;282(5397):2258–61.

79. Bochner BS, Klunk DA, Sterbinsky SA, et al. IL-13 selectively induces vascular cell adhesion molecule-1 expression in human endothelial cells. J Immunol 1995;154(2):799–803.

80. Defrance T, Carayon P, Billian G, et al. Interleukin 13 is a B cell stimulating factor. J Exp Med 1994; 179(1):135–43.

81. Punnonen J, Aversa G, Cocks BG, et al. Interleukin 13 induces interleukin 4-independent IgG4 and IgE synthesis and CD23 expression by human B cells. Proc Natl Acad Sci U S A 1993;90(8):3730–4.

82. Huang SK, Xiao HQ, Kleine-Tebbe J, et al. IL-13 expression at the sites of allergen challenge in patients with asthma. J Immunol 1995;155(5): 2688–94.

83. Kroegel C, Julius P, Matthys H, et al. Endobronchial secretion of interleukin-13 following local allergen challenge in atopic asthma: relationship to interleukin-4 and eosinophil counts. Eur Respir J 1996;9(5):899–904.

84. Humbert M, Durham SR, Kimmitt P, et al. Elevated expression of messenger ribonucleic acid encoding IL-13 in the bronchial mucosa of atopic and nonatopic subjects with asthma. J Allergy Clin Immunol 1997;99(5):657–65.

85. Spahn JD, Szefler SJ, Surs W, et al. A novel action of IL-13: induction of diminished monocyte glucocorticoid receptor-binding affinity. J Immunol 1996;157(6):2654–9.

86. Woodruff PG, Modrek B, Choy DF, et al. T-helper type 2-driven inflammation defines major subphenotypes of asthma. Am J Respir Crit Care Med 2009;180(5):388–95.

87. Corren J, Lemanske RF, Hanania NA, et al. Lebrikizumab treatment in adults with asthma. N Engl J Med 2011;365(12):1088–98.

88. Hanania NA, Noonan M, Corren J, et al. Lebrikizumab in moderate-to-severe asthma: pooled data from two randomised placebo-controlled studies. Thorax 2015;70(8):748–56.

89. Hanania NA, Korenblat P, Chapman KR, et al. Efficacy and safety of lebrikizumab in patients with

uncontrolled asthma (LAVOLTA I and LAVOLTA II): replicate, phase 3, randomised, double-blind, placebo-controlled trials. Lancet Respir Med 2016; 4(10):781–96.

90. Korenblat P, Kerwin E, Leshchenko I, et al. Efficacy and safety of lebrikizumab in adult patients with mild-to-moderate asthma not receiving inhaled corticosteroids. Respir Med 2018;134:143–9.

91. Borish LC, Nelson HS, Lanz MJ, et al. Interleukin-4 receptor in moderate atopic asthma. A phase I/II randomized, placebo-controlled trial. Am J Respir Crit Care Med 1999;160(6):1816–23.

92. Borish LC, Nelson HS, Corren J, et al. Efficacy of soluble IL-4 receptor for the treatment of adults with asthma. J Allergy Clin Immunol 2001;107(6): 963–70.

93. Wenzel S, Wilbraham D, Fuller R, et al. Effect of an interleukin-4 variant on late phase asthmatic response to allergen challenge in asthmatic patients: results of two phase 2a studies. Lancet 2007;370(9596):1422–31.

94. Corren J, Busse W, Meltzer EO, et al. A randomized, controlled, phase 2 study of AMG 317, an IL-4Ralpha antagonist, in patients with asthma. Am J Respir Crit Care Med 2010;181(8): 788–96.

95. Wenzel S, Ford L, Pearlman D, et al. Dupilumab in persistent asthma with elevated eosinophil levels. N Engl J Med 2013;368(26):2455–66.

96. Wenzel S, Castro M, Corren J, et al. Dupilumab efficacy and safety in adults with uncontrolled persistent asthma despite use of medium-to-high-dose inhaled corticosteroids plus a long-acting beta2 agonist: a randomised double-blind placebo-controlled pivotal phase 2b dose-ranging trial. Lancet 2016;388(10039):31–44.

97. Krug N, Hohlfeld JM, Kirsten AM, et al. Allergen-induced asthmatic responses modified by a GATA3-specific DNAzyme. N Engl J Med 2015; 372(21):1987–95.

98. Braddock M, Hanania NA, Sharafkhaneh A, et al. Potential risks related to modulating interleukin-13 and interleukin-4 signalling: a systematic review. Drug Saf 2018;41(5):489–509.

99. Paul WE. History of interleukin-4. Cytokine 2015; 75(1):3–7.

100. Coffman RL, Ohara J, Bond MW, et al. B cell stimulatory factor-1 enhances the IgE response of lipopolysaccharide-activated B cells. J Immunol 1986;136(12):4538–41.

101. Sutherland GR, Baker E, Callen DF, et al. Interleukin 4 is at 5q31 and interleukin 6 is at 7p15. Hum Genet 1988;79(4):335–7.

102. Russell SM, Keegan AD, Harada N, et al. Interleukin-2 receptor gamma chain: a functional component of the interleukin-4 receptor. Science 1993;262(5141):1880–3.

103. Swain SL, Weinberg AD, English M, et al. IL-4 directs the development of Th2-like helper effectors. J Immunol 1990;145(11):3796–806.

104. Zhu J, Yamane H, Cote-Sierra J, et al. GATA-3 promotes Th2 responses through three different mechanisms: induction of Th2 cytokine production, selective growth of Th2 cells and inhibition of Th1 cell-specific factors. Cell Res 2006;16(1):3–10.

105. Brown MA, Pierce JH, Watson CJ, et al. B cell stimulatory factor-1/interleukin-4 mRNA is expressed by normal and transformed mast cells. Cell 1987; 50(5):809–18.

106. Moqbel R, Ying S, Barkans J, et al. Identification of messenger RNA for IL-4 in human eosinophils with granule localization and release of the translated product. J Immunol 1995;155(10):4939–47.

107. Nonaka M, Nonaka R, Woolley K, et al. Distinct immunohistochemical localization of IL-4 in human inflamed airway tissues. IL-4 is localized to eosinophils in vivo and is released by peripheral blood eosinophils. J Immunol 1995;155(6):3234–44.

108. Plaut M, Pierce JH, Watson CJ, et al. Mast cell lines produce lymphokines in response to cross-linkage of Fc epsilon RI or to calcium ionophores. Nature 1989;339(6219):64–7.

109. Seder RA, Paul WE, Dvorak AM, et al. Mouse splenic and bone marrow cell populations that express high-affinity Fc epsilon receptors and produce interleukin 4 are highly enriched in basophils. Proc Natl Acad Sci U S A 1991;88(7): 2835–9.

110. Yoshimoto T, Bendelac A, Watson C, et al. Role of NK1.1+ T cells in a TH2 response and in immunoglobulin E production. Science 1995;270(5243):1845–7.

111. Doherty TA, Khorram N, Lund S, et al. Lung type 2 innate lymphoid cells express cysteinyl leukotriene receptor 1, which regulates TH2 cytokine production. J Allergy Clin Immunol 2013;132(1):205–13.

112. Bochner BS, Luscinskas FW, Gimbrone MA Jr, et al. Adhesion of human basophils, eosinophils, and neutrophils to interleukin 1-activated human vascular endothelial cells: contributions of endothelial cell adhesion molecules. J Exp Med 1991; 173(6):1553–7.

113. Masinovsky B, Urdal D, Gallatin WM. IL-4 acts synergistically with IL-1 beta to promote lymphocyte adhesion to microvascular endothelium by induction of vascular cell adhesion molecule-1. J Immunol 1990;145(9):2886–95.

114. Temann UA, Prasad B, Gallup MW, et al. A novel role for murine IL-4 in vivo: induction of MUC5AC gene expression and mucin hypersecretion. Am J Respir Cell Mol Biol 1997;16(4):471–8.

115. Brusselle GG, Kips JC, Tavernier JH, et al. Attenuation of allergic airway inflammation in IL-4 deficient mice [see comments]. Clin Exp Allergy 1994;24(1):73–80.

116. Coyle AJ, Le Gros G, Bertrand C, et al. Interleukin-4 is required for the induction of lung Th2 mucosal immunity. Am J Respir Cell Mol Biol 1995;13(1):54–9.

117. Corry DB, Folkesson HG, Warnock ML, et al. Interleukin 4, but not interleukin 5 or eosinophils, is required in a murine model of acute airway hyperreactivity [see comments]. J Exp Med 1996;183(1):109–17.

118. Robinson DS, Hamid Q, Ying S, et al. Predominant TH2-like bronchoalveolar T-lymphocyte population in atopic asthma. N Engl J Med 1992;326(5):298–304.

119. Walker C, Bode E, Boer L, et al. Allergic and nonallergic asthmatics have distinct patterns of T-cell activation and cytokine production in peripheral blood and bronchoalveolar lavage. Am Rev Respir Dis 1992;146(1):109–15.

120. Robinson D, Hamid Q, Ying S, et al. Prednisolone treatment in asthma is associated with modulation of bronchoalveolar lavage cell interleukin-4, interleukin-5, and interferon-gamma cytokine gene expression. Am Rev Respir Dis 1993;148(2):401–6.

121. Robinson D, Hamid Q, Bentley A, et al. Activation of CD4+ T cells, increased TH2-type cytokine mRNA expression, and eosinophil recruitment in bronchoalveolar lavage after allergen inhalation challenge in patients with atopic asthma. J Allergy Clin Immunol 1993;92(2):313–24.

122. Holgate ST. Innate and adaptive immune responses in asthma. Nat Med 2012;18(5):673–83.

123. Veldhoen M. Interleukin 17 is a chief orchestrator of immunity. Nat Immunol 2017;18(6):612–21.

124. Newcomb DC, Peebles RS Jr. Th17-mediated inflammation in asthma. Curr Opin Immunol 2013;25(6):755–60.

125. Cua DJ, Tato CM. Innate IL-17-producing cells: the sentinels of the immune system. Nat Rev Immunol 2010;10(7):479–89.

126. Miossec P, Kolls JK. Targeting IL-17 and TH17 cells in chronic inflammation. Nat Rev Drug Discov 2012;11(10):763–76.

127. Tamassia N, Arruda-Silva F, Calzetti F, et al. A reappraisal on the potential ability of human neutrophils to express and produce IL-17 family members in vitro: failure to reproducibly detect it. Front Immunol 2018;9:795.

128. Toy D, Kugler D, Wolfson M, et al. Cutting edge: interleukin 17 signals through a heteromeric receptor complex. J Immunol 2006;177(1):36–9.

129. Ghoreschi K, Laurence A, Yang XP, et al. Generation of pathogenic T(H)17 cells in the absence of TGF-beta signalling. Nature 2010;467(7318):967–71.

130. Korn T, Bettelli E, Oukka M, et al. IL-17 and Th17 cells. Annu Rev Immunol 2009;27:485–517.

131. Veldhoen M, Hocking RJ, Atkins CJ, et al. TGFbeta in the context of an inflammatory cytokine milieu supports de novo differentiation of IL-17-producing T cells. Immunity 2006;24(2):179–89.

132. Schnyder-Candrian S, Togbe D, Couillin I, et al. Interleukin-17 is a negative regulator of established allergic asthma. J Exp Med 2006;203(12):2715–25.

133. Lajoie S, Lewkowich IP, Suzuki Y, et al. Complement-mediated regulation of the IL-17A axis is a central genetic determinant of the severity of experimental allergic asthma. Nat Immunol 2010;11(10):928–35.

134. McKinley L, Alcorn JF, Peterson A, et al. TH17 cells mediate steroid-resistant airway inflammation and airway hyperresponsiveness in mice. J Immunol 2008;181(6):4089–97.

135. Barlow JL, Flynn RJ, Ballantyne SJ, et al. Reciprocal expression of IL-25 and IL-17A is important for allergic airways hyperreactivity. Clin Exp Allergy 2011;41(10):1447–55.

136. Molet S, Hamid Q, Davoine F, et al. IL-17 is increased in asthmatic airways and induces human bronchial fibroblasts to produce cytokines. J Allergy Clin Immunol 2001;108(3):430–8.

137. Doe C, Bafadhel M, Siddiqui S, et al. Expression of the T helper 17-associated cytokines IL-17A and IL-17F in asthma and COPD. Chest 2010;138(5):1140–7.

138. Bullens DM, Truyen E, Coteur L, et al. IL-17 mRNA in sputum of asthmatic patients: linking T cell driven inflammation and granulocytic influx? Respir Res 2006;7:135.

139. Saleh A, Shan L, Halayko AJ, et al. Critical role for STAT3 in IL-17A-mediated CCL11 expression in human airway smooth muscle cells. J Immunol 2009;182(6):3357–65.

140. Inoue D, Numasaki M, Watanabe M, et al. IL-17A promotes the growth of airway epithelial cells through ERK-dependent signaling pathway. Biochem Biophys Res Commun 2006;347(4):852–8.

141. Chen Y, Thai P, Zhao YH, et al. Stimulation of airway mucin gene expression by interleukin (IL)-17 through IL-6 paracrine/autocrine loop. J Biol Chem 2003;278(19):17036–43.

142. Fujisawa T, Velichko S, Thai P, et al. Regulation of airway MUC5AC expression by IL-1beta and IL-17A; the NF-kappaB paradigm. J Immunol 2009;183(10):6236–43.

143. Chang Y, Al-Alwan L, Risse PA, et al. Th17-associated cytokines promote human airway smooth muscle cell proliferation. FASEB J 2012;26(12):5152–60.

144. Chang Y, Al-Alwan L, Risse PA, et al. TH17 cytokines induce human airway smooth muscle cell migration. J Allergy Clin Immunol 2011;127(4):1046–53.e1-2.

145. Rusta-Sallehy S, Gooderham M, Papp K. Brodalumab: a review of safety. Skin Ther Lett 2018; 23(2):1–3.

146. Harizi H, Juzan M, Moreau JF, et al. Prostaglandins inhibit 5-lipoxygenase-activating protein expression and leukotriene B4 production from dendritic cells via an IL-10-dependent mechanism. J Immunol 2003;170(1):139–46.

147. Peebles RS Jr, Boyce JA. Lipid mediators of hypersensitivity and inflammation. In: Adkinson NF Jr, Bochnor BS, Burks AW, et al, editors. Middleton's allergy principles and practice, vol. 1, 8th edition. Philadelphia: Elsevier; 2014. p. 139–61.

148. Smith WL, Urade Y, Jakobsson PJ. Enzymes of the cyclooxygenase pathways of prostanoid biosynthesis. Chem Rev 2011;111(10):5821–65.

149. Luna-Gomes T, Magalhaes KG, Mesquita-Santos FP, et al. Eosinophils as a novel cell source of prostaglandin D2: autocrine role in allergic inflammation. J Immunol 2011;187(12):6518–26.

150. Mutalithas K, Guillen C, Day C, et al. CRTH2 expression on T cells in asthma. Clin Exp Immunol 2010;161(1):34–40.

151. Barnig C, Cernadas M, Dutile S, et al. Lipoxin A4 regulates natural killer cell and type 2 innate lymphoid cell activation in asthma. Sci Transl Med 2013;5(174):174ra126.

152. Xue L, Salimi M, Panse I, et al. Prostaglandin D2 activates group 2 innate lymphoid cells through chemoattractant receptor-homologous molecule expressed on TH2 cells. J Allergy Clin Immunol 2014;133(4):1184–94.

153. Salimi M, Stoger L, Liu W, et al. Cysteinyl leukotriene E4 activates human group 2 innate lymphoid cells and enhances the effect of prostaglandin D2 and epithelial cytokines. J Allergy Clin Immunol 2017;140(4):1090–100.e1.

154. Murray M, Webb MS, O'Callaghan C, et al. Respiratory status and allergy after bronchiolitis. Arch Dis Child 1992;67(4):482–7.

155. Fajt ML, Gelhaus SL, Freeman B, et al. Prostaglandin D(2) pathway upregulation: relation to asthma severity, control, and TH2 inflammation. J Allergy Clin Immunol 2013;131(6):1504–12.

156. Naclerio RM, Meier HL, Kagey-Sobotka A, et al. Mediator release after nasal airway challenge with allergen. Am Rev Respir Dis 1983;128(4):597–602.

157. Proud D, Sweet J, Stein P, et al. Inflammatory mediator release on conjunctival provocation of allergic subjects with allergen. J Allergy Clin Immunol 1990;85(5):896–905.

158. Charlesworth EN, Kagey-Sobotka A, Schleimer RP, et al. Prednisone inhibits the appearance of inflammatory mediators and the influx of eosinophils and basophils associated with the cutaneous late-phase response to allergen. J Immunol 1991; 146(2):671–6.

159. Barnes N, Pavord I, Chuchalin A, et al. A randomized, double-blind, placebo-controlled study of the CRTH2 antagonist OC000459 in moderate persistent asthma. Clin Exp Allergy 2012; 42(1):38–48.

160. Straumann A, Hoesli S, Bussmann C, et al. Anti-eosinophil activity and clinical efficacy of the CRTH2 antagonist OC000459 in eosinophilic esophagitis. Allergy 2013;68(3):375–85.

161. Krug N, Gupta A, Badorrek P, et al. Efficacy of the oral chemoattractant receptor homologous molecule on TH2 cells antagonist BI 671800 in patients with seasonal allergic rhinitis. J Allergy Clin Immunol 2014;133(2):414–9.

162. Hall IP, Fowler AV, Gupta A, et al. Efficacy of BI 671800, an oral CRTH2 antagonist, in poorly controlled asthma as sole controller and in the presence of inhaled corticosteroid treatment. Pulm Pharmacol Ther 2015;32:37–44.

163. Miller D, Wood C, Bateman E, et al. A randomized study of BI 671800, a CRTH2 antagonist, as add-on therapy in poorly controlled asthma. Allergy Asthma Proc 2017;38(2):157–64.

164. Erpenbeck VJ, Popov TA, Miller D, et al. The oral CRTh2 antagonist QAW039 (fevipiprant): a phase II study in uncontrolled allergic asthma. Pulm Pharmacol Ther 2016;39:54–63.

165. Gonem S, Berair R, Singapuri A, et al. Fevipiprant, a prostaglandin D2 receptor 2 antagonist, in patients with persistent eosinophilic asthma: a single-centre, randomised, double-blind, parallel-group, placebo-controlled trial. Lancet Respir Med 2016;4(9):699–707.

166. Kuna P, Bjermer L, Tornling G. Two phase II randomized trials on the CRTH2 antagonist AZD1981 in adults with asthma. Drug Des Dev Ther 2016; 10:2759–70.

167. Hsieh FH, Lam BK, Penrose JF, et al. T helper cell type 2 cytokines coordinately regulate immunoglobulin E-dependent cysteinyl leukotriene production by human cord blood-derived mast cells: profound induction of leukotriene C(4) synthase expression by interleukin 4. J Exp Med 2001; 193(1):123–33.

168. Figueroa DJ, Breyer RM, Defoe SK, et al. Expression of the cysteinyl leukotriene 1 receptor in normal human lung and peripheral blood leukocytes. Am J Respir Crit Care Med 2001;163(1): 226–33.

169. Lynch KR, O'Neill GP, Liu Q, et al. Characterization of the human cysteinyl leukotriene CysLT1 receptor. Nature 1999;399(6738):789–93.

170. Mellor EA, Frank N, Soler D, et al. Expression of the type 2 receptor for cysteinyl leukotrienes (CysLT2R) by human mast cells: functional distinction from CysLT1R. Proc Natl Acad Sci U S A 2003; 100(20):11589–93.

171. Matsuda M, Tabuchi Y, Nishimura K, et al. Increased expression of CysLT2 receptors in the lung of asthmatic mice and role in allergic responses. Prostaglandins Leukot Essent Fatty Acids 2018;131:24–31.

172. Kanaoka Y, Maekawa A, Austen KF. Identification of GPR99 protein as a potential third cysteinyl leukotriene receptor with a preference for leukotriene E4 ligand. J Biol Chem 2013;288(16):10967–72.

173. Bankova LG, Lai J, Yoshimoto E, et al. Leukotriene E4 elicits respiratory epithelial cell mucin release through the G-protein-coupled receptor, GPR99. Proc Natl Acad Sci U S A 2016;113(22):6242–7.

174. Dube LM, Swanson LJ, Awni W. Zileuton, a leukotriene synthesis inhibitor in the management of chronic asthma. Clinical pharmacokinetics and safety. Clin Rev Allergy Immunol 1999;17(1–2):213–21.

175. Findlay SR, Barden JM, Easley CB, et al. Effect of the oral leukotriene antagonist, ICI 204,219, on antigen-induced bronchoconstriction in subjects with asthma. J Allergy Clin Immunol 1992;89(5):1040–5.

176. Taylor IK, O'Shaughnessy KM, Fuller RW, et al. Effect of cysteinyl-leukotriene receptor antagonist ICI 204.219 on allergen-induced bronchoconstriction and airway hyperreactivity in atopic subjects. Lancet 1991;337(8743):690–4.

177. Calhoun WJ, Lavins BJ, Minkwitz MC, et al. Effect of zafirlukast (Accolate) on cellular mediators of inflammation: bronchoalveolar lavage fluid findings after segmental antigen challenge. Am J Respir Crit Care Med 1998;157(5 Pt 1):1381–9.

178. Kane GC, Pollice M, Kim CJ, et al. A controlled trial of the effect of the 5-lipoxygenase inhibitor, zileuton, on lung inflammation produced by segmental antigen challenge in human beings. J Allergy Clin Immunol 1996;97(2):646–54.

179. Finnerty JP, Wood-Baker R, Thomson H, et al. Role of leukotrienes in exercise-induced asthma.

Inhibitory effect of ICI 204219, a potent leukotriene D4 receptor antagonist. Am Rev Respir Dis 1992;145(4 Pt 1):746–9.

180. Leff JA, Busse WW, Pearlman D, et al. Montelukast, a leukotriene-receptor antagonist, for the treatment of mild asthma and exercise-induced bronchoconstriction. N Engl J Med 1998;339(3):147–52.

181. Meltzer SS, Hasday JD, Cohn J, et al. Inhibition of exercise-induced bronchospasm by zileuton: a 5-lipoxygenase inhibitor. Am J Respir Crit Care Med 1996;153(3):931–5.

182. Reiss TF, Hill JB, Harman E, et al. Increased urinary excretion of LTE4 after exercise and attenuation of exercise-induced bronchospasm by montelukast, a cysteinyl leukotriene receptor antagonist. Thorax 1997;52(12):1030–5.

183. Sladek K, Szczeklik A. Cysteinyl leukotrienes overproduction and mast cell activation in aspirin-provoked bronchospasm in asthma. Eur Respir J 1993;6(3):391–9.

184. Christie PE, Smith CM, Lee TH. The potent and selective sulfidopeptide leukotriene antagonist, SK&F 104353, inhibits aspirin-induced asthma. Am Rev Respir Dis 1991;144(4):957–8.

185. Fischer AR, Rosenberg MA, Lilly CM, et al. Direct evidence for a role of the mast cell in the nasal response to aspirin in aspirin-sensitive asthma. J Allergy Clin Immunol 1994;94(6 Pt 1):1046–56.

186. Israel E, Fischer AR, Rosenberg MA, et al. The pivotal role of 5-lipoxygenase products in the reaction of aspirin-sensitive asthmatics to aspirin. Am Rev Respir Dis 1993;148(6 Pt 1):1447–51.

187. Kumlin M, Dahlen B, Bjorck T, et al. Urinary excretion of leukotriene E4 and 11-dehydro-thromboxane B2 in response to bronchial provocations with allergen, aspirin, leukotriene D4, and histamine in asthmatics. Am Rev Respir Dis 1992;146(1):96–103.

Modulation of Bronchomotor Tone Pathways in Airway Smooth Muscle Function and Bronchomotor Tone in Asthma

Cynthia J. Koziol-White, PhD[a],*,
Reynold A. Panettieri Jr, MD[b]

KEYWORDS

- Asthma • Airway remodeling • Bronchoconstriction • Bronchodilation • Airway obstruction

KEY POINTS

- Airway smooth muscle serves as the pivotal tissue regulating bronchomotor tone.
- Evidence suggests a hypercontractile phenotype in the airway smooth muscle of patients with asthma that in part is driven by intrinsic abnormalities in excitation–contraction signaling pathways in airway smooth muscle.
- Airway smooth muscle shortening occurs through activation of mechanisms that are calcium dependent and that are partially calcium independent.
- The modulation of airway smooth muscle contractility is achieved through independent mechanisms of inhibiting receptor-mediated bronchoconstriction or stimulating bronchodilation.

INTRODUCTION

Airway smooth muscle (ASM) is the primary cell modulating airway resistance and hyperreactivity, hallmark features of asthma and exacerbations of the disease. The inflammatory milieu generated in allergic asthma modulates contractility of ASM; however, antiinflammatory therapies often inadequately control asthma morbidity and mortality. A study of patients with and without asthma examining inspiratory volume noted that patients without asthma dilate their airways to baseline measurements after methacholine provocation, whereas those with asthma were unable to reverse methacholine-induced bronchospasm after deep inspiration.[1] Additionally, the airways of the patients without asthma recovered faster than those of patients with asthma. The differences between patients with and without asthma may be attributable to characteristic differences in the ASM phenotypes. A study of isolated human ASM also noted an increased velocity of force generation in asthma-derived ASM as compared with non–asthma-derived ASM (see review[2]). In some patients with asthma, airway hyperresponsiveness (AHR) exists even in the absence of airway inflammation.[3,4] Taken together, such findings suggest that there is an

This article is funded by NIH (P01-HL081064) and NIH (P01-HL114471).
[a] Department of Pharmacology, Robert Wood Johnson Medical School, Rutgers Institute for Translational Medicine and Science, Rutgers University, State University of New Jersey, 89 French Street, Suite 4268, New Brunswick, NJ 08901, USA; [b] Department of Medicine, Rutgers Institute for Translational Medicine and Science, Rutgers University, State University of New Jersey, 89 French Street, Room 4210, New Brunswick, NJ 08901, USA
* Corresponding author.
E-mail address: cjk167@rbhs.rutgers.edu

underlying intrinsic abnormality in ASM that evokes the hyperresponsiveness and airway narrowing associated with asthma. Mechanisms underlying a hypercontractile phenotype have only been investigated more recently.[2,5–9] Current evidence is derived from animal models of allergic airways disease, airway biopsies from asthma and patients without asthma, ASM cells derived from patients with and without asthma, and from an ex vivo tissue model of precision cut lung slices derived from donors with and without asthma. To date, there exists no method to study ASM in vivo; thus, the evidence suggesting that there are intrinsic differences in ASM have only been observed in in vitro models.

PATHWAYS MODULATING CONTRACTILITY IN AIRWAY SMOOTH MUSCLE

Shortening of ASM is primarily induced by GPCR agonists, and modulated by downstream pathways that are calcium (Ca^{2+})-dependent and -independent (**Fig. 1**). In the canonical Ca^{2+} mobilization pathway, phospholipase β (PLCβ) activation generates inositol triphosphate that then binds to the inositol triphosphate (IP3) receptor on the sarcoplasmic reticulum (SR) to elicit $[Ca^{2+}]_i$ release. The increased $[Ca^{2+}]_i$ activates calmodulin and myosin light chain kinase (MLCK) to phosphorylate myosin light chain (MLC) and induce actin-myosin cross-bridge cycling and ASM shortening. In parallel, increased expression of CD38 evokes generation of cyclic ADP-ribose, which binds to the ryanodine receptor to promote sarcoplasmic reticulum (SR) $[Ca^{2+}]_i$ release. The sarco/endoplasmic reticulum Ca^{2+}-ATPase (SERCA) refills the SR with the cytosolic $[Ca^{2+}]_i$, inhibiting ASM shortening (as reviewed in[10]). Contractile agonists such as methacholine, thrombin, histamine, and leukotriene D_4 elicit $[Ca^{2+}]_i$ release in ASM. After the release of intracellular stores of Ca^{2+} from the SR, there is an activation of cell

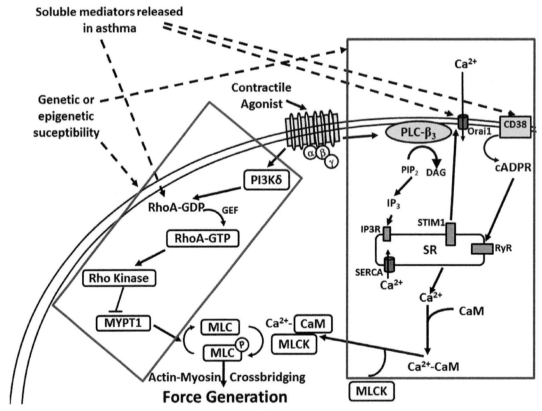

Fig. 1. Calcium-dependent (*blue box*) and calcium sensitization (*red box*) pathways that modulate ASM contraction. cADPR, cyclic adenosine phosphate ribose; CaM, calmodulin; CD38, cluster of differentiation 38; DAG, diacylglycerol; GEF, guanine nucleotide exchange factor; IP_3, inositol triphosphate; IP3R, IP_3 receptor; MLC, myosin light chain; MLCK, myosin light chain kinase; MYPT1, myosin phosphatase target subunit; Orai1, calcium release-activated calcium modulator 1; PI3Kδ, phosphoinositide 3-kinase δ; PIP_2, phosphatidylinositol 4,5-bisphosphate; PLC β, phospholipase β; RyR, ryanodine receptor; SERCA, sarco/endoplasmic reticulum calcium-ATPase; SR, sarcoplasmic reticulum; STIM1, stromal interaction molecule 1.

surface channels to facilitate extracellular Ca^{2+} refilling of cytosolic stores. This occurs through activation of the Orai/STIM pathway, modulating store-operated Ca^{2+} entry (SOCE) through plasma membrane channels when intracellular stores of Ca^{2+} are depleted after IP3 receptor-mediated $[Ca^{2+}]_i$ release from the SR. Calcium sensitization pathways that are relatively Ca^{2+} independent are mediated by activation of RhoA, stimulating Rho kinase (ROCK), which phosphorylates the myosin light chain phosphatase target subunit (MYTP1) to inactivate it. Under resting conditions, the MYPT1 is active and limits ASM shortening; upon its phosphorylation and hence its inhibition, ASM shortening is enhanced. Components of each of these pathways can be modulated by the inflammatory environment present in asthma. **Table 1** illustrates signaling molecules that differ between asthma and non–asthma-derived ASM that may contribute to the enhanced contractile phenotype observed in asthma.

MODULATION OF AIRWAY SMOOTH MUSCLE PROCONTRACTILE PATHWAYS IN ASTHMA

At first glance, changes in the expression of components of signaling pathways modulating constriction of the airways could explain the contractile differences between asthma-derived and non–asthma-derived ASM. Studies have shown that components of contractile signaling pathways are increased in ASM derived from patients with asthma compared with those from patients without asthma.[11–13] Ma and colleagues[12] noted that, in asthma-derived ASM, there was increased expression of MLCK that is the kinase that phosphorylates MLC to promote actin-myosin cross-bridging. Other investigators showed that the fast myosin isoform was found to be more highly expressed in bronchial biopsies from patients with asthma compared with patients without asthma.[13] Similar results were observed in human ASM derived from patients with severe asthma and age- and gender-matched patients without asthma.[11] However, in addition to studies examining gene expression in ASM from biopsies, the intrinsic differences in contractile pathways in patients with asthma may not be at the level of gene expression, but rather at the level of translation, posttranslational modification of proteins, or alterations in enzymatic activity of proteins.

Underlying changes in sensitivity to Ca^{2+} may also modulate contractile responses in ASM in

Table 1
Signaling proteins involved in contraction and relaxation of ASM that are altered between asthma and non–asthma-derived ASM

	Signaling Protein	Expression/Activity	AHR/Responsiveness to Bronchodilator	Reference(s)
Procontractile signaling	MLC	↑ Expression/phosphorylation	↑	11–13,23
	Rho kinase	↑ Activity	↑	6,23,27–30
	CysLT1 receptor	↑ Expression	↑	38
	PGD$_2$, TXB	↑ Expression/release	↑	36–38
	IL-13	↑ Expression/release	↑	18,19,21
	TGFβ1	↑ Expression/release	↑	23–25
	SERCA	↑ Expression/activity	↓	8
	MLCK	↑ Expression/activity	↑	12
	TNFα	↑ Expression/release	↑	14,15,18
	CD38/cADPR	↑ Expression/activity	↑	16,17
	Orai/STIM	↑ Expression/activity	↑	26
Relaxation signaling	TNFα/IL1β	↑ Expression/release	↓	21,41
	PGE$_2$	↑ Expression/release	↑	43
	IL-13	↑ Expression/release	↓	18,21,41
	IL-1β	↑ Expression/release	↓	21,41
	Corticosteroid	Stimulation with	↑	6,42
	PI3K	Inhibition	↑	6
	sGC	↑ Expression/activity	↑	44
	NO	↑ Expression/stimulation	↑	44
	RhoA	↓ Expression/activity	↑	35

Abbreviations: ↑, increased; ↓, decreased; ASM, airway smooth muscle; MLC, myosin light chain; MLCK, myosin light chain kinase; PG, prostaglandin; SERCA, sarco/endoplasmic reticulum Ca^{2+} ATPase; TGF, transforming growth factor; TNF, tumor necrosis factor; TXB, thromboxane.

asthma. Consistent with this concept, Mahn and colleagues[8] showed that ASM derived from patients with asthma manifest a sustained $[Ca^{2+}]_i$ release in response to contractile agonists and an attenuated expression of SERCA2, a protein that negatively regulates changes in $[Ca^{2+}]_i$ levels. These data suggest that the inflammatory milieu of asthma alters the contractile phenotype of ASM. Inflammatory cytokines released in asthma and exacerbations of asthma increase the sensitivity of ASM to contractile agonists. Tumor necrosis factor (TNF)α, a prominent cytokine present in the airways during allergic airway inflammation,[14] evokes AHR.[15] Recently, evidence suggests that ASM derived from patients with asthma expresses higher levels of TNFα-induced CD38 in comparison with ASM derived from patients without asthma.[16] TNFα increases CD38 expression/cyclic ADP-ribose activity and augments contractile agonist-induced $[Ca^{2+}]_i$ release in ASM.[16,17] IL-13 produced by T helper type 2 cells, mast cells, basophils, and eosinophils induces hyperresponsiveness of rabbit tracheal smooth muscle, increases contractility of human ASM, and augments the narrowing of human small airways to methacholine.[18,19] Additionally, TNFα augments methacholine-induced airway narrowing in a model of human small airways.[18] Antagonism of other cytokine receptors that modulate contractile and noncontractile properties of ASM have also been investigated as potential therapies in asthma. Etanercept, a TNFα receptor/IgG fusion protein that is a TNF receptor antagonist, significantly improved methacholine-induced AHR, increased the forced expiratory volume in 1 second, and improved quality-of-life scores.[20] IL-13 augmented $[Ca^{2+}]_i$ release in ASM induced by bradykinin, histamine, and methacholine.[21] IL-13 and TNFα stimulation also enhance aggregation of STIM1 and increase SOCE after SR $[Ca^{2+}]_i$ depletion.[22] Unfortunately, neither anti-TNFα nor IL-13 monoclonal antibodies were effective in preventing asthma exacerbations and as such have been abandoned as potential asthma therapies.

Although transforming growth factor (TGF)β1 is generally thought to be important in remodeling of the airways observed in asthma, recent evidence suggests that it also directly induces AHR in asthma. TGFβ1 stimulation of human ASM induces activation of contractile pathways and augments activation of agonist-induced contractile pathways.[23,24] Gao and colleagues[25] showed that TGFβ1 treatment induces expression of both STIM1 and Orai1 in human ASM, as well as enhancement of basal $[Ca^{2+}]_i$ levels and SOCE in response to thapsigargin, a compound that stimulates $[Ca^{2+}]_i$ release from the

SR. The amplitude of arachidonic acid (AA)-activated $[Ca^{2+}]_i$ oscillations is enhanced in ASM derived from patients with asthma compared with ASM from patients without asthma. AA-induced $[Ca^{2+}]_i$ oscillations in ASM are also inhibited by the knockdown of STIM1 and Orai3.[26] These data suggest a role for alterations in Orai/STIM-dependent modulation of SOCE, which may contribute to enhanced AHR with asthma.

In ASM, RhoA and ROCK-associated AHR is associated with exposure to inflammatory cytokines,[23,27–30] sphingolipids,[31,32] and mechanical stress.[33] Additionally, Koziol-White and colleagues[6] showed increased activity of Rho kinase, a component of the calcium sensitization pathway, in ASM derived from patients with severe asthma as compared with those from age- and gender-matched controls without asthma. These findings suggest that there is an intrinsic hypercontractile phenotype that occurs in ASM derived from patients with asthma. IL-13 has been shown to augment canonical calcium mobilization pathways[21] and enhance calcium sensitization pathways.[34] Additionally, inhibition of RhoA induced relaxation of methacholine-constricted human small airways.[35] TGFβ1-induced phosphorylation of myosin light chain was found to be ROCK dependent in human ASM.[23]

Cytokines and chemokines released in the airway may directly modulate ASM function, but other inflammatory mediators including lipid mediators alter the contractile status of the ASM. Prostaglandins (PG), products of metabolism of AA by cyclooxygenase enzymes, are mediators that modulate AHR associated with allergic airways disease, and in many cases can act directly on ASM. Prostaglandins like PGD_2 and thromboxane can act as bronchoconstrictors.[36] In fact, thromboxane has been found to be a more potent and effective bronchoconstrictor than methacholine, and amplifies methacholine responsiveness in patients with asthma.[37] Receptors for leukotrienes LTC4 and LTD4, including CysLT1, are expressed on ASM.[38] Interferon-γ, a mediator increased in viral exacerbations of asthma, increased cell surface expression of CysLT1 receptors and markedly increased the contraction of ASM in culture to lipid mediators.[39]

MODULATION OF RELAXATION OF AIRWAY SMOOTH MUSCLE IN ASTHMA

Agonists of the β_2 adrenergic receptor (β_2AR) induce the generation of cAMP and attenuate MLCK activity to abrogate actin–myosin cross-bridging and induce relaxation of ASM. β_2AR agonists provide the mainstays for rescue therapy to reverse the bronchoconstriction associated with airways disease. Jiang and Stephens[40] demonstrated that, in canine ASM, isolated muscle from allergen sensitized dogs showed a failure to relax after an increased maximum shortening velocity, suggesting that there may also be intrinsic differences in asthma-derived ASM that drive hyperreactivity of the muscle/hyposensitivity to a relaxant. As with contractility, the inflammatory environment of the lung in asthma modulates reversal of ASM shortening. TNFα synergizes with IL-1β to promote β2AR hyporesponsiveness that is ablated by selective cyclooxygenase-2 inhibition, thereby suggesting that AA derivatives serve to desensitize the ASM to bronchodilation. IL-13, TNFα, and IL-1β stimulation of human ASM modulated contractile agonist signaling pathways by enhancing agonist-induced calcium responses and/or inhibiting cAMP production.[21,41] Additionally, exposure to IL-13 attenuated β2 agonist-induced dilation of human small airways in an in vitro model[18] that was reversed by the inhibition of PI3Kδ and administration of budesonide.[6,42] Interestingly, an AA metabolite, PGE2, abrogates early and late phase responses to antigen challenge and serves as a bronchodilator; in murine models of allergen-induced AHR, the lack of EP3 receptors for PGE2 increases AHR to OVA.[43]

Although effective at bronchodilation, β2AR agonists induce desensitization of the β2 receptor, which that attenuates the efficacy of such treatment. Modulation of the pathways downstream of the β2AR has been an attractive approach for developing novel therapeutics. In addition to pathways activated by the β2AR, modulation of smooth muscle relaxation can also be achieved through generation of cGMP via soluble guanylate cylase (sGC) using nitric oxide (NO) or pharmacologic sGC agonists that activate sGC independently of NO. Ghosh and colleagues[44] demonstrated that an NO donor induces dilation of human small airways, and that pharmacologic agonists of sGC reversed AHR in a murine model of allergic airway disease. These investigators also noted in the murine asthma model that there was oxidative damage to sGC that rendered it unresponsive to NO. Such oxidative damage was also observed in human ASM, suggesting that the increased NO levels measured in patients with severe asthma may render their airways insensitive to NO donors for bronchodilation, but may also offer a target for pharmacologic intervention to activate sGC independently of NO. New evidence shows that the inhibition of PI3K, primarily to inhibit airway inflammation to allergen, induces bronchodilation in a human precision cut lung slice model.[6]

Interestingly, the inhibition of PI3K p110, more specifically the δ isoform, induces bronchodilation despite β2AR desensitization or IL-13 treatment.[6] Inhibition of PI3K and agonism of sGC may serve as novel targets to induce bronchodilation in a T helper type 2 inflammatory milieu characteristic of asthma, as well as during an exacerbation where a β2AR agonist may be ineffective owing to overuse.

SUMMARY AND FUTURE DIRECTIONS

Although antagonists of contractile receptors and agonists of the β2AR have been used extensively as asthma therapies, these therapeutics are restricted to specific classes of receptors and may be ineffective in severe disease. Emerging evidence suggests that the manipulation of components of contractile signaling pathways that may be altered in ASM of patients with asthma may serve as novel targets to inhibit constriction of the airways or to promote bronchodilation. Given the intrinsic differences in excitation–contraction pathways between ASM derived from patients with and without asthma, specific signaling molecules whose activity is altered by the disease state may offer unique therapeutic opportunities. Such opportunities leverage intrinsic functional differences in ASM to enhance therapeutic responses while potentially minimizing systemic off-target or adverse effects.

REFERENCES

1. Koziol-White CJ, Damera G, Panettieri RA Jr. Targeting airway smooth muscle in airways diseases: an old concept with new twists. Expert Rev Respir Med 2011;5(6):767–77.
2. An SS, Bai TR, Bates JH, et al. Airway smooth muscle dynamics: a common pathway of airway obstruction in asthma. Eur Respir J 2007;29(5):834–60.
3. Brusasco V, Crimi E, Pellegrino R. Airway hyperresponsiveness in asthma: not just a matter of airway inflammation. Thorax 1998;53(11):992–8.
4. Howarth PH, Knox AJ, Amrani Y, et al. Synthetic responses in airway smooth muscle. J Allergy Clin Immunol 2004;114(2 Suppl):S32–50.
5. An SS, Mitzner W, Tang WY, et al. An inflammation-independent contraction mechanophenotype of airway smooth muscle in asthma. J Allergy Clin Immunol 2016;138(1):294–7.e4.
6. Koziol-White CJ, Yoo EJ, Cao G, et al. Inhibition of PI3K promotes dilation of human small airways in a rho kinase-dependent manner. Br J Pharmacol 2016;173(18):2726–38.

7. Mahn K, Hirst SJ, Ying S, et al. Diminished sarco/endoplasmic reticulum Ca2+ ATPase (SERCA) expression contributes to airway remodelling in bronchial asthma. Proc Natl Acad Sci U S A 2009;106(26):10775–80.

8. Mahn K, Ojo OO, Chadwick G, et al. Ca(2+) homeostasis and structural and functional remodelling of airway smooth muscle in asthma. Thorax 2010;65(6):547–52.

9. Roth M, Johnson PR, Borger P, et al. Dysfunctional interaction of C/EBPalpha and the glucocorticoid receptor in asthmatic bronchial smooth-muscle cells. N Engl J Med 2004;351(6):560–74.

10. Jude JA, Wylam ME, Walseth TF, et al. Calcium signaling in airway smooth muscle. Proc Am Thorac Soc 2008;5(1):15–22.

11. Himes BE, Koziol-White C, Johnson M, et al. Vitamin D modulates expression of the airway smooth muscle transcriptome in fatal asthma. PLoS One 2015;10(7):e0134057.

12. Ma X, Cheng Z, Kong H, et al. Changes in biophysical and biochemical properties of single bronchial smooth muscle cells from asthmatic subjects. Am J Physiol Lung Cell Mol Physiol 2002;283(6):L1181–9.

13. Woodruff PG. Gene expression in asthmatic airway smooth muscle. Proc Am Thorac Soc 2008;5(1):113–8.

14. Hackett TL, Holloway R, Holgate ST, et al. Dynamics of pro-inflammatory and anti-inflammatory cytokine release during acute inflammation in chronic obstructive pulmonary disease: an ex vivo study. Respir Res 2008;9:47.

15. Thomas PS, Heywood G. Effects of inhaled tumour necrosis factor alpha in subjects with mild asthma. Thorax 2002;57(9):774–8.

16. Jude JA, Solway J, Panettieri RA Jr, et al. Differential induction of CD38 expression by TNF-{alpha} in asthmatic airway smooth muscle cells. Am J Physiol Lung Cell Mol Physiol 2010;299(6):L879–90.

17. Jude JA, Tirumurugaan KG, Kang BN, et al. Regulation of CD38 expression in human airway smooth muscle cells: role of class I phosphatidylinositol 3 kinases. Am J Respir Cell Mol Biol 2012;47(4):427–35.

18. Cooper PR, Lamb R, Day ND, et al. TLR3 activation stimulates cytokine secretion without altering agonist-induced human small airway contraction or relaxation. Am J Physiol Lung Cell Mol Physiol 2009;297(3):L530–7.

19. Cooper PR, Poll CT, Barnes PJ, et al. Involvement of IL-13 in tobacco smoke-induced changes in the structure and function of rat intrapulmonary airways. Am J Respir Cell Mol Biol 2010;43(2):220–6.

20. Howarth PH, Babu KS, Arshad HS, et al. Tumour necrosis factor (TNFalpha) as a novel therapeutic target in symptomatic corticosteroid dependent asthma. Thorax 2005;60(12):1012–8.

21. Tliba O, Deshpande D, Chen H, et al. IL-13 enhances agonist-evoked calcium signals and contractile responses in airway smooth muscle. Br J Pharmacol 2003;140(7):1159–62.

22. Jia L, Delmotte P, Aravamudan B, et al. Effects of the inflammatory cytokines TNF-alpha and IL-13 on stromal interaction molecule-1 aggregation in human airway smooth muscle intracellular Ca(2+) regulation. Am J Respir Cell Mol Biol 2013;49(4):601–8.

23. Ojiaku CA, Cao G, Zhu W, et al. TGF-β1 evokes human airway smooth muscle cell shortening and hyperresponsiveness via Smad3. Am J Respir Cell Mol Biol 2018;58(5):575–84.

24. Shaifta Y, MacKay CE, Irechukwu N, et al. Transforming growth factor-β enhances Rho-kinase activity and contraction in airway smooth muscle via the nucleotide exchange factor ARHGEF1. J Physiol 2018;596(1):47–66.

25. Gao YD, Zheng JW, Li P, et al. Store-operated Ca2+ entry is involved in transforming growth factor-beta1 facilitated proliferation of rat airway smooth muscle cells. J Asthma 2013;50(5):439–48.

26. Thompson MA, Prakash YS, Pabelick CM. Arachidonate-regulated Ca(2+) influx in human airway smooth muscle. Am J Respir Cell Mol Biol 2014;51(1):68–76.

27. Hunter I, Cobban HJ, Vandenabeele P, et al. Tumor necrosis factor-alpha-induced activation of RhoA in airway smooth muscle cells: role in the Ca2+ sensitization of myosin light chain20 phosphorylation. Mol Pharmacol 2003;63(3):714–21.

28. Parris JR, Cobban HJ, Littlejohn AF, et al. Tumour necrosis factor-alpha activates a calcium sensitization pathway in Guinea-pig bronchial smooth muscle. J Physiol 1999;518(Pt 2):561–9.

29. Sakai H, Otogoto S, Chiba Y, et al. Involvement of p42/44 MAPK and RhoA protein in augmentation of ACh-induced bronchial smooth muscle contraction by TNF-alpha in rats. J Appl Physiol (1985) 2004;97(6):2154–9.

30. Sakai H, Otogoto S, Chiba Y, et al. TNF-alpha augments the expression of RhoA in the rat bronchus. J Smooth Muscle Res 2004;40(1):25–34.

31. Kume H, Takeda N, Oguma T, et al. Sphingosine 1-phosphate causes airway hyper-reactivity by rho-mediated myosin phosphatase inactivation. J Pharmacol Exp Ther 2007;320(2):766–73.

32. Rosenfeldt HM, Amrani Y, Watterson KR, et al. Sphingosine-1-phosphate stimulates contraction of human airway smooth muscle cells. FASEB J 2003;17(13):1789–99.

33. Smith PG, Hoy C, Zhang YN, et al. Mechanical stress increases RhoA activation in airway smooth muscle cells. Am J Respir Cell Mol Biol 2003;28(4):436–42.

34. Chiba Y, Nakazawa S, Todoroki M, et al. Interleukin-13 augments bronchial smooth muscle contractility

with an up-regulation of RhoA protein. Am J Respir Cell Mol Biol 2009;40(2):159–67.

35. Yoo EJ, Cao G, Koziol-White CJ, et al. Galpha12 facilitates shortening in human airway smooth muscle by modulating phosphoinositide 3-kinase-mediated activation in a RhoA-dependent manner. Br J Pharmacol 2017;174(23):4383–95.

36. Boyce JA. Eicosanoids in asthma, allergic inflammation, and host defense. Curr Mol Med 2008;8(5):335–49.

37. Jones GL, Saroea HG, Watson RM, et al. Effect of an inhaled thromboxane mimetic (U46619) on airway function in human subjects. Am Rev Respir Dis 1992;145(6):1270–4.

38. Panettieri RA, Tan EM, Ciocca V, et al. Effects of LTD4 on human airway smooth muscle cell proliferation, matrix expression, and contraction in vitro: differential sensitivity to cysteinyl leukotriene receptor antagonists. Am J Respir Cell Mol Biol 1998;19(3):453–61.

39. Amrani Y, Moore PE, Hoffman R, et al. Interferon-gamma modulates cysteinyl leukotriene receptor-1 expression and function in human airway myocytes. Am J Respir Crit Care Med 2001;164(11):2098–101.

40. Jiang H, Stephens NL. Isotonic relaxation of sensitized bronchial smooth muscle. Am J Physiol 1992;262(3 Pt 1):L344–50.

41. Amrani Y, Syed F, Huang C, et al. Expression and activation of the oxytocin receptor in airway smooth muscle cells: regulation by TNFalpha and IL-13. Respir Res 2010;11:104.

42. Koziol-White CJ, Cooper PR, Zhang J, et al. Budesonide reverses IL-13-induced airway hyperresponsiveness but has little effect on β2 agonist response in human small airways. Eur Respir J 2012;40.

43. Kunikata T, Yamane H, Segi E, et al. Suppression of allergic inflammation by the prostaglandin E receptor subtype EP3. Nat Immunol 2005;6(5):524–31.

44. Ghosh A, Koziol-White CJ, Asosingh K, et al. Soluble guanylate cyclase as an alternative target for bronchodilator therapy in asthma. Proc Natl Acad Sci U S A 2016;113(17):E2355–62.

Systematic Approach to Asthma of Varying Severity

Sandhya Khurana, MD[a],*, Nizar N. Jarjour, MD[b]

KEYWORDS

- Systematic approach • Structured approach • Asthma management • Asthma pharmacotherapy
- Asthma severity • Asthma control

KEY POINTS

- The goals of asthma management are to control symptoms and mitigate future risk. Contemporary guidelines recommend a stepwise approach to pharmacotherapy with ongoing adjustment based on asthma control.
- Apart from severity of asthma itself, there are several factors that contribute to poor control of asthma, including nonadherence, alternate diagnoses, triggers, and comorbidities.
- A structured approach to the evaluation of asthma severity and management allows for more appropriate and cost-effective utilization of advanced asthma therapies while decreasing risk of treatment-related adverse effects.
- Referral to a severe asthma clinic should be considered in asthmatics requiring steps 4 or 5 of therapy, especially those considered for novel and biologic therapies.

INTRODUCTION

Asthma is a serious global health issue affecting 235 million people worldwide.[1] Approximately 25 million people suffer from asthma in the United States, and 47% reported having at least 1 asthma attack in the past year.[2] Both the Global Initiative for Asthma (GINA) and the National Asthma Education and Prevention Program guidelines recommend a stepwise approach to management of asthma, with the goal of achieving control and minimizing future risk.[3,4] Several studies have shown that asthma is both overdiagnosed and underdiagnosed.[5–9] Prior to escalation of pharmacotherapy, the importance of confirming accurate diagnosis as well as addressing comorbidities and triggers cannot be overstated. Once the diagnosis of asthma is confirmed, contemporary guidelines recommend control-based asthma management with adjustment of pharmacologic and nonpharmacologic therapy based on ongoing assessment.[3]

GENERAL PRINCIPLES OF ASTHMA MANAGEMENT

The goals of asthma management generally relate to 2 domains[3,4]:

- Impairment: this is reduced by achieving good control of symptoms so as to allow normal activities without limitation.

Disclosure Statement: Dr N.N. Jarjour received honorarium from Astra Zeneca Pharmaceuticals (a total of $10,000–15,000 in 2016–2017). This work is supported, in part, by grants from National Institutes of Health Awards (U10 HL 109168 & P01 HL 088594; PI: N.N. Jarjour). Dr S. Khurana has participated in clinical trials funded by GlaxoSmithKline, Sanofi, Astra Zeneca, and Teva Pharmaceuticals.
a Division of Pulmonary and Critical Care Medicine, Department of Medicine, Mary Parkes Center for Asthma, Allergy and Pulmonary Care, University of Rochester Medical Center, 601 Elmwood Avenue, Box 692, Rochester, NY 14642, USA; b University of Wisconsin School of Medicine and Public Health, K4/914 Clinical Science Center, 600 Highland Avenue, Madison, WI 53792-9988, USA
* Corresponding author.
E-mail address: sandhya_khurana@urmc.rochester.edu

chestmed.theclinics.com

- Risk: minimize future risk of exacerbations and loss of lung function.

These goals can be achieved through an effective asthma management strategy that includes several key components:

- Ongoing assessment of symptoms and lung function
- Patient education and engagement
- Control of triggers and comorbidities
- Pharmacologic therapy

Current asthma guidelines, based on best available evidence, recommend a stepwise approach to adjusting pharmacotherapy guided by disease severity and control. A stepped model for asthma management has been recommended for decades (**Fig. 1**); however, these recommendations are population based and require modifications based on patient and health system factors.

RATIONALE FOR SYSTEMATIC APPROACH

Most patients with asthma respond well to judicious use of inhaled corticosteroids (ICSs), long-acting β_2-agonists (LABAs), and leukotriene modifiers. However, 5% to 10% remain uncontrolled despite these therapies and require further step-up in their management. Apart from severity of asthma itself, there are several factors that can make asthma poorly controlled, including nonadherence with treatment, alternate diagnosis, unidentified triggers, and uncontrolled comorbidities. Differentiating uncontrolled or difficult-to-control asthma from severe therapy-resistant asthma, before stepping up pharmacotherapy, allows appropriate and cost-effective utilization of novel therapies while decreasing the risk of treatment-related adverse effects.[10–14] Using a structured approach, Tay and colleagues[11] demonstrated improved control of comorbidities and asthma outcomes. They used validated questionnaires to identify potential comorbidities and provided the primary care physicians with treatment recommendations based on GINA guidelines. The authors recommend a systematic approach to evaluation of uncontrolled asthma, as illustrated in **Fig. 2**.

DIAGNOSTIC CONSIDERATIONS IN ASTHMA

GINA guidelines define asthma as a "heterogeneous disease, usually characterized by chronic airway inflammation. It is defined by the history of respiratory symptoms such as wheeze, shortness of breath, chest tightness and cough that vary over time and in intensity, together with variable expiratory airflow limitation."[3] Initial diagnosis is usually based on a combination of characteristic symptoms and evidence of airflow obstruction with bronchodilator reversibility or airway hyperreactivity on lung function testing. Aaron and colleagues[5] evaluated 701 patients with physician-diagnosed asthma and, using a systematic approach, were able to rule out asthma in 33%, thereby confirming that asthma is commonly over-diagnosed. Similarly, studies have found that asthma is often underdiagnosed across all age groups.[7–9] Myriad conditions can present with similar symptoms (**Table 1**), the so-called asthma mimics, and establishing a correct diagnosis upfront with objective testing is critical to effective management. Clinical assessment of patients with asthma includes a thorough history and physical examination as well as assessment of reversible airflow limitation or airway responsiveness.

Clues from History and Physical Examination

The presence of episodic wheeze, chest tightness, shortness of breath, and cough, particularly at night and early morning, is suggestive of asthma. Symptoms are variable over time and in intensity and are often triggered by cold air, environmental allergens, exercise, or laughter. Presence of this combination of symptoms increase the likelihood of asthma. Sistek and colleagues[15] evaluated predictive value of respiratory symptoms in a large New Zealand study and found "wheezing with dyspnea" the single best predictor with sensitivity of 82% and specificity of 90%. Similarly, a large Swiss Study on Air Pollution and Lung Diseases in Adults (SAPALDIA) found a combination of wheezing with daily dyspnea at rest to have the best positive predictive value, almost double that of any 1 symptom alone.[16] Additional clues from history that increase confidence in diagnosis of asthma include early age of onset, atopic features, family history of asthma or atopy, and environmental exposures. Physical examination in a patient with stable well-controlled asthma can be normal. In poorly controlled asthma, expiratory wheeze on auscultation may be elicited. Some additional features that can support the diagnosis of asthma include presence of allergic rhinitis or conjunctivitis, allergic shiners, atopic dermatitis, and prolonged expiratory phase on forced exhalation.

Pulmonary Function Tests

Patients with suspected asthma should undergo spirometry before and after inhaled short-acting bronchodilator administration. These tests can be used to determine presence of baseline airflow limitation (reduced forced

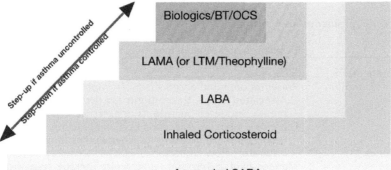

Fig. 1. Example of stepped approach to pharmacotherapy of asthma. The recommended stepwise approach to asthma pharmacotherapy is illustrated. Step-up in treatment is indicated if asthma control remains poor at current level of therapy. Step-down to lowest effective treatment level if asthma is well controlled. BT, bronchial thermoplasty; LAMA, long-acting muscarinic antagonist; LTM, leukotriene modifier; OCS, oral corticosteroid; SABA, short-acting β-agonist.

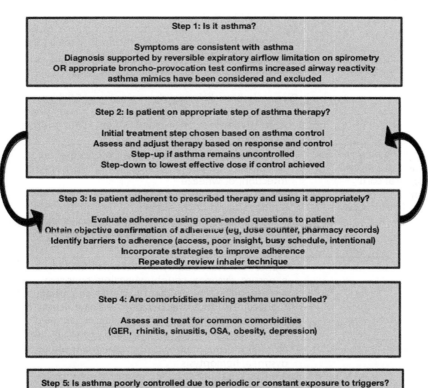

Fig. 2. Structured approach to asthma management.

Table 1
Differential diagnostic considerations in asthma

Conditions	Evaluation and Management
Conditions with overlapping symptoms	
Paradoxic vocal fold motion	Presentation: rapid onset/offset of symptoms. Inspiratory wheeze. Associated cough, throat tightness, dysphonia, shortness of breath. Triggered by irritants or exercise. Diagnosis: laryngoscopy alone or in conjunction with bronchoprovocation testing. Flow volume loop may show inspiratory flow limitation. Management: behavioral speech/voice therapy, respiratory retraining, reassurance, education, minimize laryngeal irritation by treating postnasal drip and acid reflux.
Dysfunctional breathing[72]	Presentation: episodic dyspnea, uncomfortable breathing, general sense of distress. May be associated with light-headedness, paresthesia, chest tightness or pain. Diagnosis: this is a diagnosis of exclusion, reserved for patients with episodic symptoms where no other explanation has been found after careful and meticulous evaluation; Nijmegen Questionnaire.[73] Management: reassurance, education, removal of stressors, cognitive behavioral therapy, respiratory retraining, pharmacotherapy
Tracheobronchomalacia	Presentation: severe paroxysmal cough, dyspnea, sputum retention, recurrent infections, wheeze Diagnosis: bronchoscopy, dynamic airway CT chest Management: airway clearance, positive airway pressure therapy, stent trial, surgery in selected patients with good response to stent trial
Upper or central airway obstruction (subglottic stenosis, vocal cord paralysis, stricture, tumor, or foreign body)	Presentation: acute or subacute symptoms that are constant and progressive, including dyspnea, cough, hemoptysis, recurrent infection, or wheeze Diagnosis: chest and neck imaging, flow volume loop, laryngoscopy/bronchoscopy Management: airway management, endoscopic or surgical intervention, appropriate treatment of underlying condition
Conditions associated with airflow obstruction	
COPD	Presentation: older adult with history of smoking or other noxious exposure, dyspnea, cough, wheezing, hypoxemia Diagnosis: airflow obstruction that may be partially reversible; reduced diffusing capacity; emphysema on chest imaging Management: long-acting bronchodilators, inhaled steroids, oxygen supplementation, pulmonary rehabilitation
Bronchiectasis	Presentation: cough, daily sputum, frequent respiratory infections, dyspnea, hemoptysis Diagnosis: chest imaging, laboratory testing to evaluate for associated conditions (eg, immune deficiency, cystic fibrosis, α_1-antitrypsin deficiency), pulmonary function tests Management: prevention and treatment of infections, airway clearance regimen, bronchodilators
Sarcoidosis	Presentation: cough, wheeze, dyspnea, fatigue, fever, night sweats, weight loss. May be accompanied by extrapulmonary symptoms. Diagnosis: chest imaging, pulmonary function tests, biopsy Management: observation, systemic corticosteroids or other immunomodulatory drugs

(continued on next page)

Table 1 (continued)	
Conditions	**Evaluation and Management**
Bronchiolitis	Presentation: progressive dyspnea and cough. May be associated with a variety of conditions—rheumatoid arthritis and other autoimmune disorders, lung or hematopoietic transplant, infection, toxic inhalation, cigarettes, medications. Diagnosis: evidence of small airways dysfunction on pulmonary function tests, dynamic CT chest with evidence of mosaic air trapping, lung biopsy Management: bronchodilator therapy, removal of causative agent, immunosuppressive therapy, steroids, macrolides in some, lung transplant
Conditions associated with asthma: asthma-plus	
Allergic bronchopulmonary aspergillosis	Presentation: poorly controlled asthma with frequent exacerbations, expectoration of thick mucus plugs, fever, malaise, or hemoptysis. Diagnosis: blood eosinophilia, very high IgE level, specific IgE and IgG antibodies to aspergillus; central bronchiectasis, mucus plugging, atelectasis on chest imaging Management: systemic corticosteroids, itraconazole, omalizumab
Eosinophilic granulomatosis with polyangitis	Presentation: long-standing poorly controlled asthma, need for systemic corticosteroids to maintain control, extrapulmonary manifestations (skin, sinuses, cardiovascular, neurologic, and renal) Diagnosis: blood eosinophilia, myeloperoxidase–antineutrophil cytoplasmic antibodies positive in 30%–60%, pulmonary infiltrates or nodules on chest imaging. Pulmonary function tests with airflow limitation and/or reduced diffusing capacity of the lungs for carbon monoxide; biopsy of involved organ Management: systemic corticosteroids, cyclophosphamide, other steroids sparing drugs, anti–interleukin 5 antibodies

expiratory volume in the first second of expiration [FEV_1]/forced vital capacity [FVC]) as well as bronchodilator reversibility (200 mL and 12% improvement in FEV_1 and/or FVC postbronchodilator).[17] The likelihood of capturing reversible airflow obstruction on spirometry is increased if a patient is symptomatic and not on controller therapy. Testing reversibility requires that patients withhold long-acting bronchodilator therapy; otherwise, the reversibility test may be falsely negative. Variability in twice-daily peak expiratory flow rates of greater than 10% over 2 weeks or increase in FEV_1 by greater than 12% and 200 mL after 4 weeks of controller therapy can also assist with diagnosing asthma. Variable airflow obstruction and airway hyper-responsiveness are considered cardinal features of asthma; however, these are not specific for asthma. Patients with hay fever or acute respiratory tract infections and smokers can have bronchial hyper-responsiveness, whereas bronchodilator reversibility can be observed in a majority of patients with chronic obstructive pulmonary disease (COPD).[18–20]

In symptomatic patients where reversible airflow obstruction cannot be documented, In the absence of any contraindication, the authors recommend confirmation of airway hyper-responsiveness with bronchoprovocation testing using a direct or indirect challenge.[21,22] Methacholine is commonly used for direct challenge testing and has a high sensitivity. A provocative concentration causing a 20% fall in FEV_1 (PC20) greater than 16 mg/mL or provocative dose causing a 20% fall in FEV_1 (PD20) greater than 400 μg (provocative dose causing a 20% fall in FEV_1) indicates normal airway reactivity. Recently updated European Respiratory Society statement favors the use of PD20 over PC20, because it takes into account the differences between available devices and protocols.[21] Presence of normal airway reactivity can be used to exclude a diagnosis of asthma but with certain caveats. False-negative results can occur in asymptomatic patients, exercise-induced bronchoconstriction (EIB), or failure to withhold medications for appropriate duration. Use of ICSs can improve airway reactivity by 1 to 2 doubling doses but should not result in a completely negative test.[23–25] When inducible laryngeal obstruction is considered an alternative diagnosis, full-flow volume-loop maneuvers, including inspiration, can provide valuable information if performed throughout the test.[21] Patients with extrathoracic upper airway obstruction typically show reduced inspiratory flow while their expiratory flows are minimally affected.

Exercise challenge can be used for indirect challenge testing, especially if symptoms suggest primarily EIB.[22] Breathing cold air during the exercise challenge increases the chances of eliciting a positive response. Serial lung function measurements after a specific exercise challenge protocol are used to assess for EIB. A decrease from baseline of greater than or equal to 10% in FEV_1 within 30 minutes after exercise is used to diagnose EIB. In patients with work-related symptoms where occupational asthma is a concern, evaluation can be initiated with serial measurement of lung functions (at work and home) or airway responsiveness along with testing for the immunologic response to the suspected agent (if appropriate). If these objective methods fail to provide a definitive diagnosis, or a patient is no longer exposed to the suspect agent and there is a need to identify the agent and confirm the diagnosis, a specific inhalation challenge can be useful.[26] A positive response is defined by a fall in FEV_1 greater than or equal to 15% from baseline. Specific inhalation challenge testing should be carried only out in facilities where health care professionals have appropriate expertise. It is more widely used in Europe and Canada, where several centers with such expertise are present. The experience of a specialized center is necessary to perform the appropriate testing and reduce the risk of complications, including acute attacks and exacerbation of occupational asthma.[26]

ASSESSING ASTHMA SEVERITY AND CONTROL

Historically, guidelines have described asthma severity as the intrinsic intensity of the disease process measured in patients not on controller therapy, taking into account both impairment and risk.[4,27,28] The concept of asthma severity has evolved substantially over the years. Inherent in the process of severity assessment is the assumption that a diagnosis of asthma has been confirmed, confounders addressed, and comorbidities treated. Asthma severity is then assessed based on lowest effective level of treatment required to control symptoms and exacerbations, after a patient has been on controller therapy for

several months and appropriate step-down in treatment attempted (**Fig. 3**).[3,29]

Level of asthma control is the degree to which therapeutic interventions minimize the manifestations of asthma in terms of impairment (symptoms and lung function) and risk (exacerbations). Asthma control should be assessed regularly at every visit and used to adjust treatment. Validated questionnaires, such as asthma control questionnaire and asthma control test, provide numerical scores to assess level of control and are useful in assessing patient progress.[30–32] Although apparent poor asthma control may be due to severity of underlying disease, it is often a result of suboptimal adherence, incorrect diagnosis, undertreated comorbidities, and unrecognized triggers. Hence, difficult-to-control asthma is not synonymous with severe treatment-resistant asthma, and poor performance on the asthma control test or asthma control questionnaire should not automatically prompt a step-up in asthma therapy.

STEPWISE APPROACH TO PHARMACOTHERAPY

Guidelines recommend a stepped approach to asthma pharmacotherapy with initial treatment based on degree of impairment and risk.[3,4] Treatment with at least a low-dose ICS is recommended in almost all patients with confirmed diagnosis of asthma except those with very infrequent symptoms (less than twice a month) and no other risk factors, such as impaired lung function or history of exacerbation. Additional treatment steps include low-dose ICS/LABA (step 3), medium-high dose ICS/LABA (step 4), and high-dose ICS/LABA plus tiotropium and/or biologics (step 5). A long-acting bronchodilator should not be prescribed to asthma patients without an accompanying ICS.

For most controller medications, improvement begins within days but full effect may not be evident for 3 months or even longer.[33] Subsequent adjustment to therapy should be based on ongoing assessment of asthma control. Guidelines recommend a preferred controller therapy for each treatment step based on population studies and taking into consideration treatment efficacy, safety, and access. At the individual level, treatment should be tailored to each patient based on patient preference, phenotypic characteristics, and practicality through a shared decision-making process.

If symptoms persist at a patient's current therapy, stepping up treatment should be considered after excluding other issues that may be contributing to poor control, including medication

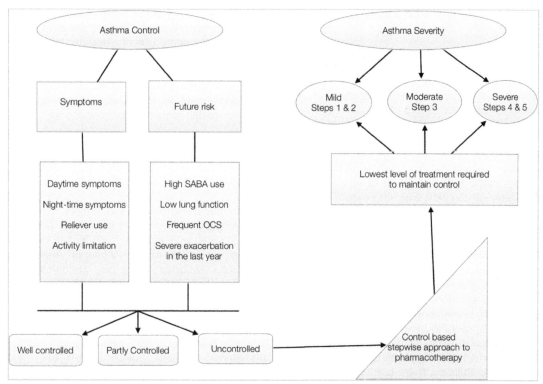

Fig. 3. Assessing asthma control and severity. Level of asthma control is the degree to which therapeutic interventions minimize the manifestations of asthma in terms of impairment and risk. Asthma severity is assessed based on lowest effective level of treatment required to maintain asthma control, after a patient has been on controller therapy for several months and appropriate step-down in treatment attempted. OCS, oral corticosteroid; SABA, short-acting β-agonist.

nonadherence, poor inhaler technique, unrecognized triggers, and uncontrolled comorbidities. There is an increasing body of evidence in favor of adding LABA to ICS over increasing the dose of ICS alone in uncontrolled asthma.[33,34] A recent publication provides practical approach for stepping up therapy in patients with poorly controlled asthma.[35]

Once asthma control is achieved and maintained for 3 months, consideration should be given to stepping down therapy to the lowest effective level. Studies have shown that patients with asthma in the community are generally overtreated and, in a supervised setting, tolerate up to 37% reduction in ICS dose without loss of asthma control.[36,37] In a recent study by Rogers and colleagues,[38] patients on stable medium-dose ICS/LABA were randomized to receive low-dose ICS/LABA, medium-dose ICS, or continued current therapy for 48 weeks. No significant differences in treatment failures were observed between the 3 strategies. The group with LABA step-off, however, was associated with greater lung function decline and hospitalization rates. Again, it is important to consider patient preference, potential

treatment-related adverse effects, and access to medication when discussing step-up or step-down therapy. In patients who are not well controlled on high-dose ICS/LABA (with and without other therapies, such as montelukast and tiotropium), referral to an asthma specialist is recommended to facilitate evaluation of the patient for potential biologic therapy or bronchial thermoplasty. Despite these advances in asthma therapy, there continues to be a gap in knowledge regarding the proper selection of specific therapies for a given patient and certainly a need exists for new therapies for patients who lack evidence of type 2 immune response (noneosinophilic severe asthma). To address this gap, the National Institutes of Health recently launched the Precision Interventions for Severe and/or Exacerbation-Prone Asthma Network to examine this issue. Similarly, the Efficacy and Mechanism Evaluation program established by the National Institute for Health Research has recently funded a similar network in the United Kingdom to examine new approaches to management of severe asthma. Therefore, over the next few years, more evidence supporting personalized approach to caring for these patients with difficult-to-control asthma is expected.

ADHERENCE ISSUES IN ASTHMA

As in most chronic diseases, medication nonadherence is a major problem in asthma, with reported nonadherence rates of 30% to 70%.[39–42] There is also robust evidence that incorrect inhaler technique is pervasive, with 30% of patients demonstrating poor technique, and requires repeated review. Disconcertingly, a recent meta-analysis found that frequency of inhaler errors has remained constant over 40 years.[43] Nonadherence in asthma is associated with increased morbidity and mortality.[44–47] Barriers to adherence can generally be identified as relating to 1 or more of the following factors: patient, disease, prescribed therapy, socioeconomics, and health care system. Nonadherence can be classified into 2 broad categories: intentional and unintentional (**Fig. 4**). Unintentional nonadherence occurs when patient wants to take the medication but is unable to, due to issues with access to the medication, misunderstanding of instructions, health literacy, or forgetfulness. These barriers are easier to overcome than intentional nonadherence, where a patient knowingly decides not to take the medication for any number of reasons, including denial of the disease, personal beliefs, or secondary gain. Accurate assessment of medication adherence can be difficult. Self-reporting tends to overestimate adherence when compared with objective

monitoring. Prescription refill monitoring and dose counters are helpful but not definitive surrogates of adherence. Use of electronic monitoring devices can provide objective evidence of adherence data to help inform clinical decision making.[48] Overcoming barriers to adherence requires a multipronged approach with patient-provider communication at its center.

ADDRESSING COMORBIDITIES AND TRIGGERS

Individuals with uncontrolled asthma should undergo a careful and systematic assessment of contributing comorbidities and triggers.

Several population-based studies have shown that patients with asthma have higher rates of myriad comorbidities.[49–51] Although the most frequently reported comorbid conditions are rhinosinusitis, dysfunctional breathing, obesity, obstructive sleep apnea (OSA), psychopathologies, and gastroesophageal reflux disease, other illnesses are also found to have higher prevalence in asthma, including cardiovascular and hypertensive diseases, diabetes mellitus, and osteoporosis. For many of these conditions, the relationship seems bidirectional. For example, uncontrolled gastroesophageal reflux (GER) can have an impact on asthma through reflux (direct microaspiration of acidic gastric contents into the lower airways) or reflex (stimulation of shared vagal innervation) mechanism.[52,53] On the other hand, asthma and asthma therapies can promote

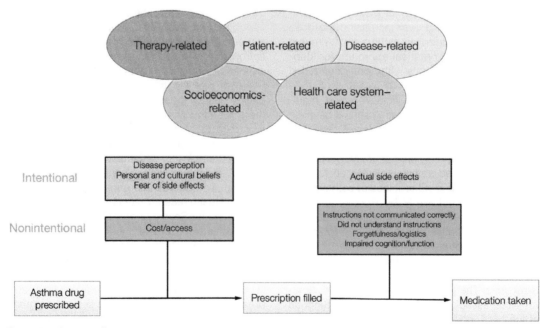

Fig. 4. Barriers to adherence.

GERby having an impact on lower esophageal sphincter tone.[54,55] Similarly, bidirectional relationships have been observed between asthma and OSA, rhinitis, rhinosinusitis, and depression.[56–60] Presence of comorbidities is associated with poor asthma control, excess medical cost, and productivity loss.[61–63] Evidence suggests that systematic evaluation and management of potential comorbidities may help improve asthma control in these patients.[11]

Identification and avoidance of asthma triggers is critical to successful asthma management (**Table 2**). These triggers may be allergic or nonallergic; occupational or domestic; and irritant or infectious. Exposure to these triggers may be episodic or continuous and successful remediation may lead to reduced medication needs for asthma control. A detailed history should include evaluation of possible triggers and, for patients with predictable exposures, interventions ranging from complete avoidance of trigger to pretreatment with short-acting bronchodilator recommended. Sources of common inhaled allergens include animals, house dust mites, cockroaches, molds, and outdoor plants. Symptomatic patients with suspected allergic triggers should undergo further evaluation with either allergen skin testing or serum assays for specific IgE. Once sensitization to specific allergens has been confirmed, a comprehensive environmental control plan can be implemented.[64–67] Common irritant exposures, such as cigarette smoke and indoor/outdoor air pollution, are also important triggers and associated with increased morbidity.[68,69] Questions about workplace exposures are particularly important because they account for up to 25% of adult-onset asthma.[70] Work-related asthma should be suspected if a patient reports symptoms that progress through the workweek or improve during periods

Table 2	
Common environmental triggers	
Triggers	**Mitigation Strategies**
Indoor triggers	
House dust mite	Keep relative humidity in home at 35%–50%. Wash bedding weekly to decrease mite allergen level. Vacuum regularly using a vacuum cleaner with high-efficiency particulate air filter. Use mite allergen–proof encasings. Use physical measures to kill mites: heat, freezing, and desiccation.
Pets (cats and dogs)	Remove pet from the home If removal of pet from home is not feasible, at least limit pet's access to the bedroom. Frequently vacuum. Consider removal of carpets because they are allergen reservoirs.
Pests (roaches and rodents)	Mitigate factors that facilitate infestation (access to food/water and paths of ingress). Incorporate an integrated pest management (IPM) program by a professional.
Mold	Removal of visible mold using appropriate protection. Eliminate dampness and repair leaks. Improve home ventilation. Avoid use of organic building materials in the home.
Air pollutants (tobacco, smoke)	Eliminate indoor smoking and other pollutant sources. Use exhaust fans and high-efficiency particulate air filters Replace wood burning/gas stoves with electric stoves.
Workplace triggers	
Immunologic triggers (high or low molecular weight)	Prompt and complete avoidance of exposure is strongly recommended. If complete removal from exposure is not possible, exposure reduction is a significantly less satisfactory strategy. In this situation, close surveillance and re-evaluation is recommended.
Irritant triggers	Use appropriate respiratory protective devices. Minimize all exposure, if possible. Change workplace environment and patient responsibilities to avoid high level exposure.

away from work. Rapid and proper confirmation of diagnosis and reduction of exposure to sensitizers or irritants at work are critical to effective management of work-related asthma.[71]

Referral to a severe asthma clinic should be considered if

- Asthma symptoms persist at steps 3 or controlled at steps 4/5 of GINA-guided therapy. Patient is likely to require additional evaluation including phenotyping for consideration of advanced therapies or participation in clinical trials evaluating novel therapies.
- Patient continues to experience frequent exacerbations or has history of near-fatal asthma.
- Diagnostic uncertainty exists, and additional diagnostics are required to confirm asthma and/or exclude an alternate diagnosis.
- Work-related asthma is suspected. This requires detailed evaluation of workplace exposures and diagnostic testing that may include specific inhalation challenge.

SUMMARY

Asthma, a global health problem, can be controlled in most patients with currently available therapies. An important subset of patients with asthma, however, remains uncontrolled despite the use of available treatment options. In addition to intrinsic disease severity, many other factors contribute to suboptimal control of asthma, including incorrect diagnosis, poor adherence, untreated comorbidities, and unrecognized triggers. A systematic approach to evaluation and management of asthma would allow for appropriate pharmacotherapy as well as recognition of these barriers to achieving good control, especially in patients who do not respond to treatment steps 3 or higher. This approach has the potential to improve asthma related morbidity while simultaneously reducing health care costs.

REFERENCES

1. Asthma. 2017. Available at: http://www.who.int/mediacentre/factsheets/fs307/en/. Accessed March 17, 2018.
2. CDC most recent asthma data. 2017. Available at: https://www.cdc.gov/asthma/most_recent_data.htm. Accessed March 17, 2018.
3. Global Initiative for Asthma. Global strategy for asthma management and prevention, 2018. Available at: www.ginasthma.org/. Accessed March 17, 2018.
4. National, Asthma Education Prevention, Program. Expert panel report 3 (EPR-3): guidelines for the diagnosis and management of asthma-summary report 2007. J Allergy Clin Immunol 2007;120(5 Suppl):S94–138.
5. Aaron SD, Vandemheen KL, FitzGerald JM, et al. Reevaluation of diagnosis in adults with physician-diagnosed asthma. JAMA 2017;317(3):269–79.
6. van Huisstede A, Castro Cabezas M, van de Geijn GJ, et al. Underdiagnosis and overdiagnosis of asthma in the morbidly obese. Respir Med 2013;107(9):1356–64.
7. Enright PL, McClelland RL, Newman AB, et al. Underdiagnosis and undertreatment of asthma in the elderly. Cardiovascular health study Research group. Chest 1999;116(3):603–13.
8. Brozek GM, Farnik M, Lawson J, et al. Underdiagnosis of childhood asthma: a comparison of survey estimates to clinical evaluation. Int J Occup Med Environ Health 2013;26(6):900–9.
9. Jose BP, Camargos PA, Cruz Filho AA, et al. Diagnostic accuracy of respiratory diseases in primary health units. Rev Assoc Med Bras (1992) 2014; 60(6):599–612.
10. Irwin RS, Curley FJ, French CL. Difficult-to-control asthma. Contributing factors and outcome of a systematic management protocol. Chest 1993;103(6): 1662–9.
11. Tay TR, Lee J, Radhakrishna N, et al. A structured approach to specialist-referred difficult asthma patients improves control of comorbidities and enhances asthma outcomes. J Allergy Clin Immunol Pract 2017;5(4):956–64.e3.
12. Hekking PP, Wener RR, Amelink M, et al. The prevalence of severe refractory asthma. J Allergy Clin Immunol 2015;135(4):896–902.
13. Athanazio R, Carvalho-Pinto R, Fernandes FLA, et al. Can severe asthmatic patients achieve asthma control? A systematic approach in patients with difficult to control asthma followed in a specialized clinic. BMC Pulm Med 2016;16(1):153.
14. Robinson DS, Campbell DA, Durham SR, et al. Systematic assessment of difficult-to-treat asthma. Eur Respir J 2003;22(3):478–83.
15. Sistek D, Wickens K, Amstrong R, et al. Predictive value of respiratory symptoms and bronchial hyperresponsiveness to diagnose asthma in New Zealand. Respir Med 2006;100(12):2107–11.
16. Sistek D, Tschopp JM, Schindler C, et al. Clinical diagnosis of current asthma: predictive value of respiratory symptoms in the SAPALDIA study. Swiss study on air pollution and lung diseases in adults. Eur Respir J 2001;17(2):214–9.
17. Pellegrino R, Viegi G, Brusasco V, et al. Interpretative strategies for lung function tests. Eur Respir J 2005;26(5):948–68.
18. Bleecker ER, Emmett A, Crater G, et al. Lung function and symptom improvement with fluticasone propionate/salmeterol and ipratropium

bromide/albuterol in COPD: response by beta-agonist reversibility. Pulm Pharmacol Ther 2008; 21(4):682–8.

19. Mahler DA, Donohue JF, Barbee RA, et al. Efficacy of salmeterol xinafoate in the treatment of COPD. Chest 1999;115(4):957–65.

20. Tashkin D, Celli B, Decramer M, et al. Bronchodilator responsiveness in patients with COPD (data from the UPLIFT trial). Rev Port Pneumol 2008;14(4):584–7.

21. Coates AL, Wanger J, Cockcroft DW, et al. ERS technical standard on bronchial challenge testing: general considerations and performance of methacholine challenge tests. Eur Respir J 2017;49(5) [pii:1601526].

22. Parsons JP, Hallstrand TS, Mastronarde JG, et al. An official American Thoracic Society clinical practice guideline: exercise-induced bronchoconstriction. Am J Respir Crit Care Med 2013;187(9):1016–27.

23. Sumino K, Sugar EA, Irvin CG, et al. Variability of methacholine bronchoprovocation and the effect of inhaled corticosteroids in mild asthma. Ann Allergy Asthma Immunol 2014;112(4):354–60.e1.

24. Currie GP, Fowler SJ, Lipworth BJ. Dose response of inhaled corticosteroids on bronchial hyperresponsiveness: a meta-analysis. Ann Allergy Asthma Immunol 2003;90(2):194–8.

25. van Grunsven PM, van Schayck CP, Molema J, et al. Effect of inhaled corticosteroids on bronchial responsiveness in patients with "corticosteroid naive" mild asthma: a meta-analysis. Thorax 1999; 54(4):316–22.

26. Vandenplas O, Suojalehto H, Aasen TB, et al. Specific inhalation challenge in the diagnosis of occupational asthma: consensus statement. Eur Respir J 2014;43(6):1573–87.

27. National Asthma Education and Prevention Program Expert Panel Report 2. Guidelines for the diagnosis and management of asthma. Bethesda (MD): National Heart, Lung, and Blood Institute; 1997.

28. Global Initiative for Asthma. Asthma management and prevention. NIH Publication number 95-3659A. Bethesda (MD): National Institutes of Health; 1995.

29. Taylor DR, Bateman ED, Boulet LP, et al. A new perspective on concepts of asthma severity and control. Eur Respir J 2008;32(3):545–54.

30. Schatz M, Sorkness CA, Li JT, et al. Asthma control test: reliability, validity, and responsiveness in patients not previously followed by asthma specialists. J Allergy Clin Immunol 2006;117(3):549–56.

31. Jia CE, Zhang HP, Lv Y, et al. The Asthma Control Test and Asthma Control Questionnaire for assessing asthma control: systematic review and meta-analysis. J Allergy Clin Immunol 2013;131(3): 695–703.

32. Juniper EF, O'Byrne PM, Guyatt GH, et al. Development and validation of a questionnaire to measure asthma control. Eur Respir J 1999;14(4):902–7.

33. Bateman ED, Boushey HA, Bousquet J, et al. Can guideline-defined asthma control be achieved? The Gaining Optimal Asthma ControL study. Am J Respir Crit Care Med 2004;170(8):836–44.

34. Pauwels RA, Lofdahl CG, Postma DS, et al. Effect of inhaled formoterol and budesonide on exacerbations of asthma. Formoterol and Corticosteroids Establishing Therapy (FACET) international study group. N Engl J Med 1997;337(20):1405–11.

35. Chipps BE, Corren J, Israel E, et al. Asthma yardstick: practical recommendations for a sustained step-up in asthma therapy for poorly controlled asthma. Ann Allergy Asthma Immunol 2017;118(2): 133–42.e3.

36. Clearie KL, Jackson CM, Fardon TC, et al. Supervised step-down of inhaled corticosteroids in the community–an observational study. Respir Med 2011;105(4):558–65.

37. Hawkins G, McMahon AD, Twaddle S, et al. Stepping down inhaled corticosteroids in asthma: randomised controlled trial. BMJ 2003;326(7399):1115.

38. Rogers L, Sugar EA, Blake K, et al. Step-down therapy for asthma well controlled on inhaled corticosteroid and long-acting beta-agonist: a randomized clinical trial. J Allergy Clin Immunol Pract 2018; 6(2):633–43.e1.

39. Bidwal M, Lor K, Yu J, et al. Evaluation of asthma medication adherence rates and strategies to improve adherence in the underserved population at a Federally Qualified Health Center. Res Social Adm Pharm 2017;13(4):759–66.

40. Clatworthy J, Price D, Ryan D, et al. The value of self-report assessment of adherence, rhinitis and smoking in relation to asthma control. Prim Care Respir J 2000;18(4):300–5.

41. Latry P, Pinet M, Labat A, et al. Adherence to anti-inflammatory treatment for asthma in clinical practice in France. Clin Ther 2008;30 Spec No:1058–68.

42. Onyirimba F, Apter A, Reisine S, et al. Direct clinician-to-patient feedback discussion of inhaled steroid use: its effect on adherence. Ann Allergy Asthma Immunol 2003;90(4):411–5.

43. Sanchis J, Gich I, Pedersen S. (ADMIT) ADMIT. Systematic review of errors in inhaler use: has patient technique improved over time? Chest 2016;150(2): 394–406.

44. Suissa S, Ernst P, Benayoun S, et al. Low-dose inhaled corticosteroids and the prevention of death from asthma. N Engl J Med 2000;343(5):332–6.

45. Suissa S, Ernst P, Kezouh A. Regular use of inhaled corticosteroids and the long term prevention of hospitalisation for asthma. Thorax 2002;57(10):880–4.

46. Gamble J, Stevenson M, McClean E, et al. The prevalence of nonadherence in difficult asthma. Am J Respir Crit Care Med 2009;180(9):817–22.

47. Murphy AC, Proeschal A, Brightling CE, et al. The relationship between clinical outcomes and

medication adherence in difficult-to-control asthma. Thorax 2012;67(8):751–3.

48. Chan AH, Harrison J, Black PN, et al. Using electronic monitoring devices to measure inhaler adherence: a practical guide for clinicians. J Allergy Clin Immunol Pract 2015;3(3):335–49.e1-5.

49. Cazzola M, Calzetta L, Bettoncelli G, et al. Asthma and comorbid medical illness. Eur Respir J 2011; 38(1):42–9.

50. Heck S, Al-Shobash S, Rapp D, et al. High probability of comorbidities in bronchial asthma in Germany. NPJ Prim Care Respir Med 2017;27(1):28.

51. Dudeney J, Sharpe L, Jaffe A, et al. Anxiety in youth with asthma: a meta-analysis. Pediatr Pulmonol 2017;52(9):1121–9.

52. Mansfield LE, Stein MR. Gastroesophageal reflux and asthma: a possible reflex mechanism. Ann Allergy 1978;41(4):224–6.

53. Ghaed N, Stein M. Assessment of a technique for scintigraphic monitoring of pulmonary aspiration of gastric contents in asthmatics with gastroesophageal reflux. Ann Allergy 1979;42(5):306–8.

54. Turbyville JC. Applying principles of physics to the airway to help explain the relationship between asthma and gastroesophageal reflux. Med Hypotheses 2010;74(6):1075–80.

55. Crowell MD, Zayat EN, Lacy BE, et al. The effects of an inhaled beta(2)-adrenergic agonist on lower esophageal function: a dose-response study. Chest 2001;120(4):1184–9.

56. Guilleminault C, Quera-Salva MA, Powell N, et al. Nocturnal asthma: snoring, small pharynx and nasal CPAP. Eur Respir J 1988;1(10):902–7.

57. Aihara K, Oga T, Chihara Y, et al. Analysis of systemic and airway inflammation in obstructive sleep apnea. Sleep Breath 2013;17(2):597–604.

58. Trojan TD, Khan DA, Defina LF, et al. Asthma and depression: the Cooper center longitudinal study. Ann Allergy Asthma Immunol 2014;112(5):432–6.

59. Brunner WM, Schreiner PJ, Sood A, et al. Depression and risk of incident asthma in adults. The CARDIA study. Am J Respir Crit Care Med 2014;189(9): 1044–51.

60. Khan DA. Allergic rhinitis and asthma: epidemiology and common pathophysiology. Allergy Asthma Proc 2014;35(5):357–61.

61. Chen W, Lynd LD, FitzGerald JM, et al. Excess medical costs in patients with asthma and the role of comorbidity. Eur Respir J 2016;48(6):1584–92.

62. Ehteshami-Afshar S, FitzGerald JM, Carlsten C, et al. The impact of comorbidities on productivity loss in asthma patients. Respir Res 2016;17(1):106.

63. Braido F, Brusselle G, Guastalla D, et al. Determinants and impact of suboptimal asthma control in Europe: the International Cross-Sectional and Longitudinal Assessment on Asthma Control (LIAISON) study. Respir Res 2016;17(1):51.

64. Phipatanakul W, Matsui E, Portnoy J, et al. Environmental assessment and exposure reduction of rodents: a practice parameter. Ann Allergy Asthma Immunol 2012;109(6):375–87.

65. Portnoy J, Kennedy K, Sublett J, et al. Environmental assessment and exposure control: a practice parameter–furry animals. Ann Allergy Asthma Immunol 2012;108(4):223.e1-5.

66. Portnoy J, Chew GL, Phipatanakul W, et al. Environmental assessment and exposure reduction of cockroaches: a practice parameter. J Allergy Clin Immunol 2013;132(4):802–8.e1-5.

67. Portnoy J, Miller JD, Williams PB, et al. Environmental assessment and exposure control of dust mites: a practice parameter. Ann Allergy Asthma Immunol 2013;111(6):465–507.

68. Siroux V, Pin I, Oryszczyn MP, et al. Relationships of active smoking to asthma and asthma severity in the EGEA study. Epidemiological study on the genetics and environment of asthma. Eur Respir J 2000; 15(3):470–7.

69. Strickland MJ, Darrow LA, Klein M, et al. Short-term associations between ambient air pollutants and pediatric asthma emergency department visits. Am J Respir Crit Care Med 2010;182(3):307–16.

70. Kogevinas M, Zock JP, Jarvis D, et al. Exposure to substances in the workplace and new-onset asthma: an international prospective population-based study (ECRHS-II). Lancet 2007;370(9584):336–41.

71. Malo JL, Tarlo SM, Sastre J, et al. An official American Thoracic Society Workshop Report: presentations and discussion of the fifth Jack Pepys Workshop on asthma in the workplace. Comparisons between asthma in the workplace and non-work-related asthma. Ann Am Thorac Soc 2015; 12(7):S99–110.

72. Boulding R, Stacey R, Niven R, et al. Dysfunctional breathing: a review of the literature and proposal for classification. Eur Respir Rev 2016;25(141): 287–94.

73. Veidal S, Jeppegaard M, Sverrild A, et al. The impact of dysfunctional breathing on the assessment of asthma control. Respir Med 2017;123: 42–7.

Nonallergic Triggers and Comorbidities in Asthma Exacerbations and Disease Severity

Octavian C. Ioachimescu, MD, PhD, MBA[a,1],
Nikita S. Desai, MD[b,*]

KEYWORDS

- Asthma • Allergy • Nonallergic triggers • Exacerbation • Severity

KEY POINTS

- Patients with asthma typically have more than one trigger.
- Optimal identification and management of triggers require an effective clinician-patient partnership and may lead to better outcomes.
- Common triggers for asthma may be inhaled from the environment, may be ingested as food, or may start with exposure to the skin or via medications.
- Comorbidities that exacerbate asthma include obesity, gastroesophageal reflux, obstructive sleep apnea, and chronic rhinitis.
- Obesity can result in more frequent, severe symptoms and disease exacerbations, poorer control with medications, and more altered asthma-related quality of life.

INTRODUCTION

Asthma is a heterogeneous chronic disease of the respiratory system that affects approximately 300 million people of all ages worldwide. More than half of the patients living with chronic asthma are poorly controlled, presenting with frequent and burdensome symptoms, significant limitation in their daily activities, work absenteeism or presenteeism (ie, unproductive work days), unplanned health care visits, and decreased quality of life (QOL). Asthma exacerbations are largely responsible for the overall disease burden, leading to hospitalizations, mechanical ventilation, decline in lung function, and sometimes, death.[1,2] In 1993, the Global Initiative for Asthma (GINA) was developed to provide guidelines for asthma management and to help incorporate advances in asthma therapy into clinical practice.[3] Prompt and accurate diagnosis, regular monitoring in clinic visits, engaging patient-clinician relationships, and adherence to appropriate therapies are essential for effective management. Furthermore, trigger identification and avoidance are equally important for symptom control and prevention of exacerbations. Although for most cases asthma is a chronic disease without a cure, a combined approach entailing improved therapeutic adherence and trigger avoidance can dramatically improve disease manifestation and progression.

ASTHMA TRIGGERS
Definitions and General Frameworks

An *asthma trigger* is a stimulus that causes an increase in asthma symptoms and/or airflow

[a] Pulmonary, Critical Care and Sleep Medicine, Emory University, Atlanta VA Medical Center, Atlanta, GA, USA;
[b] Pulmonary and Critical Care, Respiratory Institute, Cleveland Clinic, Cleveland, OH, USA
[1] Present address: 35 Plantation Drive Northeast, Atlanta, GA 30324.
* Corresponding author. 400 Park Avenue East Drive, Apartment 313, Beachwood, OH 44122.
E-mail address: nikitasdesai@gmail.com

Clin Chest Med 40 (2019) 71–85
https://doi.org/10.1016/j.ccm.2018.10.005
0272-5231/19/© 2018 Elsevier Inc. All rights reserved.

limitation.[4] GINA guidelines discuss triggers as environmental factors that put a subject at risk for transient acute worsening of asthma symptoms.[3] Others define asthma triggers as chemical, physical, or biologic agents (substances or events) that last hours to days, and which could lead to acute symptomatic deterioration.[5] In contrast, exposures or stimuli that may *cause* or *contribute to development* of asthma are typically called *risk factors*. Traditional risk factors for asthma development include genetic predisposition, age, gender, environmental allergies, obesity, socioeconomic status, urbanization status, and exposure to tobacco smoke.

Although this differentiation may seem clear and easy, some overlap does exist, because some events or agents could be risk factors for the development of asthma (eg, early life exposure to tobacco smoke) and simultaneously be asthma symptom triggers (eg, primary or secondary exposure to cigarette smoke). Unfortunately, beyond this overlap phenomenon, the literature abounds in confusing terminologies for asthma triggers and risk factors, at times using them interchangeably. Triggers of poor asthma control vary greatly from patient to patient, from perceived (known) to nonperceived (occult) triggers, and this may be a helpful distinction. The latter category makes therapeutic interventions more challenging and sometimes destined to fail. Better characterization of disease phenotypes may help target therapies for asthma patients.[6] This article aims to guide clinicians to identify nonallergic triggers and comorbid associations relevant for asthma's disease control.

A potentially useful framework for asthma trigger analysis is the so-called 3P schema developed by Arthur J. Spielman for the pathogenesis of insomnia: predisposing, precipitating, and perpetuating factors.[7] In this case, although very few asthma triggers are in the predisposing factors' category (most being actually risk factors for disease development), most triggers belong to the precipitating category (and responsible for acute exacerbations and lack of control), whereas perpetuating domain is best represented by comorbidities, that is, medical conditions that could lead to disease progression, loss of lung function, and remodeling process (**Fig. 1**). This framework also highlights the importance of environmental factors and comorbidities for chronic symptoms, inflammation, airflow limitation, disease "flare-ups," and progression.

Trigger Characterization

Asthma, with its pathogenesis rooted in atopy and airway hyperresponsiveness, can be best addressed by knowledge and subsequent avoidance of the various triggers.

Triggers described by adult asthma patients are either allergic (pollens, dust or dust mites, mold, animal dander, cockroaches, food allergens, and similar) or nonallergic (**Table 1**). Nonallergic triggers include air pollution and irritants, respiratory infections, strong odors, exercise, cold air, medications, and emotional factors.[5] Triggers can also be categorized as endogenous (eg, psychological factors) or exogenous (all other allergens, irritants, and so forth), as outlined in **Table 2**.

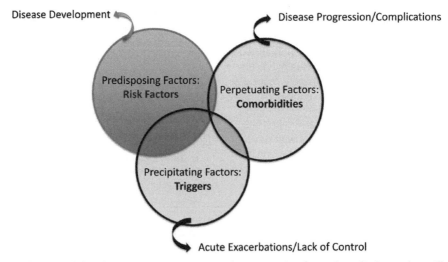

Fig. 1. The 3P framework (predisposing, precipitating and perpetuating factors) applied to asthma, illustrated as a nonproportional Venn diagram of factors of importance for disease development (risk factors), exacerbations and disease control (triggers), progression, and complications (comorbidities).

Table 1
Allergic versus nonallergic triggers

Allergic Triggers	Nonallergic Triggers
Pollens	Air pollution or irritants
Mold	(including tobacco smoke)
Dust or	Respiratory infections
dust mites	Strong odors
Animal dander	Medications
Food allergens	Exercise
	Weather-related (cold or
	dry air, and so forth)
	Emotional factors
	(anxiety, stress)

Ingredients or chemicals in food (sulfites, gastric acid/enzymes) and medications (eye drops) are often overlooked.

Table 3 illustrates a proposed new framework for a standardized characterization of asthma triggers that includes environmental factors, quantitative and qualitative assessments, as well as associated symptoms.

Awareness of triggers can better identify phenotype or endotype characterizations. For example, most patients with disease precipitated by aeroallergens such as dust mites (allergic phenotype) have an inflammatory response centered on CD4$^+$ T-helper cell types 2, with eosinophilic inflammation, elevated levels of type 2 cytokines, such as interleukin-4 (IL-4), IL-5, and IL-13, and increased production of immunoglobulin E (IgE) (Th2^{high} endotype).[8,9]

Allergic triggers

Although asthma is often associated with an allergic diathesis, allergic triggers can be identified only in a subset or a minority of patients. Interestingly, most of the investigative work published focuses on the relationship between allergic triggers and asthma. This association will not be addressed, because this article focuses on nonallergic triggers of asthma.

Infectious triggers

Viral infections Identification of infectious triggers can be useful in guiding treatment of acute asthma exacerbations as well as predicting resolution of symptoms. Childhood respiratory infections have been implicated in the *development* of reactive airways disease (ie, risk factors), and viral infections are the most frequent cause of acute asthma exacerbations. Differentiating between true viral infection versus colonization (epiphenomenon) is only one of the challenges in establishing the clear role of viral infection in exacerbations.[10]

Rhinovirus The most prevalent infectious trigger in adults is the rhinovirus, which is detected in about two-thirds of asthma exacerbations caused by viruses.[10] Rhinovirus infection is typically associated with an exaggerated Th2 response, with higher numbers of serum eosinophils and neutrophils, in both asthmatic and nonasthmatic patients.[11] This response is associated with an increase in airway hyperresponsiveness, decreases in forced expiratory volume in 1 second (FEV$_1$), and peak expiratory flow rates in asthmatic patients versus healthy subjects.[12] Viral infections can result in worsening cough, but no difference in recovery of lung function at 4 weeks' follow-up, when compared with exacerbations without viral coinfection.[13] Rhinovirus infections can be resistant to the anti-inflammatory effects of corticosteroids, which may be due to the virus' ability to

Table 2
General classification of exogenous asthma triggers by general type and route of exposure

Respiratory or Inhalant Triggers	Digestive or Oral Triggers	Oculocutaneous Triggers
Indoor or workplace allergens (dust or dust mites, pet dander, mold, and others)	Food allergens	Skin contact (allergens)
	Medications (oral)	Medications (skin or intraocular
	Sulfite sensitivity	application)
Indoor or workplace irritants (tobacco smoke, fumes, paints, cleaning agents, sprays, perfumes, heaters, fireplaces, stoves, and similar)	Gastroesophageal reflux	Ocular contact (allergens)
Outdoor allergens (dust, pollens, animal dander, mold, and others)		
Outdoor irritants (tobacco smoke, particulate pollution, fumes, strong odors, weather-related)		
Respiratory infections (rhinosinusitis, bronchitis)		

Table 3
PQRSTU framework of trigger exposure characterization

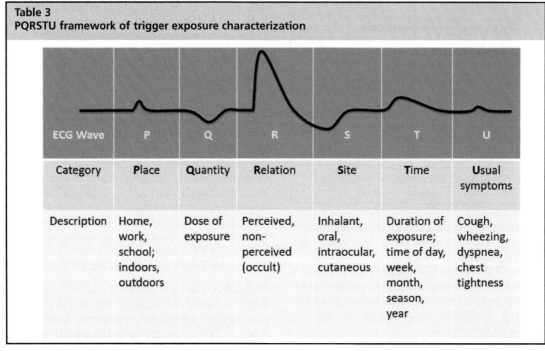

ECG Wave	P	Q	R	S	T	U
Category	Place	Quantity	Relation	Site	Time	Usual symptoms
Description	Home, work, school; indoors, outdoors	Dose of exposure	Perceived, non-perceived (occult)	Inhalant, oral, intraocular, cutaneous	Duration of exposure; time of day, week, month, season, year	Cough, wheezing, dyspnea, chest tightness

Abbreviation: ECG, electrocardiogram.

induce transforming growth factor-β in the airway epithelium. Glucocorticoids may also enhance viral replication, which may explain the worsening of respiratory symptoms, specifically in rhinovirus-induced exacerbations.[14–16] Emerging evidence suggests that macrolide antibiotics may play a role in the reduction of rhinovirus titers.[17]

Influenza The "flu" is an acute respiratory illness caused by infection with influenza viruses, which can be severe and, especially in high-risk subjects, may result in significant morbidity and mortality. In a recent systematic review and meta-analysis on the outcomes of vaccination in asthma,[18] it was found (1) that the overall quality of evidence is poor for all studied outcomes; (2) that the pooled vaccine effectiveness in subjects with asthma was 45% (95% confidence interval [CI], 31%–56%) for laboratory-confirmed influenza; (3) that pooled efficacy of live vaccines in reducing influenza was 81% (95% CI, 33%– 94%); (4) that live vaccine reduced febrile illness by 72% (95% CI, 20%–90%); and, importantly, (5) that influenza vaccine prevented 59% to 78% of asthma attacks leading to emergency visits or hospitalizations.[18]

Bacterial infections Infections, especially "atyp-ical" bacterial infections, can herald the onset of asthma diagnosis. Of these bacterial organisms, both *Chlamydophila pneumoniae* and *Myco-plasma pneumoniae* have been detected at higher rates in asthmatics versus normal controls, with up

to two-thirds of patients with refractory asthma testing positive for *Mycoplasma*.[19] Nevertheless, it is difficult to distinguish between "innocent bystander" colonization with "atypical" bacteria in chronic stable asthma and an exacerbation-causative agent.[20,21] Although there are no estab-lished guidelines for "atypical" bacterial infection testing in an acute asthma exacerbation, clinicians should consider a more targeted therapy with mac-rolides when there is a strong index of suspicion. Macrolides have shown promise in improving asthma control, likely due to their antibacterial as well as their anti-inflammatory properties. Treatment with azithromycin led to a reduction in frequency of exacerbations in patients with symptomatic persis-tent asthma (the AMAZES trial[22]) and an improve-ment in the asthma-related QOL.[23]

Fungal infections Fungal organisms have also been implicated as triggers for asthma exacerba-tions. The most well-known example is that of *Aspergillus* species, which trigger an IgE response in allergic bronchopulmonary aspergillosis; other mycoses (eg, with *Candida*) can cause allergic bronchopulmonary mycosis. A review of these allergic-mediated triggers is outside the scope of this article.

With the emerging importance of the micro-biome in various pathologic conditions, including in patients with lung conditions, it is likely that asthma presents a unique, complex, and possibly pathogenic interaction between microbiome and the airways that needs further investigation.[24]

Exercise

Although many individuals may experience dyspnea with exercise, people who experience $\geq 10\%$ reduction in FEV_1 during exercise are classified as having exercise-induced bronchospasm (EIB).[25] The prevalence is especially increased in "elite" athletes.[26,27] Identification of exercise as an asthma trigger is crucial for improving asthma-related QOL as well as severity control. Although the precise mechanism is still unclear, EIB is thought to be due to narrowing and hyperresponsiveness of a "dehydrated" airway, leading to upregulation of inflammatory mechanisms.[28–30] Neural dysregulation (ie, an increase in parasympathetic tone) may also play a role in bronchoconstriction during exercise.[31] Although a survey of practice patterns revealed that most clinicians start these patients empirically on beta-agonists for presumed EIB, a recent review revealed that a third of patients treated for presumed EIB have no evidence of asthma when confirmatory testing is performed.[32,33] Bronchoprovocation testing, including eucapnic voluntary hyperpnea, exercise, mannitol, or methacholine challenge, may be helpful in establishing a diagnosis. Because patients may have variable, individualized response to each test, multiple tests may be necessary to confirm EIB.[34] Because athletes with EIB typically do not have eosinophilic airway inflammation, their response to inhaled corticosteroid controller medications is typically diminished. The mainstay of therapy remains short-acting beta-agonist therapy; however, patients should be cautioned to use it less than 3 times per week, because tolerance has been reported.[35] Although the pathogenesis of EIB remains unconfirmed, mast cell activation has also been demonstrated; therefore, anti-inflammatory medications, including antihistamines and antileukotriene inhibitors, may have a role as well.[28]

Smoking

Self-smoking When compared with non-smokers, asthma patients who are active smokers have higher rates of exacerbation, including life-threatening flares and higher mortality. More frequent exacerbations lead to increased health care utilization through unscheduled clinic visits and hospital admissions. With higher rates of life-threatening exacerbations, mortality is also increased in smokers with asthma.[36] Risk of worsening asthma is especially pronounced in patients with greater than 20 pack-year smoking history.[37] In pregnant patients, smokers are more likely to have worsening of asthma symptoms versus never-smokers.[38] Smokers with asthma are more likely to have neutrophil-predominant sputum and decreased responsiveness to both oral and inhaled corticosteroids versus non-smoking patients with asthma.[39,40] Fractional exhaled nitric oxide (FeNO) levels appear to be decreased in subjects with either active or passive tobacco exposure, with or without asthma. When clinicians adjust asthma control therapies, these facts should be taken into consideration in conjunction with disease control questionnaires and patient-reported symptoms.[41] For example, asthma patients who smoke may have improved symptomatic control with addition of long-acting bronchodilators, rather than increasing the dose of inhaled corticosteroids. Adult-onset asthma patients with greater than 10 pack-year smoking history had accelerated decline in lung function versus those with less than 10 pack-year histories even in those patients who quit smoking.[42]

Environmental tobacco smoke Passive smoking is also a trigger for acute asthma exacerbations. Although only 11.6% to 15.4% of patients report at least an hour of passive smoking, a study that quantified nicotine exposure found that the actual number approaches 72% of subjects. Patients with higher levels of nicotine and cotinine in their hair follicles were found to have higher risk of hospitalization, whereas elevated levels of nicotine were associated with higher rates of admission to intensive care.[43] In pregnant non-smoking women with asthma, passive smoking exposure is also associated with increased episodes of uncontrolled asthma.[44]

Multiple population-based studies found that smoking interdiction in public areas was associated with decreased visits for uncontrolled asthma and lower health care utilization.[45,46] Smoking cessation in asthma patients is associated with decreases in sputum neutrophils over time and restoration of corticosteroid responsiveness. Patients who quit smoking see an improvement in disease-related QOL, reduction in use and dosage of controller and rescue medications, as well as improvements in FEV_1.[47–49] Furthermore, there is also evidence to support an initial worsening of respiratory symptoms in individuals with asthma who attempt smoking cessation; therefore, patients should be counseled about potential initial symptomatic deterioration, and potentially have their controller medication dosages increased during their cessation attempts.

Other smoking Although data are limited, adolescents with asthma have higher rates of e-cigarette use, and more studies are clearly warranted to evaluate their effects on asthma control.[50,51] Although smoking both marijuana and tobacco has been associated with worsening respiratory symptoms, more studies are needed to determine the effects of marijuana smoking alone on asthma control. Cocaine and heroin insufflation have been directly correlated with worsening asthma symptoms and increased rates of exacerbation and should be avoided in all asthma patients.[52]

Psychological factors/stress

Anxiety and depression are very common comorbidities in patients with asthma[53–56] and associated with increased health care utilization and high indirect costs from work-related absence (absenteeism).[57,58] Patients with preexisting asthma are just as likely to suffer from worsening anxiety, whereas anxiety is likely to trigger asthma symptoms. Given this bidirectional relationship, patients with asthma should be screened and appropriately referred and treated for underlying anxiety disorders.

A variety of psychogenic factors can act as asthma triggers. Emotional triggers such as stress and depression are well known to influence the level of asthma control.[59] For example, children who grow up in more stressful environments seem to have higher prevalence of asthma.[60,61] Interestingly, the association seems to be stronger between stress, anxiety, or depression and atopic asthma.[62] In a recent article, anxiety and depression were associated with patient trigger reports, particularly nonallergic triggers.[63] Asthma trigger reports were also strongly correlated with disease outcomes, and asthma triggers explained more than a third of the variance for asthma-related QOL. Nonallergic triggers explained almost 20% of the variance, whereas allergic triggers played only a minor role in this relationship.[63]

Medications

Beta-blockers Because symptoms of bronchoconstriction are primarily mediated by $\beta2$-adrenoreceptors in the airways, β-blockers have been traditionally avoided in patients with severe asthma, likely leading to unopposed cholinergic tone. A systematic review analyzed the effect of oral β-blockers on the respiratory system and found that β-blockers caused a mean decrease in FEV_1 of 6.9% with initiation of selective $\beta1$-blockade, and 10.2% with nonselective β-blockers. Up to 13% of patients had an FEV_1 decrease of more than 20%, and this effect was largely dependent on the dose of β-blockers administered. The Arginine-16 $\beta2$-adrenoceptor polymorphism has been pathogenically implicated in hyperresponsive patients who may have exaggerated cholinergic tone.[64] Interestingly, acute administration of topical nonselective β-blockers for the treatment of ophthalmologic conditions has also been associated with an increase in moderate asthma exacerbations; however, this risk does not persist with chronic administration.[65] These data suggest that β-blockers should be avoided in patients with poorly controlled asthma in the absence of significant cardiovascular risk factors. In patients with cardiovascular indications for β-blockers, the dose should be cautiously titrated and patients should be closely monitored for worsening asthma control.

Nonsteroidal anti-inflammatory drugs Nonsteroidal anti-inflammatory drug-exacerbated airway disease (NERD) has an estimated prevalence of 9% of all patients with asthma, and acetylsalicylic acid (ASA or aspirin) is the most frequently implicated medication. In NERD, ASA inhibits cyclo-oxygenase-1 (COX-1) enzyme, which increases proinflammatory cysteinyl leukotrienes and decreases anti-inflammatory prostaglandins to cause bronchoconstriction in the airways. The COX-2 inhibitors have not demonstrated the same effects on the respiratory system as COX-1 inhibitors and are generally better tolerated. Patients with NERD are twice as likely to have poorly controlled asthma symptoms. Oral provocation studies have demonstrated that the average clinically significant dose of ASA to provoke respiratory symptoms is ~ 85 mg; however, individual reaction to ASA in patients with NERD varies considerably by dose. Further studies are needed to determine whether higher ASA doses can be safely tolerated in patients with NERD, whereas existing studies suggest worsening respiratory symptoms in a dose-dependent fashion. In patients who have cardiovascular imperatives for ASA treatment, consultation with allergy experts is advised to guide protocols for ASA desensitization to attenuate asthma symptoms.[66]

ASTHMA COMORBIDITIES AND CONDITIONS
Chronic Obstructive Pulmonary Disease

Although a discussion about the coexistence of chronic obstructive pulmonary disease (COPD) and asthma is beyond the scope of this article, the authors mention briefly the most salient features of this condition.

Asthma-COPD overlap (ACO) is characterized by persistent airflow limitation combined with several features of asthma and a few traits usually associated with COPD.[67] Patients with coexisting asthma and COPD, "asthma-COPD overlap syndrome (ACOS)"[68] or "obstructive lung disease overlap syndrome,"[69] have accelerated decline in lung function, decreased responsiveness to conventional treatments such as corticosteroids, and higher rates of exacerbations and health care resource utilization.[67,70–73] In 2017, ACOS was renamed Asthma-COPD Overlap "in order to avoid the perception that this is a single disease," somehow ignoring the distinct connotations of syndrome and disease.[68] The estimated prevalence of ACO ranges from 12% to 55% among patients with COPD and from 13% to 61% in patients with asthma alone,[74] with significant variability by gender and age.[70,75,76] Concurrent doctor-diagnosed asthma and COPD have been reported in 15% to 20% of patients.[77–80] FeNO is a frequently used marker of eosinophilic airway inflammation that could help determine a patient's responsiveness to corticosteroid therapy. A value greater than 50 ppb is predictive of eosinophilic inflammation and corticosteroid responsiveness.[81] Higher doses of inhaled corticosteroids may be beneficial in patients with elevated FeNO.[82–84]

The current guidelines for ACO treatment suggest treating the dominant phenotype, with first-line therapy being inhaled corticosteroids with the addition of a long-acting bronchodilator or anticholinergic agent with increasing clinical symptoms or radiographic COPD abnormalities.[68] Aggressive risk factor modification, including smoking cessation, pulmonary rehabilitation, and trigger avoidance, is warranted. Further studies in this specific patient population are definitely needed to develop evidence-based, targeted therapies.

In conclusion, ACO is a heterogeneous condition, including patients with several forms of airway and parenchymal disease (phenotypes) and caused by a range of different underlying mechanisms (endo types), including a neutrophilic-predominant, relatively corticosteroid-unresponsive inflammatory form.[67]

Obesity

Obesity is a very important comorbidity in asthma. In lean adults, prevalence of asthma is 7.1%, whereas in obese adults, asthma is noted in 11.1% of people. The discrepancy is even more significant in women, where a diagnosis of asthma is encountered in 7.9% of lean and in 14.6% of obese individuals, and may double the odds of asthma.[85,86] When asthma is complicated by obesity, patients are likely to have more frequent exacerbations and to have increased asthma severity and increased incidence of mechanical ventilator support.[87–90]

The diagnosis of asthma can be challenging in obese individuals, because low exercise tolerance can mirror symptoms of asthma. Because of worsening chest wall restriction from truncal obesity (mechanical loading), a near-normal or normal FEV_1/forced vital capacity (FVC) on spirometry can mask the presence of airflow limitation or obstruction; FEV_1 may be more useful for monitoring asthma in obese patients.[91] Interestingly, in children with asthma who become obese later in early adulthood, the FEV_1/FVC ratio progressively declines without any change in FVC, suggesting that obesity is responsible for worsening airflow limitation.[92] FeNO in obesity is reduced and may be less useful as a diagnostic test for asthma.[93]

There is evidence of an obesity-asthma endophenotype due to multiple pathophysiologic mechanisms. A physical reason for obesity worsening asthma is the incongruence between lung parenchyma size and airway caliber (known as airway dysanapsis), which can reduce the treatment response to albuterol and inhaled corticosteroids.[94] There is a clear association between neutrophil-mediated inflammation and obesity in asthma, and women with a neutrophilic asthma phenotype are more likely to be obese.[93,95–97] Inflammatory pathways in obesity and asthma are complementary; increased secretion of leptin and adiponectin results in downstream upregulation of inflammatory cytokines IL-6 and tumor necrosis factor-α (TNF-α), which may result in airway hyperresponsiveness.[98] Serum levels of IL-6 (a cytokine also produced by adipose tissue macrophages and a surrogate marker of metabolic dysregulation) are correlated with asthma severity, although some subjects with nonobese body mass indices (BMI) can also have increased IL-6 levels.[99] Adipose tissue inflammation is increased in obese patients with asthma versus obese controls. These facts suggest that BMI and metabolic dysfunction in asthma are not synonymous and that metabolic dysregulation may be more important in this condition than body weight.[100,101]

Nutrition

Although adipose tissue has effects on airway inflammation, an unhealthy diet may also impact asthma control. High-fat diets have been associated with an increase in sputum neutrophils as well as decreased response to inhaled beta-agonists.[102,103] Similarly, worsening dietary standards by decreasing intake of fruit and vegetables is associated with an increase in sputum neutrophils and an increased risk of exacerbations.[104,105] High-fat diets have also shown upregulation of CHI3L1, which could lead to worsening Th2 inflammation.[106] Although a few single nucleotide polymorphisms have been associated with asthma and obesity, these genetic connections have limited treatment implications so far.[107]

Management of asthma in obese patients is also challenging, because they tend to be less responsive to beta-agonists, inhaled or oral corticosteroids, or montelukast.[108–110] Despite the weight-based dosing for omalizumab and other "biologic" agents in asthma, obese patients are less likely to have a significant response to therapy. However, obese patients who respond to omalizumab tend to improve to the same degree as nonobese responders.[111] Treatment with systemic glucocorticoids is further complicated by the increased incidence of insulin resistance and diabetes mellitus in the obese population.

Weight loss and lifestyle interventions are of paramount importance in the management of the obese-asthma phenotype. Up to 10% weight loss is associated with improvement in QOL in up to 83% of patients, with better asthma control in 58% of patients. Exercise has also demonstrated reduction in sputum eosinophils by 50%.[19] As an adjunct to diet and exercise, weight loss medications have also shown promise in improving weight, QOL, and FVC.[112] Bariatric surgery can also improve asthma symptoms in obese patients; these patients not only had improved asthma-related QOL and asthma control scores but also had improvement of airway hyperresponsiveness based on methacholine challenge testing.[113]

Gastroesophageal Reflux Disease

Although the coexistence of asthma with gastroesophageal reflux disease (GERD, also called laryngopharyngeal reflux) has been linked to both earlier onset of asthma symptoms and poorer asthma control, a pathophysiologic mechanism has yet to be established.[11] There are 2 main working theories on the coexisting of asthma and GERD: *reflux theory*, which posits that direct exposure to acid and nonacid gastric content could lead to damage of the airways and possibly of the pulmonary parenchyma, whereas *reflex theory* suggests hyper-bronchoconstriction as a result of vagal stimulation.[114]

Prevalence of GERD in patients with asthma has been estimated from 35% to 82%, with a greater likelihood for coexisting GERD in patients with severe or difficult-to-control asthma.[115] Conversely, patients with GERD also have an increased prevalence of asthma versus controls.[116] Several trials suggested that treatment of GERD in patients with asthma could improve lung function and reduce the use of controller medications.[117,118]

Despite the increased incidence of GERD in asthma patients, based on several randomized trials, empiric treatment with proton pump inhibitors in all patients or just in patients with mild to moderate asthma is currently not recommended.[119–121] In addition to aggressive gastric acid suppression therapy with medical therapy, procedures to improve competency of the lower esophageal sphincter, including Nissen fundoplication or laparoscopic attachment of magnetic beads around the lower esophageal sphincter, have shown improvement in refractory asthma.[122] Some medications for asthma can worsen reflux, therefore reducing duration of corticosteroid therapy, and judicial use of beta-agonists, which relax the lower esophageal sphincter, can improve reflux symptoms.[123,124] Patients with severe asthma with self-reported GERD symptoms and individuals found to have reflux when evaluated by gastroenterologists are likely to benefit from aggressive antiacid therapy. The role for treating coexistent GERD and asthma as well as the impact of nonacid reflux in asthma management is still being debated.

Obstructive Sleep Apnea

Obstructive sleep apnea (OSA) is an important comorbid condition in asthma ("alternative overlap syndrome"[69]), because these patients often have well-described nocturnal symptoms, including nighttime asthma attacks, poor sleep quality, snoring, and excessive daytime sleepiness.[125–127] Patients with fatigue and daytime sleepiness experience worsening scores on respiratory QOL questionnaires, and subjects with asthma and OSA experience a higher rate of decline in FEV_1.[128,129] Furthermore, higher Apnea Hypopnea Index (AHI) values have also been associated with increasing frequency of exacerbations.[130] A recent systematic review estimates the prevalence of OSA in asthma to be 19% to 60%, with an even higher prevalence of 50% to 95% in patients with severe or difficult-to-treat asthma.

Several mechanisms have been proposed to connect OSA with asthma. The mechanical stress from snoring as well as repeated, intermittent hypoxemia have been suggested as activators of proinflammatory pathways, heightened downstream sympathetic tone, and endothelial dysfunction, which could result in bronchoconstriction and nighttime asthma attacks. Apnea in OSA may also trigger activation of the muscarinic receptors in the central airways, resulting in higher airway resistance and worse asthma symptoms.[131,132] Proinflammatory cytokines, such as TNF-α, C-reactive protein, IL-6, as well as the adipokine leptin, have been found elevated in OSA patients, which may contribute to bronchoconstriction and subsequent disease exacerbations.[133]

Similarly, vascular endothelial growth factor (VEGF) may be elevated in patients with recurrent hypoxemia; however, there are no data to connect elevated VEGF levels in coexistent asthma and OSA.[131] Worsening respiratory symptoms during rapid eye movement sleep may be secondary to increased cholinergic outflow, which could heighten lower airway reactivity, whereas frequent arousals from sleep may cause a nocturnal increase in airway resistance.[131,134] Diagnosis of OSA can be suggested with in-office tools, such as Berlin and STOP-BANG questionnaires, but ultimately must be confirmed by polysomnogram.[135]

The mainstay of OSA treatment in adults is implementation of nocturnal positive airway pressure, which improves both patient-reported QOL and asthma control, whereas expected improvements in pulmonary function are still unclear. One study showed no improvement in lung function, despite having improved nocturnal asthma control scores, whereas another study showed a reduction in the rate of decline in FEV_1 of asthmatic patients with OSA.[129,136]

Chronic Rhinosinusitis

Approximately half of patients with poorly controlled asthma have chronic rhinosinusitis. Although the provocation of asthma symptoms by allergic rhinitis is well documented, nonallergic rhinitis (NAR) is also a significant trigger for asthma exacerbations. A diagnosis of NAR is made once infectious and allergic causes for rhinitis are excluded; these patients do not have a clinically significant IgE response to aeroallergens. There are several proposed phenotypes for NAR, including idiopathic NAR (formerly known as vasomotor rhinitis), NAR with eosinophilia syndrome, hormonal rhinitis associated with pregnancy, drug-induced rhinitis (also known as rhinitis medicamentosa), gustatory rhinitis, senile rhinitis, atrophic rhinitis, and the cerebrospinal fluid leak–related rhinitis.[137,138]

To date, intranasal saline irrigation and topical steroids represent the main medical therapy for chronic rhinosinusitis. Multiple randomized studies have shown efficacy of nasal saline irrigation in rhinosinusitis, improving symptoms of nasal congestion.[139] Both medical and surgical treatment modalities seemed to improve asthma control scores; however, a sustained improvement was seen in the medical therapy group, particularly in those with nasal polyposis.[140]

Low-dose macrolide therapy has shown some promise in chronic rhinosinusitis and in patients who underwent endoscopic sinus surgery for nasal polyposis. With further study, macrolides may be a consideration for patients with chronic rhinosinusitis refractory to saline irrigation and intranasal steroids.[141]

Samter's triad describes the syndrome of bronchial asthma, ASA sensitivity, and chronic sinusitis associated with nasal polyposis. In patients with chronic rhinosinusitis, the prevalence of Samter's triad has been estimated to be approximately 13% and is more common in patients with poorly controlled asthma. Endoscopic nasal surgery has improved asthma control in patients with severe nasal polyposis when medical therapy fails. Notably, there is a high rate of recurrence in nasal polyposis, and both leukotriene antagonists and antieosinophilic therapy with monoclonal antibodies have shown promise in reducing the need for surgery.[137,142–144]

Paradoxic Vocal Fold Motion Disorder

Paradoxic vocal fold motion disorder (PVFM) is a paradoxic adduction of the vocal cords during inspiration, associated with episodic dyspnea, wheezing, or stridor. One small study noted the prevalence of PVFM in asthmatics to be 19% versus only 5% in a control group; interestingly, patients with PVFM also had more laryngopharyngeal reflux and allergies.[145] Patients with PVFM and asthma have higher health care resource utilization than those without PVFM.[146] Not only is there an increased prevalence of PVFM in asthmatic patients, but also a primary diagnosis of PVFM should be considered in patients previously diagnosed with asthma who have not responded to standard therapy. Patients with coexisting PVFM are more likely to be younger and women. Although most patients have "psychogenic PVFM," it is important to recognize that exertion, rhinitis, and chemical irritants have all been identified as triggers for PVFM.[147]

Diagnostic inquiries into PVFM begin first with a thorough history and physical examination, because both asthma and PVFM present with episodic, sudden symptoms. Inciting factors frequently include emotional stress or exposure to noxious fumes, and symptoms of wheezing can often be localized to an upper airway inspiratory stridor. Although spirometry should classically have truncation of the inspiratory limb of the flow-volume loop, less than 25% of patients with PVFM actually present with this finding. When patients underwent bronchial provocation testing with a methacholine challenge test, more than 60% of patients had truncation of the inspiratory limb of the flow-volume loop. If a strong clinical suspicion for PVFM is present, laryngoscopic evaluation is required.[148–150] Speech language pathology referral may be helpful in alleviating symptoms of PVFM through breathing relaxation techniques and biofeedback mechanisms. Some patients with exercise-induced PVFM may also respond to aerosolized anticholinergic medications before activity.[151]

SUMMARY

Asthma is a chronic, incurable respiratory disease with high burden of health care utilization and impact on patient QOL. Although asthma has traditionally been classified as an allergic disease, nonallergic triggers have been increasingly identified as worsening asthma management. In addition to ensuring adherence to medical therapies, diligent identification of asthma triggers is essential in disease management, and identification of asthma risk factors can prevent disease progression. In addition to disease triggers, common comorbidities, such as obesity, gastroesophageal reflux, OSA, and COPD, could exert significant effects on asthma control, persistence of symptoms, and even the natural history of the disease.

REFERENCES

1. National Asthma Education and Prevention Program. Expert panel report 3: guidelines for the diagnosis and management of asthma. Bethesda (MD): National Heart, Lung, and Blood Institute; 2007. Available at: https://www.nhlbi.nih.gov/science/national-asthma-education-and-prevention-program-naepp. Accessed May 2, 2018.

2. Bahadori K, Doyle-Waters MM, Marra C, et al. Economic burden of asthma: a systematic review. BMC Pulm Med 2009;9:24.

3. Global Initiative for Asthma - GINA. Global strategy for asthma management and prevention. Available at: http://www.ginasthma.com. Accessed May 2, 2018.

4. McGraw-Hill concise dictionary of modern medicine. Columbus (OH): McGraw-Hill Companies, Inc; 2002. Available at: http://medical-dictionary.thefreedictionary.com/trigger. Accessed May 2, 2018.

5. Vernon MK, Wiklund I, Bell JA, et al. What do we know about asthma triggers? a review of the literature. J Asthma 2012;49(10):991–8.

6. Moore WC, Meyers DA, Wenzel SE, et al. Identification of asthma phenotypes using cluster analysis in the Severe Asthma Research Program. Am J Respir Crit Care Med 2010;181(4):315–23.

7. Spielman AJ, Caruso LS, Glovinsky PB. A behavioral perspective on insomnia treatment. Psychiatr Clin North Am 1987;10(4):541–53.

8. Woodruff PG, Modrek B, Choy DF, et al. T-helper type 2-driven inflammation defines major subphenotypes of asthma. Am J Respir Crit Care Med 2009;180(5):388–95.

9. Froidure A, Mouthuy J, Durham SR, et al. Asthma phenotypes and IgE responses. Eur Respir J 2016;47(1):304–19.

10. Jackson DJ, Johnston SL. The role of viruses in acute exacerbations of asthma. J Allergy Clin Immunol 2010;125(6):1178–87 [quiz: 1188–9].

11. Ciprandi G, Gallo F, Gelardi M. Impact of gastric reflux on asthma in clinical practice. Respirology 2018;23(2):230–1.

12. Message SD, Laza-Stanca V, Mallia P, et al. Rhinovirus-induced lower respiratory illness is increased in asthma and related to virus load and Th1/2 cytokine and IL-10 production. Proc Natl Acad Sci U S A 2008;105(36):13562–7.

13. Liao H, Yang Z, Yang C, et al. Impact of viral infection on acute exacerbation of asthma in out-patient clinics: a prospective study. J Thorac Dis 2016; 8(3):505–12.

14. Hayward G, Thompson MJ, Perera R, et al. Corticosteroids for the common cold. Cochrane Database Syst Rev 2015;(10):CD008116.

15. Xia YC, Radwan A, Keenan CR, et al. Glucocorticoid insensitivity in virally infected airway epithelial cells is dependent on transforming growth factor-beta activity. PLoS Pathog 2017;13(1):e1006138.

16. Thomas BJ, Porritt RA, Hertzog PJ, et al. Glucocorticosteroids enhance replication of respiratory viruses: effect of adjuvant interferon. Sci Rep 2014; 4:7176.

17. Yamaya M, Nomura K, Arakawa K, et al. Clarithromycin decreases rhinovirus replication and cytokine production in nasal epithelial cells from subjects with bronchial asthma: effects on IL-6, IL-8 and IL-33. Arch Pharm Res 2017. https://doi.org/10.1007/s12272-017-0950-x.

18. Vasileiou E, Sheikh A, Butler C, et al. Effectiveness of influenza vaccines in asthma: a systematic review and meta-analysis. Clin Infect Dis 2017; 65(8):1388–95.

19. Scott HA, Gibson PG, Garg ML, et al. Dietary restriction and exercise improve airway inflammation and clinical outcomes in overweight and obese asthma: a randomized trial. Clin Exp Allergy 2013;43(1):36–49.

20. Johnston SL, Martin RJ. Chlamydophila pneumoniae and Mycoplasma pneumoniae: a role in asthma pathogenesis? Am J Respir Crit Care Med 2005;172(9):1078–89.

21. Carr TF, Kraft M. Chronic infection and severe asthma. Immunol Allergy Clin North Am 2016; 36(3):483–502.

22. Gibson PG, Yang IA, Upham JW, et al. Effect of azithromycin on asthma exacerbations and quality of

life in adults with persistent uncontrolled asthma (AMAZES): a randomised, double-blind, placebo-controlled trial. Lancet 2017;390(10095):659–68.

23. Tojima I, Shimizu S, Ogawa T, et al. Anti-inflammatory effects of a novel non-antibiotic macrolide, EM900, on mucus secretion of airway epithelium. Auris Nasus Larynx 2015;42(4):332–6.

24. Webley WC, Hahn DL. Infection-mediated asthma: etiology, mechanisms and treatment options, with focus on Chlamydia pneumoniae and macrolides. Respir Res 2017;18(1):98.

25. Crapo RO, Casaburi R, Coates AL, et al. Guidelines for methacholine and exercise challenge testing-1999. This official statement of the American Thoracic Society was adopted by the ATS Board of Directors, July 1999. Am J Respir Crit Care Med 2000;161(1):309–29.

26. Carlsen KH, Anderson SD, Bjermer L, et al. Exercise-induced asthma, respiratory and allergic disorders in elite athletes: epidemiology, mechanisms and diagnosis: part I of the report from the Joint Task Force of the European Respiratory Society (ERS) and the European Academy of Allergy and Clinical Immunology (EAACI) in cooperation with GA2LEN. Allergy 2008;63(4):387–403.

27. Bonini M, Gramiccioni C, Fioretti D, et al. Asthma, allergy and the Olympics: a 12-year survey in elite athletes. Curr Opin Allergy Clin Immunol 2015; 15(2):184–92.

28. Hallstrand TS, Moody MW, Wurfel MM, et al. Inflammatory basis of exercise-induced bronchoconstriction. Am J Respir Crit Care Med 2005;172(6): 679–86.

29. Gauvreau GM, Ronnen GM, Watson RM, et al. Exercise-induced bronchoconstriction does not cause eosinophilic airway inflammation or airway hyperresponsiveness in subjects with asthma. Am J Respir Crit Care Med 2000;162(4 Pt 1): 1302–7.

30. Crimi E, Balbo A, Milanese M, et al. Airway inflammation and occurrence of delayed bronchoconstriction in exercise-induced asthma. Am Rev Respir Dis 1992;146(2):507–12.

31. Canning BJ, Fischer A. Neural regulation of airway smooth muscle tone. Respir Physiol 2001;125(1–2): 113–27.

32. Simpson AJ, Romer LM, Kippelen P. Self-reported symptoms after induced and inhibited bronchoconstriction in athletes. Med Sci Sports Exerc 2015;47(10):2005–13.

33. Aaron SD, Vandemheen KL, FitzGerald JM, et al. Reevaluation of diagnosis in adults with physician-diagnosed asthma. JAMA 2017;317(3): 269–79.

34. Boulet LP, O'Byrne PM. Asthma and exercise-induced bronchoconstriction in athletes. N Engl J Med 2015;372(7):641–8.

35. Cote A, Turmel J, Boulet LP. Exercise and asthma. Semin Respir Crit Care Med 2018;39(1):19–28.

36. Ulrik CS, Frederiksen J. Mortality and markers of risk of asthma death among 1,075 outpatients with asthma. Chest 1995;108(1):10–5.

37. Polosa R, Russo C, Caponnetto P, et al. Greater severity of new onset asthma in allergic subjects who smoke: a 10-year longitudinal study. Respir Res 2011;12:16.

38. Murphy VE, Clifton VL, Gibson PG. The effect of cigarette smoking on asthma control during exacerbations in pregnant women. Thorax 2010;65(8): 739–44.

39. Shimoda T, Obase Y, Kishikawa R, et al. Influence of cigarette smoking on airway inflammation and inhaled corticosteroid treatment in patients with asthma. Allergy Asthma Proc 2016;37(4):50–8.

40. Chaudhuri R, Livingston E, McMahon AD, et al. Cigarette smoking impairs the therapeutic response to oral corticosteroids in chronic asthma. Am J Respir Crit Care Med 2003; 168(11):1308–11.

41. Nadif R, Matran R, Maccario J, et al. Passive and active smoking and exhaled nitric oxide levels according to asthma and atopy in adults. Ann Allergy Asthma Immunol 2010;104(5):385–93.

42. Tommola M, Ilmarinen P, Tuomisto LE, et al. The effect of smoking on lung function: a clinical study of adult-onset asthma. Eur Respir J 2016;48(5): 1298–306.

43. Eisner MD, Klein J, Hammond SK, et al. Directly measured second hand smoke exposure and asthma health outcomes. Thorax 2005;60(10): 814–21.

44. Grarup PA, Janner JH, Ulrik CS. Passive smoking is associated with poor asthma control during pregnancy: a prospective study of 500 pregnancies. PLoS One 2014;9(11):e112435.

45. Croghan IT, Ebbert JO, Hays JT, et al. Impact of a countywide smoke-free workplace law on emergency department visits for respiratory diseases: a retrospective cohort study. BMC Pulm Med 2015;15:6.

46. Menzies D, Nair A, Williamson PA, et al. Respiratory symptoms, pulmonary function, and markers of inflammation among bar workers before and after a legislative ban on smoking in public places. JAMA 2006;296(14):1742–8.

47. Tonnesen P, Pisinger C, Hvidberg S, et al. Effects of smoking cessation and reduction in asthmatics. Nicotine Tob Res 2005;7(1):139–48.

48. Chaudhuri R, Livingston E, McMahon AD, et al. Effects of smoking cessation on lung function and airway inflammation in smokers with asthma. Am J Respir Crit Care Med 2006;174(2):127–33.

49. Piccillo G, Caponnetto P, Barton S, et al. Changes in airway hyperresponsiveness following smoking

cessation: comparisons between Mch and AMP. Respir Med 2008;102(2):256–65.

50. Larsen K, Faulkner GEJ, Boak A, et al. Looking beyond cigarettes: are Ontario adolescents with asthma less likely to smoke e-cigarettes, marijuana, waterpipes or tobacco cigarettes? Respir Med 2016;120:10–5.

51. Kim SY, Sim S, Choi HG. Active, passive, and electronic cigarette smoking is associated with asthma in adolescents. Sci Rep 2017;7(1):17789.

52. Self TH, Shah SP, March KL, et al. Asthma associated with the use of cocaine, heroin, and marijuana: a review of the evidence. J Asthma 2017; 54(7):714–22.

53. Goodwin RD, Jacobi F, Thefeld W. Mental disorders and asthma in the community. Arch Gen Psychiatry 2003;60(11):1125–30.

54. Lavoie KL, Cartier A, Labrecque M, et al. Are psychiatric disorders associated with worse asthma control and quality of life in asthma patients? Respir Med 2005;99(10):1249–57.

55. Wood BL, Lim J, Miller BD, et al. Family emotional climate, depression, emotional triggering of asthma, and disease severity in pediatric asthma: examination of pathways of effect. J Pediatr Psychol 2007;32(5):542–51.

56. Trojan TD, Khan DA, Defina LF, et al. Asthma and depression: the Cooper Center Longitudinal Study. Ann Allergy Asthma Immunol 2014;112(5):432–6.

57. Hutter N, Knecht A, Baumeister H. Health care costs in persons with asthma and comorbid mental disorders: a systematic review. Gen Hosp Psychiatry 2011;33(5):443–53.

58. Del Giacco SR, Cappai A, Gambula L, et al. The asthma-anxiety connection. Respir Med 2016;120: 44–53.

59. Miller, R. Trigger control to enhance asthma management. In: Bochner BS, editor. UpToDate 2018. Available at: https://www.uptodate.com/contents/trigger-control-to-enhance-asthma-management?search=miller%20asthma%20trigger%20control&source=search_result&selectedTitle=1~127&usage_type=default&display_rank=1. Accessed November 14, 2018.

60. Gupta RS, Zhang X, Springston EE, et al. The association between community crime and childhood asthma prevalence in Chicago. Ann Allergy Asthma Immunol 2010;104(4):299–306.

61. Pittman TP, Nykiforuk CI, Mignone J, et al. The association between community stressors and asthma prevalence of school children in Winnipeg, Canada. Int J Environ Res Public Health 2012;9(2): 579–95.

62. Lind N, Nordin M, Palmquist E, et al. Psychological distress in asthma and allergy: the Vasterbotten Environmental Health Study. Psychol Health Med 2014;19(3):316–23.

63. Ritz T, Wittchen HU, Klotsche J, et al. Asthma trigger reports are associated with low quality of life, exacerbations, and emergency treatments. Ann Am Thorac Soc 2016;13(2):204–11.

64. Morales DR, Jackson C, Lipworth BJ, et al. Adverse respiratory effect of acute beta-blocker exposure in asthma: a systematic review and meta-analysis of randomized controlled trials. Chest 2014;145(4):779–86.

65. Morales DR, Dreischulte T, Lipworth BJ, et al. Respiratory effect of beta-blocker eye drops in asthma: population-based study and meta-analysis of clinical trials. Br J Clin Pharmacol 2016;82(3): 814–22.

66. Morales DR, Guthrie B, Lipworth BJ, et al. NSAID-exacerbated respiratory disease: a meta-analysis evaluating prevalence, mean provocative dose of aspirin and increased asthma morbidity. Allergy 2015;70(7):828–35.

67. Gibson PG, Simpson JL. The overlap syndrome of asthma and COPD: what are its features and how important is it? Thorax 2009;64(8):728–35.

68. Diagnosis and Initial Treatment of Asthma, COPD and Asthma - COPD Overlap (a joint project of GINA and GOLD, updated April 2017). Global Initiative for Asthma (GINA, ginasthma.org) 2017. Available at: https://ginasthma.org/. Accessed November 14, 2018.

69. Ioachimescu OC, Teodorescu M. Integrating the overlap of obstructive lung disease and obstructive sleep apnoea: OLDOSA syndrome. Respirology 2013;18(3):421–31.

70. Kauppi P, Kupiainen H, Lindqvist A, et al. Overlap syndrome of asthma and COPD predicts low quality of life. J Asthma 2011;48(3):279–85.

71. Shaya FT, Dongyi D, Akazawa MO, et al. Burden of concomitant asthma and COPD in a Medicaid population. Chest 2008;134(1):14–9.

72. Blanchette CM, Broder M, Ory C, et al. Cost and utilization of COPD and asthma among insured adults in the US. Curr Med Res Opin 2009;25(6): 1385–92.

73. Rhee CK, Yoon HK, Yoo KH, et al. Medical utilization and cost in patients with overlap syndrome of chronic obstructive pulmonary disease and asthma. COPD 2014;11(2):163–70.

74. Wurst KE, Kelly-Reif K, Bushnell GA, et al. Understanding asthma-chronic obstructive pulmonary disease overlap syndrome. Respir Med 2016;110: 1–11.

75. Marsh SE, Travers J, Weatherall M, et al. Proportional classifications of COPD phenotypes. Thorax 2008;63(9):761–7.

76. Weatherall M, Travers J, Shirtcliffe PM, et al. Distinct clinical phenotypes of airways disease defined by cluster analysis. Eur Respir J 2009; 34(4):812–8.

77. Mannino DM, Gagnon RC, Petty TL, et al. Obstructive lung disease and low lung function in adults in the United States: data from the National Health and Nutrition Examination Survey, 1988-1994. Arch Intern Med 2000;160(11):1683–9.

78. Soriano JB, Davis KJ, Coleman B, et al. The proportional Venn diagram of obstructive lung disease: two approximations from the United States and the United Kingdom. Chest 2003;124(2):474–81.

79. McDonald VM, Simpson JL, Higgins I, et al. Multidimensional assessment of older people with asthma and COPD: clinical management and health status. Age Ageing 2011;40(1):42–9.

80. Louie S, Zeki AA, Schivo M, et al. The asthma-chronic obstructive pulmonary disease overlap syndrome: pharmacotherapeutic considerations. Expert Rev Clin Pharmacol 2013;6(2):197–219.

81. Dweik RA, Boggs PB, Erzurum SC, et al. An official ATS clinical practice guideline: interpretation of exhaled nitric oxide levels (FENO) for clinical applications. Am J Respir Crit Care Med 2011;184(5):602–15.

82. Tamada T, Sugiura H, Takahashi T, et al. Biomarker-based detection of asthma-COPD overlap syndrome in COPD populations. Int J Chron Obstruct Pulmon Dis 2015;10:2169–76.

83. Kitaguchi Y, Komatsu Y, Fujimoto K, et al. Sputum eosinophilia can predict responsiveness to inhaled corticosteroid treatment in patients with overlap syndrome of COPD and asthma. Int J Chron Obstruct Pulmon Dis 2012;7:283–9.

84. Chen FJ, Huang XY, Liu YL, et al. Importance of fractional exhaled nitric oxide in the differentiation of asthma-COPD overlap syndrome, asthma, and COPD. Int J Chron Obstruct Pulmon Dis 2016;11:2385–90.

85. Akinbami LJ, Moorman JE, Liu X, National Center for Health Statistics (U.S.). Asthma prevalence, health care use, and mortality : United States, 2005-2009. Hyattsville (MD): U.S. Dept. of Health and Human Services, Centers for Disease Control and Prevention, National Center for Health Statistics; 2011.

86. Beuther DA, Sutherland ER. Overweight, obesity, and incident asthma: a meta-analysis of prospective epidemiologic studies. Am J Respir Crit Care Med 2007;175(7):661–6.

87. Braido F, Brusselle G, Guastalla D, et al. Determinants and impact of suboptimal asthma control in Europe: the International Cross-Sectional And Longitudinal Assessment on Asthma ControL (LIAISON) study. Respir Res 2016;17(1):51.

88. Tay TR, Radhakrishna N, Hore-Lacy F, et al. Comorbidities in difficult asthma are independent risk factors for frequent exacerbations, poor control and diminished quality of life. Respirology 2016;21(8):1384–90.

89. Baltieri L, Claudio Martins L, Cazzo E, et al. Analysis of quality of life among asthmatic individuals with obesity and its relationship with pulmonary function: cross-sectional study. Sao Paulo Med J 2017;135(4):332–8.

90. Okubo Y, Nochioka K, Hataya H, et al. Burden of obesity on pediatric inpatients with acute asthma exacerbation in the United States. J Allergy Clin Immunol Pract 2016;4(6):1227–31.

91. King GG, Brown NJ, Diba C, et al. The effects of body weight on airway calibre. Eur Respir J 2005;25(5):896–901.

92. Strunk RC, Colvin R, Bacharier LB, et al. Airway obstruction worsens in young adults with asthma who become obese. J Allergy Clin Immunol Pract 2015;3(5):765–71.e762.

93. Holguin F, Comhair SA, Hazen SL, et al. An association between L-arginine/asymmetric dimethyl arginine balance, obesity, and the age of asthma onset phenotype. Am J Respir Crit Care Med 2013;187(2):153–9.

94. Forno E, Weiner DJ, Mullen J, et al. Obesity and airway dysanapsis in children with and without asthma. Am J Respir Crit Care Med 2017;195(3):314–23.

95. Forno E, Acosta-Perez E, Brehm JM, et al. Obesity and adiposity indicators, asthma, and atopy in Puerto Rican children. J Allergy Clin Immunol 2014;133(5):1308–14, 1314.e1-5.

96. Visness CM, London SJ, Daniels JL, et al. Association of childhood obesity with atopic and nonatopic asthma: results from the national health and nutrition examination survey 1999-2006. J Asthma 2010;47(7):822–9.

97. Telenga ED, Tideman SW, Kerstjens HA, et al. Obesity in asthma: more neutrophilic inflammation as a possible explanation for a reduced treatment response. Allergy 2012;67(8):1060–8.

98. Fantuzzi G. Adipose tissue, adipokines, and inflammation. J Allergy Clin Immunol 2005;115(5):911–9 [quiz: 920].

99. Peters MC, McGrath KW, Hawkins GA, et al. Plasma interleukin-6 concentrations, metabolic dysfunction, and asthma severity: a cross-sectional analysis of two cohorts. Lancet Respir Med 2016;4(7):574–84.

100. Peters U, Dixon AE, Forno E. Obesity and asthma. J Allergy Clin Immunol 2018;141(4):1169–79.

101. Sideleva O, Suratt BT, Black KE, et al. Obesity and asthma: an inflammatory disease of adipose tissue not the airway. Am J Respir Crit Care Med 2012;186(7):598–605.

102. Wood LG, Garg ML, Gibson PG. A high-fat challenge increases airway inflammation and impairs bronchodilator recovery in asthma. J Allergy Clin Immunol 2011;127(5):1133–40.

103. Scott HA, Gibson PG, Garg ML, et al. Airway inflammation is augmented by obesity and fatty acids in asthma. Eur Respir J 2011;38(3):594–602.

104. Wood LG, Garg ML, Powell H, et al. Lycopene-rich treatments modify noneosinophilic airway inflammation in asthma: proof of concept. Free Radic Res 2008;42(1):94–102.

105. Wood LG, Garg ML, Smart JM, et al. Manipulating antioxidant intake in asthma: a randomized controlled trial. Am J Clin Nutr 2012;96(3):534–43.

106. Ahangari F, Sood A, Ma B, et al. Chitinase 3-like-1 regulates both visceral fat accumulation and asthma-like Th2 inflammation. Am J Respir Crit Care Med 2015;191(7):746–57.

107. Butsch Kovacic M, Martin LJ, Biagini Myers JM, et al. Genetic approach identifies distinct asthma pathways in overweight vs normal weight children. Allergy 2015;70(8):1028–32.

108. Boulet LP, Franssen E. Influence of obesity on response to fluticasone with or without salmeterol in moderate asthma. Respir Med 2007;101(11):2240–7.

109. Camargo CA Jr, Boulet LP, Sutherland ER, et al. Body mass index and response to asthma therapy: fluticasone propionate/salmeterol versus montelukast. J Asthma 2010;47(1):76–82.

110. Sutherland ER, Goleva E, Strand M, et al. Body mass and glucocorticoid response in asthma. Am J Respir Crit Care Med 2008;178(7):682–7.

111. Gibson PG, Reddel H, McDonald VM, et al. Effectiveness and response predictors of omalizumab in a severe allergic asthma population with a high prevalence of comorbidities: the Australian Xolair Registry. Intern Med J 2016;46(9):1054–62.

112. Dias-Junior SA, Reis M, de Carvalho-Pinto RM, et al. Effects of weight loss on asthma control in obese patients with severe asthma. Eur Respir J 2014;43(5):1368–77.

113. Dixon AE, Pratley RE, Forgione PM, et al. Effects of obesity and bariatric surgery on airway hyperresponsiveness, asthma control, and inflammation. J Allergy Clin Immunol 2011;128(3):508–15.e1-2.

114. Castell DO, Schnatz PF. Gastroesophageal reflux disease and asthma. Reflux or reflex? Chest 1995;108(5):1186–7.

115. Liang B, Yi Q, Feng Y. Association of gastroesophageal reflux disease with asthma control. Dis Esophagus 2013;26(8):794–8.

116. Havemann BD, Henderson CA, El-Serag HB. The association between gastro-oesophageal reflux disease and asthma: a systematic review. Gut 2007;56(12):1654–64.

117. Sharma B, Sharma M, Daga MK, et al. Effect of omeprazole and domperidone on adult asthmatics with gastroesophageal reflux. World J Gastroenterol 2007;13(11):1706–10.

118. Larrain A, Carrasco E, Galleguillos F, et al. Medical and surgical treatment of nonallergic asthma associated with gastroesophageal reflux. Chest 1991;99(6):1330–5.

119. Chan WW, Chiou E, Obstein KL, et al. The efficacy of proton pump inhibitors for the treatment of asthma in adults: a meta-analysis. Arch Intern Med 2011;171(7):620–9.

120. Kiljander TO, Junghard O, Beckman O, et al. Effect of esomeprazole 40 mg once or twice daily on asthma: a randomized, placebo-controlled study. Am J Respir Crit Care Med 2010;181(10):1042–8.

121. American Lung Association Asthma Clinical Research Centers, Mastronarde JG, Anthonisen NR, et al. Efficacy of esomeprazole for treatment of poorly controlled asthma. N Engl J Med 2009;360(15):1487–99.

122. Sriratanaviriyakul N, Kivler C, Vidovszky TJ, et al. LINX(R), a novel treatment for patients with refractory asthma complicated by gastroesophageal reflux disease: a case report. J Med Case Rep 2016;10(1):124.

123. Lazenby JP, Guzzo MR, Harding SM, et al. Oral corticosteroids increase esophageal acid contact times in patients with stable asthma. Chest 2002;121(2):625–34.

124. Gupta S, Lodha R, Kabra SK. Asthma, GERD and obesity: triangle of inflammation. Indian J Pediatr 2018;85(10):887–92.

125. Teodorescu M, Consens FB, Bria WF, et al. Correlates of daytime sleepiness in patients with asthma. Sleep Med 2006;7(8):607–13.

126. Kales A, Beall GN, Bajor GF, et al. Sleep studies in asthmatic adults: relationship of attacks to sleep stage and time of night. J Allergy 1968;41(3):164–73.

127. Fitzpatrick MF, Engleman H, Whyte KF, et al. Morbidity in nocturnal asthma: sleep quality and daytime cognitive performance. Thorax 1991;46(8):569–73.

128. Vinnikov D, Blanc PD, Alilin A, et al. Fatigue and sleepiness determine respiratory quality of life among veterans evaluated for sleep apnea. Health Qual Life Outcomes 2017;15(1):48.

129. Wang TY, Lo YL, Lin SM, et al. Obstructive sleep apnoea accelerates FEV1 decline in asthmatic patients. BMC Pulm Med 2017;17(1):55.

130. Wang Y, Liu K, Hu K, et al. Impact of obstructive sleep apnea on severe asthma exacerbations. Sleep Med 2016;26:1–5.

131. Puthalapattu S, Ioachimescu OC. Asthma and obstructive sleep apnea: clinical and pathogenic interactions. J Investig Med 2014;62(4):665–75.

132. Hatipoglu U, Rubinstein I. Inflammation and obstructive sleep apnea syndrome: how many ways do I look at thee? Chest 2004;126(1):1–2.

133. Nadeem R, Molnar J, Madbouly EM, et al. Serum inflammatory markers in obstructive sleep apnea: a meta-analysis. J Clin Sleep Med 2013;9(10):1003–12.

134. Khatri SB, Ioachimescu OC. The intersection of obstructive lung disease and sleep apnea. Cleve Clin J Med 2016;83(2):127–40.

135. Lu H, Fu C, Li W, et al. Screening for obstructive sleep apnea syndrome in asthma patients: a prospective study based on Berlin and STOP-Bang questionnaires. J Thorac Dis 2017;9(7):1945–58.

136. Ciftci TU, Ciftci B, Guven SF, et al. Effect of nasal continuous positive airway pressure in uncontrolled nocturnal asthmatic patients with obstructive sleep apnea syndrome. Respir Med 2005;99(5):529–34.

137. Porsbjerg C, Menzies-Gow A. Co-morbidities in severe asthma: clinical impact and management. Respirology 2017;22(4):651–61.

138. Daramola OO, Kern RC. An update regarding the treatment of nonallergic rhinitis. Curr Opin Otolaryngol Head Neck Surg 2016;24(1):10–4.

139. Chong LY, Head K, Hopkins C, et al. Saline irrigation for chronic rhinosinusitis. Cochrane Database Syst Rev 2016;(4):CD011995.

140. Ragab S, Scadding GK, Lund VJ, et al. Treatment of chronic rhinosinusitis and its effects on asthma. Eur Respir J 2006;28(1):68–74.

141. Lasso A, Masoudian P, Quinn JG, et al. Long-term low-dose macrolides for chronic rhinosinusitis in adults - a systematic review of the literature. Clin Otolaryngol 2017;42(3):637–50.

142. Samter M, Beers RF Jr. Intolerance to aspirin. Clinical studies and consideration of its pathogenesis. Ann Intern Med 1968;68(5):975–83.

143. Bachert C, Sousa AR, Lund VJ, et al. Reduced need for surgery in severe nasal polyposis with mepolizumab: randomized trial. J Allergy Clin Immunol 2017;140(4):1024–31.e14.

144. Yelverton JC, Holmes TW, Johnson CM, et al. Effectiveness of leukotriene receptor antagonism in the postoperative management of chronic rhinosinusitis. Int Forum Allergy Rhinol 2016;6(3):243–7.

145. Yelken K, Yilmaz A, Guven M, et al. Paradoxical vocal fold motion dysfunction in asthma patients. Respirology 2009;14(5):729–33.

146. Mikita J, Parker J. High levels of medical utilization by ambulatory patients with vocal cord dysfunction as compared to age- and gender-matched asthmatics. Chest 2006;129(4):905–8.

147. Morris MJ, Christopher KL. Diagnostic criteria for the classification of vocal cord dysfunction. Chest 2010;138(5):1213–23.

148. Morris MJ, Deal LE, Bean DR, et al. Vocal cord dysfunction in patients with exertional dyspnea. Chest 1999;116(6):1676–82.

149. Perkins PJ, Morris MJ. Vocal cord dysfunction induced by methacholine challenge testing. Chest 2002;122(6):1988–93.

150. Walsted ES, Hull JH, Sverrild A, et al. Bronchial provocation testing does not detect exercise-induced laryngeal obstruction. J Asthma 2017;54(1):77–83.

151. Weinberger M, Doshi D. Vocal cord dysfunction: a functional cause of respiratory distress. Breathe (Sheff) 2017;13(1):15–21.

Microbiome in Mechanisms of Asthma

Tara F. Carr, MD*, Rhonda Alkatib, MD, Monica Kraft, MD

KEYWORDS

- Microbiome • Asthma • Lung • Gut • Short-chain fatty acids • Type 2 inflammation

KEY POINTS

- The human microbiome impacts the development of asthma through direct and indirect mechanisms.
- There are independent relationships between the different microbiome niches, particularly lung and gut, and the development of asthma.
- The mechanisms through which the microbiome relate to asthma involve immune development, immune tolerance, functional metabolites, and relationship to infections.
- Further work is necessary to determine how and when manipulation of the microbiome may be implemented toward the prevention or treatment of asthma.

INTRODUCTION

The development and implementation of non-culture-based methods to identify bacteria, commonly 16s ribosomal RNA sequencing, have identified an enormous diversity and quantity of bacterial species living within and on the human host. It is estimated that more than 10,000 different microbial species live in and on humans, representing 100 trillion organisms. Importantly, this so-called human microbiome is in a commensal, symbiotic relationship with the human host, which is thought to be necessary for many host functions, including immune regulation. The microbiome may indeed impact the balance between heath and disease of many organ systems, including the respiratory, cardiovascular, gastrointestinal, and immune systems.[1–4] Specifically, in asthma, the human microbiome may contribute to the development and severity of asthma. This article describes the current knowledge of the relationship of human microbiome niches to asthma development and severity, and the mechanisms thought to contribute to this relationship.

EARLY LIFE EXPOSURES

The often-discussed "hygiene hypothesis" harbors the idea that exposure to various bacteria and other microbiota in early infancy and childhood can diminish the risk of subsequent allergy and asthma.[5] This relationship has been studied in robust population cohorts, some of which leverage geopolitics and population bottlenecking to describe differences in exposures, microbiome development, and health outcomes.

von Mutius and colleagues[6] recognized that growing up in a traditional European farm environment seemed to protect children from developing asthma and other atopic disorders, when compared with children growing up in urbanized areas. This group has subsequently described a variety of

Disclosure Statement: Dr T.F. Carr reports royalties from Wolters-Kluwer; and has provided consulting services to Sanofi-Regeneron, AstraZeneca, and Boehringer Ingelheim. Dr R. Alkatib has no disclosures to report. Dr M. Kraft reports royalties from Elsevier; has received research funds paid to the University of Arizona by National Institutes of Health, American Lung Association, Sanofi-Regeneron, and Chiesi; and has provided consulting services to Astra-Zeneca, Sanofi-Regeneron, and TEVA Pharmaceuticals.
Department of Medicine, University of Arizona, 1501 North Campbell Avenue, Tucson, AZ 85724-5030, USA
* Corresponding author.
E-mail address: tcarr@deptofmed.arizona.edu

Clin Chest Med 40 (2019) 87–96
https://doi.org/10.1016/j.ccm.2018.10.006

environmental exposures to be protective against asthma and allergic sensitization, including exposure to pet dogs and farm animals,[7] and measurable differences of endotoxin load in bedding suggested increased diversity of environmental microorganisms in those exposed populations.[8] Furthermore, ingestion of raw cow's milk is inversely correlated with asthma in this population.[9] Murine models of allergic asthma have shown that ingestion of raw cow's milk can prevent house dust mite–induced airways hyperresponsiveness (AHR) and lung eosinophilia by suppressing airway production of chemokine ligand 17 and type 2 inflammatory cytokines interleukin (IL)-5 and IL-13, suggesting altered epithelial or innate lymphoid cell responses to the raw milk.[10]

Individuals living across the Russia-Finland border in the Karelia region, although of similar ancestry, have distinctly different rates of disease and different lifestyles, the Finnish side having higher socioeconomic status and substantial urbanization. Those living on the Finnish side have substantially higher rates of asthma, allergen sensitization, and eczema compared with those living on the Russian side of the border, and the skin and nasal microbial communities differ between populations.[11] One possible explanation or contributing factor to these epidemiologic findings is that those living in Russian Karelia have significantly higher microbial burden in their drinking water compared with those in Finnish Karelia, an exposure that seems to be protective against atopy.[12] Researchers have determined that health on both sides of that international border relates more to the diversity of overall bacterial environmental exposures than any one exposure. The underlying mechanism may be attributable to immune skewing by less diverse dust to eosinophilic responses, compared with type 1 helper-T cell (Th1)-transformation of naive T lymphocytes or induction of IL-10 responses by more diverse bacterial exposure.[13]

The Amish and Hutterite communities of the United States are rural farming populations with closely related European ancestry, who share similarities in diet and family size. However, whereas the Hutterites have embraced industrialized farming, the Amish use traditional farming practices that exclude mechanization. The prevalence of asthma and allergy in the Amish population is strikingly lower than that of the Hutterites.[14] Stein and colleagues[15] made extracts from indoor dust samples collected from representative homes of each of these populations and described marked differences in allergen, endotoxin, and bacterial abundance across the sites with much higher burden in the Amish samples. Using a mouse model of allergic asthma, the authors also showed that the Amish dust extracts were protective against allergic airway inflammation in a manner dependent on innate immune signaling. These data suggest that one or many components of the dust, particularly the bacterial colonies, function through innate immune mechanisms to protect against the development of allergic inflammation and asthma.

These and other population studies strongly support that certain environmental exposures, particularly to bacterial organisms, are protective against the development of asthma and atopic diseases. Because the environment can particularly impact the composition of the lung and gut microbiota, the associations between each of these bacterial niches and development of asthma warrant close evaluation for causal relationships, mechanisms, and therapeutic opportunities.

LUNG MICROBIOME AND ASTHMA

The role of the lung microbiome in the pathogenesis of asthma is not yet fully understood. However, well described are variables during the first years of a child's life, including home environment, viral infections, and antibiotic exposures, which have been correlated with the onset of atopy and asthma.[16] Because these variables also theoretically relate to differences in respiratory exposures and to the lung microbiome, the need for more careful examination of the relationship between the lung microbiome and asthma has sparked enthusiasm on an international level.

The impact of airway bacteria on development of asthma may indeed relate to early life bacterial colony establishment. Bisgaard and colleagues[17] cultured hypopharyngeal aspirates from 1-month-old infants, finding that colonization with the encapsulated bacteria *Streptococcus pneumoniae*, *Moraxella catarrhalis*, and/or *Haemophilus influenzae* was significantly associated with persistent wheeze, hospitalization for wheeze, and asthma diagnosis at age 5. In addition, colonization with any of these bacteria related to increased blood eosinophil counts and elevated total IgE at age 4. A recent study of children with asthma showed that coincident infection of *M catarrhalis* or *S pneumoniae* and rhinovirus conferred greater severity of respiratory tract illness, including asthma exacerbations, suggesting that these, and possibly other, respiratory bacteria contribute to airway inflammation.[18]

Furthermore, infection or colonization of the airway with atypical bacteria, such as *Mycoplasma pneumoniae*, are related to asthma development and severity in epidemiologic and mechanistic studies, and this type of exposure is detected with readily available culture-based or serologic techniques.[19] For example, *M pneumoniae* infection in childhood causes acute wheezing[20] and is associated with structural changes[21] of the lung and long-term lung function deficits,[22] and to the development of asthma.[23] For individuals who already have allergic sensitization, *M pneumoniae* may contribute to the development of asthma through inducing AHR,[24] inflammation,[25] mucin expression,[26,27] and remodeling through collagen deposition.[28] For individuals with asthma, *M pneumoniae* may induce pronounced eosinophilic inflammation,[29] which may relate to severity of disease[30] or host innate immune response characteristics.[31] Treatment of the infection or related inflammation may indeed provide asthma control for the affected patient[32] and underscore the importance of bacterial exposures to asthma.

Respiratory pathogens, such as those noted previously, are easy to identify using culture-based or serologic laboratory techniques that are widely commercially available. However, with the recognition of the myriad bacterial species that are not easily cultured, more recent work has focused on using non-culture-based techniques to examine and characterize the scope of microbiota in human niches, and to relate differences in these populations to clinical outcomes. Researchers and clinicians assumed for many years that the lungs were a sterile environment; however, a plethora of common bacterial phyla are now recognized as colonizers of the entire respiratory tract, including in the lungs. Such phyla include Actinobacteria, Bacteroidetes, Firmicutes, and Proteobacteria, with estimates of almost 2000 bacterial genomes present per square centimeter of a single upper lobe of the lung.[33]

When using non-culture-based techniques to compare bacteria present in the lungs of healthy adults with patients with asthma, patients with asthma have lower proportions of Bacteroidetes and increased Proteobacteria, particularly *Haemophilus*.[34] Marri and colleagues[35] reported alterations in the microbial composition of induced sputum of patients with asthma that were similar among patients with asthma suffering from mild or severe disease but distinguished patients with asthma from normal control subjects, and which also noted increased Proteobacteria in samples from patients with asthma. Huang and colleagues[36] performed 16s sequencing for bacterial rRNA on bronchial epithelial brushing from subjects with asthma and healthy subjects. In this study, samples from patients with asthma had

significantly higher bacterial burden and bacterial diversity. Further, AHR in the patients with asthma was related to the relative abundance of members of the Comamonadaceae, Sphingomonadaceae, and Oxalobacteraceae phylotypes, and interestingly, increased bacterial diversity was related to improvement in AHR following clarithromycin therapy.

Lung microbiota may contribute not only to presence of asthma, but to asthma phenotypes and severity. Durack and colleagues[37] compared microbiota from bronchial brushings among healthy patients, patients with asthma, and patients with atopy, showing that subjects with type 2 inflammation had lower bacterial burden than other patients with asthma. A recent study by Taylor and colleagues[38] showed that asthma with prominent airway neutrophilia was characterized by lower microbial richness with enrichment of airway colonies for members of the class Gammaproteobacteria, to which *Haemophilus* and *Moraxella* belong, and that these microbiota characteristics relate to asthma severity. Green and colleagues[39] similarly identified bacterial profiles of induced sputum from patients with severe asthma, dominated by *Moraxella*, *Haemophilus*, or *Streptococcal spp*, in the airway to be associated with severe airway obstruction and airway neutrophilia.

To relate the bronchial microbiome to phenotypic and epigenetic features of asthma, Huang and colleagues[40] performed bronchial bacterial composition by 16s sequencing in patients with severe asthma and healthy control patients. These investigators found that Proteobacteria enrichment related to worsening asthma control, fewer airway eosinophils, and the induction of Th17-related genes. In contrast, Actinobacteria were prominent in patients with high epithelial gene expression for FK506 binding protein, a marker of steroid responsiveness. These findings suggest that the mechanisms relating the bacterial species enrichment and clinical outcomes relate directly to proinflammatory pathways and treatment responsiveness. Goleva and colleagues[41] compared 16s sequencing from bronchoalveolar lavage in corticosteroid-resistant and corticosteroid-responsive patients with asthma, finding relative increased abundance of Proteobacteria (including *Neisseria*, *Haemophilus spp*), Fusobacteria, Firmicutes, and Actinobacteria in the steroid-resistant patients. The authors supported these findings with *in vitro* experiments, showing *Haemophilus parainfluenzae* to activate toll-like receptor 4, subsequently activating transforming growth factor-β–associated kinase-1, which induces transcription of proinflammatory factors, such as IL-8, while inhibiting glucocorticoid-receptor-mediated mitogen-activated kinase phosphatase 1 production and conferring corticosteroid resistance. Because inhaled steroids are a mainstay of asthma therapy, this pathway to steroid resistance may help to explain severe and steroid-unresponsive asthma.

Mechanistic evaluations of these airway microbiotic influences on asthma susceptibility are largely reliant on murine models. Published literature supports the importance of early life lung microbiome development on risk of asthma. Herbst and colleagues[42] used a mouse model of allergic asthma in germ-free and control mice to show that the germ-free mice had elevated airway inflammation, type 2 cytokines, and basophils, and increased AHR on ovalbumin challenge compared with control mice. However, when the neonatal germ-free mice were recolonized with the diverse microbiota from the control mice before allergen sensitization, they exhibited reduced levels of circulating IgE and reduced AHR similar to the control mice. Gollwitzer and colleagues[3] exposed mice at both neonatal and adult stages to house dust mite antigen to compare the effect of age and microbiome development on reactivity to antigen. On antigen exposure, the neonatal mice showed a substantial increase in airway eosinophilia, blood eosinophilia, type 2 cytokine (IL-4, IL-5, and IL-13) production, mucus production, and AHR when compared with mice exposed later in development. The airway microbiome of the neonatal mice was composed of Firmicutes and Gammaproteobacteria, compared with predominance of Bacteroidetes in the adults. The authors concluded that temporal shifts in airway microbiota are associated with decreased responsiveness to aeroallergens, via the induction of T-regulatory cells in a programmed death ligand 1–mediated manner.

Some bacterial exposures may indeed be protective against a type 2 airway response. For example, in a murine model of ovalbumin-induced allergic asthma, pulmonary administration of *Escherichia coli* to the lung induced a TLR4-dependent response with induction of γδ-T cells, decreased dendritic cell activation in the lung, and diminished IL-2 cytokine production, which collectively protected the mice from allergic airway inflammation.[43]

In the aforementioned study by Durack and colleagues,[37] the investigators studied predicted bacterial functions among the differentially expressed bronchial bacteria. Sputum from subjects with asthma was enriched for members of the *Haemophilus*, *Neisseria*, *Fusobacterium*, and *Porphyromonas* species and the Sphingomonodaceae family, and depleted in members of the Mogibacteriaceae family and Lactobacillales order, when compared with healthy control subjects. *In silico*–predicted bacterial functions based on the 16s rRNA sequencing showed enrichment for short-chain fatty acid (SCFA) metabolism. SCFAs are important for epithelial barrier function and have been implicated as important for immune tolerance in the gut (discussed later).

Clearly, patterns of lung microbial dysbiosis are evident among patients with asthma, and Proteobacteria seem to consistently relate to asthma presence, cellular phenotype, and severity. Furthermore, mechanistic work suggests multiple levels of interaction of microbiota and the immune system can confer protection or risk for asthma development. Indeed, the quantity of bacteria, quality of bacteria, time course of exposure and colony establishment, and immunologic function of those bacteria all play a role in the relationship between lung microbiome and asthma (**Fig. 1**). With these findings, the mechanisms by which microbiota determine early life immunity may have great implications when applied to the prevention of both asthma and allergic diseases.

GUT MICROBIOME AND ASTHMA

The gut microbiome is vitally important for health. Evidence underscoring the fundamental need for a gut microbiome includes studies of gnotobiotic mice, where the mice born in a germ-free environment fail to develop normal intestinal structure or normal immune maturation.[44] These findings may simply confirm that an individual's gut microbiome contributes substantially to the proper digestion of foods, releasing minerals, vitamins, and digestive products, such as SCFAs. However, fascinatingly, introduction of different microbial communities into gnotobiotic mice can confer a specific phenotype, such as obesity,[45] abnormal behavior,[46] and immune development.[47] These and other data suggest that manipulation of the gut microbiome may be preventative or therapeutic for many chronic diseases and may indeed be leveraged to address allergic diseases and asthma. To do so, however, requires a better understanding of gut microbiome development and function as pertaining to asthma.

The gut microbiome develops in early life, with a rapid increase in diversity that seems necessary for health.[48] In fact, the microbiome of the gastrointestinal tract, measured by stool sampling, is present even in the first neonatal meconium stool.[49] The stool microbiome develops with time, and evidence supports critical time periods of development of that microbiome for establishing health-protective bacterial communities.

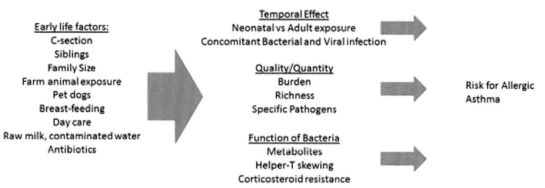

Fig. 1. Exposures and modifying factors contribute to the effect of microbiome on the risk of allergic asthma.

Longitudinal cohorts describe a relationship between establishment of the early life gut microbiome and development of allergic diseases. For example, a cohort from Canada[50] revealed that reduced stool bacterial diversity measured from samples obtained at 3 months of life was associated with risk of asthma through age 3. A study from Sweden revealed that lower microbial diversity within stool samples at 1 week and 1 month of life was related to risk for asthma development through age 7.[51] In both of these cohorts, the stool communities among those children at risk or not became more similar with time and by 12 months of age there was no relationship between stool diversity and asthma risk. In contrast, a study of the Copenhagen Prospective Studies on Asthma in Childhood 2010 cohort assessed diversity of the gut and found that relative abundance of species at 1 year of age were related to asthma at age 5, only among children born to mothers with asthma.[52] A comparison of cellular responses from neonates born in Papua New Guinea showed that antigen-presenting cells from these infants are less active than those from Australia, suggesting that the increased bacterial exposures related to the traditional lifestyle in Papua New Guinea would confer protection against immune responses.[53] Cox and colleagues[54] used a mouse model of low-dose penicillin exposure in early life to show that this exposure transiently affects the microbiota, but has lasting impact on body composition and metabolism. These and other studies support that the window for developing and impacting the gut microbiome may be limited to, or crucially important in, early life but may also relate to multifactorial asthma susceptibility and comorbidities.[49,55]

There are many potential contributing factors to the development of stool microbiome (see **Fig. 1**). Much of the neonatal microbiome conferred during birth differs by mode of delivery. That is, the microbiome of infants delivered vaginally represent that of the mother's vagina and gut. In contrast, the microbiome of infants delivered by caesarian section resembles skin flora.[56] Caesarian section, particularly when performed before membrane rupture, may indeed be a risk factor for the development of atopy and allergic diseases[57]; however, studies of this relationship show conflicting results.

Furthermore, early life exposure to livestock or domesticated pets, particularly dogs, decreases the risk of asthma development through mechanisms that may involve the gut microbiome.[58–60] Early life exposure to traditional, nonmechanized farming environments, such as in the Amish or European cohorts, is protective against asthma in a way that may strongly relate to microbiome through inhaled and ingested exposures.[15,59] Fujimura and colleagues[61] used a murine model of allergic asthma to show that dog-associated house dust exposure via oral gavage protected against asthmatic changes. Furthermore, this protection specifically related to gut microbiome profile (in particular, enrichment for *Lactobacillus johnsonii*) and supplementation of this species could confer protection against the asthma phenotype.

Dietary exposure may also contribute to gut microbiome development. Sordillo and colleagues[62] reported that among other factors, breastfeeding, when compared with bottle-feeding, substantially influenced the gut microbiome development within the first 6 years of life. Breastfed infants had lower abundance of stool Clostridales family species in this study. These are findings of interest, because prior work has shown that *Clostridium difficile* enrichment in early life may actually increase risk of wheeze and asthma in childhood.[63] Atarashi and colleagues[64] fed gnotobiotic mice a *Clostridium* mixture, noting a subsequent expansion of regulatory T cells in the colon and lower specific IgE production in a model of ova sensitization, suggesting that this mixture would protect against allergic diseases. However,

Karimi and colleagues[65] showed a similar pattern of regulatory, nonatopic immune development in a model feeding mice *Lactobacillus reuteri*. That multiple bacterial taxa are implicated in immune regulation suggests that the individual taxa of bacterium present in the gut may be less important than the presence of bacteria in general, or perhaps identifies a potential shared metabolic or immunologic function of these bacteria. Furthermore, the administration of macrolide antibiotics in childhood has been associated to persistent changes in gut microbiome and risk of asthma development in childhood, suggesting the possibility that the changes induced in the gut microbiome (presumably reduction in diversity or of specific dominant colonies) by these antibiotics put individuals at increased risk for asthma.[66]

Digestive products of the gut microbiome are important in modulating health. The metabolic functions of the gut microbiota include production of SCFAs and medium-chain fatty acids by fermentation of dietary fiber and carbohydrates (implicated in colitis, arthritis, and asthma); formation of secondary bile acids (important for reduction in liver disease and metabolic syndrome); generation of metabolites from meat-derived choline and L-carnitine (implicated in cardiovascular disease); production of vitamins K, B_{12}, and folate; and production of indole derivatives (ie, γ-aminobutyric acid, the central nervous system neurotransmitter).[67]

Of these metabolites, SCFAs have been most closely implicated in asthma risk. SCFAs can signal through G protein–coupled receptors, and can inhibit histone deacetylases, controlling gene transcription. Acetate, one SCFA produced by fermentation of fructose by Bifidobacteria, may support colonic epithelial integrity and function.[68] Additional SCFAs, butyrate and propionate, can induce regulatory T cell development, which may play an important role in protection against allergic and inflammatory diseases.[69,70] Acetate and propionate can induce regulatory T cells in the colon, resulting in increased expression of IL-10 and associated regulatory functions.[71] Consumption of dietary fiber may induce more SCFA production and induction of tolerogenic dendritic cells in the mesenteric lymph nodes.[72] Evidence supporting SCFA as protective against asthma includes a study of the gut microbiota of infants at high risk for asthma by Arrieta and colleagues.[50] These authors reported a transient gut microbial dysbiosis in the first 3 months of life, related to lower fecal acetate levels in these high-risk for asthma infants.

Fujimura and colleagues[49] have synthesized this complex relationship of gut microbiome development, metabolic products, and immunologic outcomes related to asthma. Neonatal stool samples from a diverse, longitudinal birth cohort underwent 16s ribosomal RNA sequencing and the patterns of stool microbiota were divided into three "neonatal gut microbiota composition states (NGM 1–3)." These NGM were compositionally different and conferred different risk of atopy by age 2 and asthma by age 4. The highest risk group, NGM3, had lower relative abundance of bacteria, particularly Bifidobacterium, Lactobacillaceae, and Clostridiaceae, and higher abundance of certain fungi, suggesting a substantial dysbiosis in this group. The sterile fecal water from these NGM3 samples induced significantly more IL-4 expression *in vitro* than the low-risk group, and metabolites within that sterile water were enriched for 12,13-DiHOME, a lipid metabolite that can inhibit regulatory T-cell development. In contrast, the sterile fecal water of the low-risk groups was enriched for metabolites including the polyunsaturated fatty acids docosapentaenoate and dihomo-γ-linolenate, which have anti-inflammatory properties. These findings support that differential production of immunologically active metabolites in the stool by different bacterial species, even early in life, may be an important mechanism of protection from or risk for asthma (**Fig. 2**).

THERAPEUTICS AND THE MICROBIOME

Probiotics are viable microorganisms that potentially confer health benefits on the host; however, the safety and efficacy of probiotics as organisms that can prevent or treat disease remains uncertain. Ongoing investigations on probiotic supplementation may quantify and qualify host health benefits and the long-term impact they may have on the host microbiome. If various microbial exposures are related to asthma through direct immune effects or metabolic products, could a probiotic serve a protective or therapeutic role in those diseases through influencing the host microbiota toward disrupting or redirecting immune outcomes?

Elazab and colleagues[73] performed a meta-analysis of 25 studies testing prenatal or early life probiotic administration to determine the effects on atopy and asthma in children. Variable factors among these trials included timing of supplementation and delivery method. The meta-analysis concluded that although some probiotic supplementation may reduce IgE levels and the risk of allergen sensitization, this did not affect the risk of wheezing or asthma. The decreased IgE levels were more evident with longer duration of probiotic administration. The mechanisms underlying this potential benefit against atopy have been addressed in specific trials. One randomized,

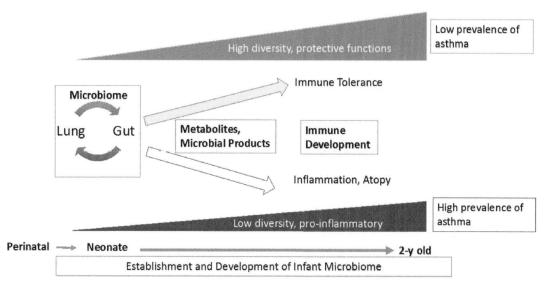

Fig. 2. The lung and gut microbiome likely impact risk for asthma through direct immune activation and metabolite effects on the immune system.

placebo-controlled clinical trial studying feedings of *Lactobacillus paracasei* F19 between 4 and 13 months of age to placebo identified more pronounced T-cell interferon-γ and IL-17 mRNA expression in the treatment group, suggesting Th1-promoting effects of this probiotic.[74] Another trial of prenatal and postnatal supplementation demonstrated a combination of *Bifidobacterium bifidum*, *Bifidobacterium lactis*, and *Lactococcus lactis* was associated with a reduction in *in vitro* lymphocyte IL-5 and IL-13 production by 3 months of age.[75] A comparison of prenatal and postnatal supplementation with *B lactis* or *Lactobacillus rhamnosus* showed differential effects of those bacteria, with cord blood interferon-γ higher in the *L rhamnosus* group. The complex host responses to probiotics likely varies based on dose, strain, treatment timing, and duration. Additionally, probiotic supplementation may contribute to protection from atopic disease include through improved epithelial barrier function.[76] Finally, although successfully implemented in severe gastrointestinal disorders,[77] the frontier of microbiome transplantation to restore health in asthma has not been well studied but may offer an interesting new approach to microbiome manipulation.

SUMMARY

Risk for asthma is strongly related to the lung and gut microbiome. Important elements of microbiome development consistent with both niches include the early life window for microbiome establishment, the diversity of bacteria, richness of bacteria, and effect of those bacteria on the local epithelium and immune system. Mechanisms through which the lung microbiome may protect against asthma include early establishment of rich, nonpathogenic bacterial colonies that are anti-inflammatory or less disposed to type 2 inflammation. Factors influencing the degree of gut microbiome protection from asthma include those that support gut microbial early development and diversity and incorporate the contribution of metabolic products and dietary exposures. With this in mind, the potential application of these findings to asthma treatment and prevention will likely include measures to broaden diversity early in life; supporting this diversity through health-protective early life exposures; and possible alteration of the microbial niche through supplementation of probiotics, bacterial products, dietary factors, or metabolites.

REFERENCES

1. Hansel TT, Johnston SL, Openshaw PJ. Microbes and mucosal immune responses in asthma. Lancet 2013;381(9869):861–73.
2. Huang YJ. The respiratory microbiome and innate immunity in asthma. Curr Opin Pulm Med 2015; 21(1):27–32.
3. Gollwitzer ES, Saglani S, Trompette A, et al. Lung microbiota promotes tolerance to allergens in neonates via PD-L1. Nat Med 2014;20(6):642–7.
4. Marsland BJ, Gollwitzer ES. Host-microorganism interactions in lung diseases. Nat Rev Immunol 2014; 14(12):827–35.
5. Strachan DP. Hay fever, hygiene, and household size. BMJ 1989;299(6710):1259–60.

6. von Mutius E, Braun-Fahrländer C, Schierl R, et al. Exposure to endotoxin or other bacterial components might protect against the development of atopy. Clin Exp Allergy 2000;30(9):1230–4.

7. Ege MJ, Frei R, Bieli C, et al. Not all farming environments protect against the development of asthma and wheeze in children. J Allergy Clin Immunol 2007;119(5):1140–7.

8. Braun-Fahrlander C, Riedler J, Herz U, et al. Environmental exposure to endotoxin and its relation to asthma in school-age children. N Engl J Med 2002;347(12):869–77.

9. Waser M, Michels KB, Bieli C, et al. Inverse association of farm milk consumption with asthma and allergy in rural and suburban populations across Europe. Clin Exp Allergy 2007;37(5):661–70.

10. Abbring S, Verheijden KAT, Diks MAP, et al. Raw cow's milk prevents the development of airway inflammation in a murine house dust mite-induced asthma model. Front Immunol 2017;8:1045.

11. Ruokolainen L, Paalanen L, Karkman A, et al. Significant disparities in allergy prevalence and microbiota between the young people in Finnish and Russian Karelia. Clin Exp Allergy 2017;47(5):665–74.

12. von Hertzen L, Laatikainen T, Pitkänen T, et al. Microbial content of drinking water in Finnish and Russian Karelia: implications for atopy prevalence. Allergy 2007;62(3):288–92.

13. Haahtela T, Laatikainen T, Alenius H, et al. Hunt for the origin of allergy: comparing the Finnish and Russian Karelia. Clin Exp Allergy 2015;45(5):891–901.

14. Holbreich M, Genuneit J, Weber J, et al. Amish children living in northern Indiana have a very low prevalence of allergic sensitization. J Allergy Clin Immunol 2012;129(6):1671–3.

15. Stein MM, Hrusch CL, Gozdz J, et al. Innate immunity and asthma risk in Amish and Hutterite farm children. N Engl J Med 2016;375(5):411–21.

16. Boutin RCT, Petersen C, Finlay BB. Microbial insights into asthmatic immunopathology. a forward-looking synthesis and commentary. Ann Am Thorac Soc 2017;14(Supplement_5):S316–25.

17. Bisgaard H, Hermansen MN, Buchvald F, et al. Childhood asthma after bacterial colonization of the airway in neonates. N Engl J Med 2007;357(15):1487–95.

18. Kloepfer KM, Lee WM, Pappas TE, et al. Detection of pathogenic bacteria during rhinovirus infection is associated with increased respiratory symptoms and asthma exacerbations. J Allergy Clin Immunol 2014;133(5):1301–7, 1307.e1-3.

19. Carr TF, Kraft M. Chronic infection and severe asthma. Immunol Allergy Clin North Am 2016;36(3):483–502.

20. Esposito S, Blasi F, Arosio C, et al. Importance of acute Mycoplasma pneumoniae and Chlamydia pneumoniae infections in children with wheezing. Eur Respir J 2000;16(6):1142–6.

21. Kim CK, Chung CY, Kim JS, et al. Late abnormal findings on high-resolution computed tomography after Mycoplasma pneumonia. Pediatrics 2000;105(2):372–8.

22. Sabato AR, Martin AJ, Marmion BP, et al. Mycoplasma pneumoniae: acute illness, antibiotics, and subsequent pulmonary function. Arch Dis Child 1984;59(11):1034–7.

23. Yano T, Ichikawa Y, Komatu S, et al. Association of Mycoplasma pneumoniae antigen with initial onset of bronchial asthma. Am J Respir Crit Care Med 1994;149(5):1348–53.

24. Chu HW, Honour JM, Rawlinson CA, et al. Effects of respiratory Mycoplasma pneumoniae infection on allergen-induced bronchial hyperresponsiveness and lung inflammation in mice. Infect Immun 2003;71(3):1520–6.

25. Martin RJ, Chu HW, Honour JM, et al. Airway inflammation and bronchial hyperresponsiveness after Mycoplasma pneumoniae infection in a murine model. Am J Respir Cell Mol Biol 2001;24(5):577–82.

26. Hao Y, Kuang Z, Jing J, et al. Mycoplasma pneumoniae modulates STAT3-STAT6/EGFR-FOXA2 signaling to induce overexpression of airway mucins. Infect Immun 2014;82(12):5246–55.

27. Wu Q, Case SR, Minor MN, et al. A novel function of MUC18: amplification of lung inflammation during bacterial infection. Am J Pathol 2013;182(3):819–27.

28. Chu HW, Rino JG, Wexler RB, et al. Mycoplasma pneumoniae infection increases airway collagen deposition in a murine model of allergic airway inflammation. Am J Physiol Lung Cell Mol Physiol 2005;289(1):L125–33.

29. Kim JH, Cho TS, Moon JH, et al. Serial changes in serum eosinophil-associated mediators between atopic and non-atopic children after Mycoplasma pneumoniae pneumonia. Allergy Asthma Immunol Res 2014;6(5):428–33.

30. Shin JE, Cheon BR, Shim JW, et al. Increased risk of refractory Mycoplasma pneumoniae pneumonia in children with atopic sensitization and asthma. Korean J Pediatr 2014;57(6):271–7.

31. Ledford JG, Mukherjee S, Kislan MM, et al. Surfactant protein-A suppresses eosinophil-mediated killing of Mycoplasma pneumoniae in allergic lungs. PLoS One 2012;7(2):e32436.

32. Kraft M, Cassell GH, Henson JE, et al. Detection of Mycoplasma pneumoniae in the airways of adults with chronic asthma. Am J Respir Crit Care Med 1998;158(3):998–1001.

33. Riiser A. The human microbiome, asthma, and allergy. Allergy Asthma Clin Immunol 2015;11:35.

34. Hilty M, Burke C, Pedro H, et al. Disordered microbial communities in asthmatic airways. PLoS One 2010;5(1):e8578.

35. Marri PR, Stern DA, Wright AL, et al. Asthma-associated differences in microbial composition of induced sputum. J Allergy Clin Immunol 2013;131(2):346–52. e1-3.

36. Huang YJ, Nelson CE, Brodie EL, et al. Airway microbiota and bronchial hyperresponsiveness in patients with suboptimally controlled asthma. J Allergy Clin Immunol 2011;127(2):372–81.e1-3.

37. Durack J, Lynch SV, Nariya S, et al. Features of the bronchial bacterial microbiome associated with atopy, asthma, and responsiveness to inhaled corticosteroid treatment. J Allergy Clin Immunol 2017; 140(1):63–75.

38. Taylor SL, Leong LEX, Choo JM, et al. Inflammatory phenotypes in patients with severe asthma are associated with distinct airway microbiology. J Allergy Clin Immunol 2018;141(1):94–103.e5.

39. Green BJ, Wiriyachaiporn S, Grainge C, et al. Potentially pathogenic airway bacteria and neutrophilic inflammation in treatment resistant severe asthma. PLoS One 2014;9(6):e100645.

40. Huang YJ, Nariya S, Harris JM, et al. The airway microbiome in patients with severe asthma: associations with disease features and severity. J Allergy Clin Immunol 2015;136(4):874–84.

41. Goleva E, Jackson LP, Harris JK, et al. The effects of airway microbiome on corticosteroid responsiveness in asthma. Am J Respir Crit Care Med 2013; 188(10):1193–201.

42. Herbst T, Sichelstiel A, Schär C, et al. Dysregulation of allergic airway inflammation in the absence of microbial colonization. Am J Respir Crit Care Med 2011;184(2):198–205.

43. Nembrini C, Sichelstiel A, Kisielow J, et al. Bacterial-induced protection against allergic inflammation through a multicomponent immunoregulatory mechanism. Thorax 2011;66(9):755–63.

44. Chung H, Pamp SJ, Hill JA, et al. Gut immune maturation depends on colonization with a host-specific microbiota. Cell 2012;149(7):1578–93.

45. Ridaura VK, Faith JJ, Rey FE, et al. Gut microbiota from twins discordant for obesity modulate metabolism in mice. Science 2013;341(6150):1241214.

46. Diaz Heijtz R, Wang S, Anuar F, et al. Normal gut microbiota modulates brain development and behavior. Proc Natl Acad Sci U S A 2011;108(7): 3047–52.

47. Yamamoto M, Yamaguchi R, Munakata K, et al. A microarray analysis of gnotobiotic mice indicating that microbial exposure during the neonatal period plays an essential role in immune system development. BMC Genomics 2012;13:335.

48. Fujimura KE, Slusher NA, Cabana MD, et al. Role of the gut microbiota in defining human health. Expert Rev Anti Infect Ther 2010;8(4):435–54.

49. Fujimura KE, Sitarik AR, Havstad S, et al. Neonatal gut microbiota associates with childhood multisensitized

50. Arrieta MC, Stiemsma LT, Dimitriu PA, et al. Early infancy microbial and metabolic alterations affect risk of childhood asthma. Sci Transl Med 2015;7(307): 307ra152.

51. Abrahamsson TR, Jakobsson HE, Andersson AF, et al. Low gut microbiota diversity in early infancy precedes asthma at school age. Clin Exp Allergy 2014;44(6):842–50.

52. Stokholm J, Blaser MJ, Thorsen J, et al. Maturation of the gut microbiome and risk of asthma in childhood. Nat Commun 2018;9(1):141.

53. Lisciandro JG, Prescott SL, Nadal-Sims MG, et al. Neonatal antigen-presenting cells are functionally more quiescent in children born under traditional compared with modern environmental conditions. J Allergy Clin Immunol 2012;130(5):1167–74.e10.

54. Cox LM, Yamanishi S, Sohn J, et al. Altering the intestinal microbiota during a critical developmental window has lasting metabolic consequences. Cell 2014;158(4):705–21.

55. Cahenzli J, Köller Y, Wyss M, et al. Intestinal microbial diversity during early-life colonization shapes long-term IgE levels. Cell Host Microbe 2013;14(5): 559–70.

56. Dominguez-Bello MG, Costello EK, Contreras M, et al. Delivery mode shapes the acquisition and structure of the initial microbiota across multiple body habitats in newborns. Proc Natl Acad Sci U S A 2010;107(26):11971–5.

57. Sevelsted A, Stokholm J, Bisgaard H. Risk of asthma from cesarean delivery depends on membrane rupture. J Pediatr 2016;171:38–42.e1-4.

58. Romeo ET, Castro-Rodriguez JA, Holberg CJ, et al. Dog exposure in infancy decreases the subsequent risk of frequent wheeze but not of atopy. J Allergy Clin Immunol 2001;108(4):509–15.

59. von Mutius E, Vercelli D. Farm living: effects on childhood asthma and allergy. Nat Rev Immunol 2010;10(12):861–8.

60. Ownby DR, Johnson CC, Peterson EL. Exposure to dogs and cats in the first year of life and risk of allergic sensitization at 6 to 7 years of age. JAMA 2002;288(8):963–72.

61. Fujimura KE, Demoor T, Rauch M, et al. House dust exposure mediates gut microbiome *Lactobacillus* enrichment and airway immune defense against allergens and virus infection. Proc Natl Acad Sci U S A 2014;111(2):805–10.

62. Sordillo JE, Zhou Y, McGeachie MJ, et al. Factors influencing the infant gut microbiome at age 3-6 months: findings from the ethnically diverse Vitamin D Antenatal Asthma Reduction Trial (VDAART). J Allergy Clin Immunol 2017;139(2):482–91.e14.

63. van Nimwegen FA, Penders J, Stobberingh EE, et al. Mode and place of delivery, gastrointestinal microbiota,

atopy and T cell differentiation. Nat Med 2016; 22(10):1187–91.

and their influence on asthma and atopy. J Allergy Clin Immunol 2011;128(5):948–55.e1-3.

64. Atarashi K, Tanoue T, Shima T, et al. Induction of colonic regulatory T cells by indigenous *Clostridium* species. Science 2011;331(6015):337–41.

65. Karimi K, Inman MD, Bienenstock J, et al. *Lactobacillus reuteri*-induced regulatory T cells protect against an allergic airway response in mice. Am J Respir Crit Care Med 2009;179(3):186–93.

66. Korpela K, Salonen A, Virta LJ, et al. Intestinal microbiome is related to lifetime antibiotic use in Finnish pre-school children. Nat Commun 2016;7:10410.

67. Abdollahi-Roodsaz S, Abramson SB, Scher JU. The metabolic role of the gut microbiota in health and rheumatic disease: mechanisms and interventions. Nat Rev Rheumatol 2016;12(8):446–55.

68. Fukuda S, Toh H, Hase K, et al. Bifidobacteria can protect from enteropathogenic infection through production of acetate. Nature 2011;469(7331):543–7.

69. Furusawa Y, Obata Y, Fukuda S, et al. Commensal microbe-derived butyrate induces the differentiation of colonic regulatory T cells. Nature 2013;504(7480): 446–50.

70. Smith-Norowitz TA, Silverberg JI, Kusonruksa M, et al. Asthmatic children have increased specific anti-*Mycoplasma pneumoniae* IgM but not IgG or IgE-values independent of history of respiratory tract infection. Pediatr Infect Dis J 2013;32(6):599–603.

71. Smith PM, Howitt MR, Panikov N, et al. The microbial metabolites, short-chain fatty acids, regulate colonic Treg cell homeostasis. Science 2013;341(6145): 569–73.

72. Goverse G, Molenaar R, Macia L, et al. Diet-derived short chain fatty acids stimulate intestinal epithelial cells to induce mucosal tolerogenic dendritic cells. J Immunol 2017;198(5):2172–81.

73. Elazab N, Mendy A, Gasana J, et al. Probiotic administration in early life, atopy, and asthma: a meta-analysis of clinical trials. Pediatrics 2013; 132(3):e666–76.

74. West CE, Hernell O, Andersson Y, et al. Probiotic effects on T-cell maturation in infants during weaning. Clin Exp Allergy 2012;42(4):540–9.

75. Niers L, Martín R, Rijkers G, et al. The effects of selected probiotic strains on the development of eczema (the PandA study). Allergy 2009;64(9): 1349–58.

76. Sonnenberg GF, Fouser LA, Artis D. Border patrol: regulation of immunity, inflammation and tissue homeostasis at barrier surfaces by IL-22. Nat Immunol 2011;12(5):383–90.

77. Eliakim-Raz N, Bishara J. Prevention and treatment of *Clostridium difficile* associated diarrhea by reconstitution of the microbiota. Hum Vaccin Immunother 2018;1–8.   https://doi.org/10.1080/21645515.2018. 1472184.

Diet and Metabolism in the Evolution of Asthma and Obesity

Anne E. Dixon, MA, BM, BCh[a],*,
Fernando Holguin, MD, MPH[b,c]

KEYWORDS

- Diet • Obesity • Asthma • Microbiome • Airway reactivity • Metabolic syndrome
- Immunometabolism

KEY POINTS

- Obesity is a major risk factor for the development of asthma, and obese patients tend to have poorly controlled asthma that does not respond as well to controller therapy as asthma in lean patients.
- The development of obesity occurs because of changes in the quality and composition of the diet: specific dietary factors can affect airway disease and might be as important as excess weight in contributing to the pathogenesis of asthma in obesity.
- Significant weight loss can improve asthma control, and changing dietary quality might also be effective for improving asthma control.
- Metabolic syndrome in obesity is associated with increased asthma severity, because metabolic dysfunction contributes to altered immune and airway function.
- Increased oxidative stress, and decreased bioavailability of nitric oxide in the airway, may result in enhanced airway closure in obese individuals.

INTRODUCTION

The world is in the midst of a major obesity epidemic, and in the United States, nearly 40% of the adult population is obese.[1] Obesity is a major risk factor for asthma and is particularly associated with poorly controlled asthma.[2] Although many different factors could contribute to the pathogenesis of asthma in obesity, changes in dietary composition and metabolic factors directly affect airway reactivity and airway inflammation.[3] This article discusses how specific changes in the western diet and metabolic changes associated with the obese state affect inflammation and airway reactivity and reviews evidence that interventions targeting weight, dietary components, lifestyle, and metabolism might improve outcomes in asthma.

DIET

The obesity epidemic is associated with a shift in the quality and composition of food in the diet, not simply increased calories. Diets that produce obesity are typically high in red and processed meats, high in fats and fried foods, low in fiber, and high in sugar. Such a dietary pattern is associated with low lung function and increased

This article is funded by NIH grants HL133920 and HL136917.
[a] Division of Pulmonary and Critical Care, University of Vermont, Given D209, 89 Beaumont Avenue, Burlington, VT 05482, USA; [b] Division of Pulmonary and Critical Care, Department of Medicine, University of Colorado, Denver, CO 80045, USA; [c] Allergy & Asthma Clinic, Anschutz 1635 Aurora Court, 6th Floor, Aurora, CO 80045, USA
* Corresponding author.
E-mail address: Anne.dixon@uvmhealth.org

Clin Chest Med 40 (2019) 97–106
https://doi.org/10.1016/j.ccm.2018.10.007

respiratory symptoms, even when controlled for body mass index (BMI).[4,5] These effects on the respiratory system are likely to occur because such nutrients can have profound effects on the immune system and the pathophysiology of asthma, as outlined in detail in later discussion.

Effects of Dietary Fiber on Asthma

Dietary fiber is metabolized by bacteria in the gut to produce short-chain fatty acids (SCFA). SCFA enter the circulation and can affect a variety of cellular processes, including the pathogenesis of asthma in obesity. Both the composition (type and amount) of fiber in the diet and the population (species and relative quantity) of the gut microbiome influence the production of SCFA. For example, diets high in soluble fiber produce high levels of the SCFA acetate, propionate, and butyrate. These SCFA enter the circulation and can signal through 2 major receptors: Free Fatty Acid Receptors 2 and 3 (also known as G-Coupled Protein Receptors 43 and 41).[6] These receptors are expressed by many cell types, including those of the immune system, and affect immune responses. The effect of dietary fiber on allergic airway disease has been studied in animal models. A low-fiber diet increased airway inflammation in a mouse model of allergic airway disease. This increased inflammation occurred because the low-fiber diet changed the gut microbiome, decreasing production of the circulating SCFA propionate; propionate inhibited the ability of dendritic cells to promote allergic inflammation, and so the lower propionate in the low-fiber diet augmented allergic airway inflammation.[7] Another study showed that a high-fiber diet increased circulating levels of acetate and suppressed allergic airway inflammation in mice: circulating acetate altered acetylation of the FoXP3 promotor, reducing Tregulatory (Treg) cell function and suppressing allergic airway inflammation. Remarkably, the high-fiber diet fed to pregnant animals produced an epigenetic change and resistance to allergic airway inflammation in offspring.[8] These elegant studies in mice suggest dietary fiber modulates allergic airway inflammation through effects on circulating SCFA and that these effects may occur as early as during in utero development.

There have, as of yet, been few studies of dietary fiber in people with asthma, and so the clinical relevance of these observations in mice remains to be determined. However, in a pilot study of 29 people with asthma randomized to either a high-fiber or a low-fiber meal challenge, there were some interesting observations: 4 hours after the meal, those who received the high-fiber challenge had decreased cellular inflammation in sputum, decreased exhaled nitric oxide (NO), and improved lung function. These changes were associated with increased expression of receptors for SCFA in sputum.[9] There have been no other interventional studies in humans targeting fiber alone, although this is often a component of the lifestyle interventions for asthma discussed later.

Effects of a High-Fat Diet on Asthma

Several publications have reported the effects of a high-fat diet sufficient to produce obesity on airway disease in animal models: whether the effects on airway disease relate directly to the dietary fat (and the specific dietary fat) or the other myriad complications induced by obesity are not entirely clear. However, these studies have shown that high-fat diet–induced obesity leads to airway reactivity even in the absence of allergen or other challenge, increases response to pollutants such as ozone, but has a variable effect on allergic airway inflammatory responses.[10–13] Some of the reported differences likely reflect strain differences in mice, but could also reflect differences in the specific composition of the high-fat diets.

Consumption of a high-fat diet increases circulating levels of free fatty acids. Free fatty acids can stimulate innate immune responses, through activation of nuclear factor k-light-chain enhancer of activated B cells, and the nucleotide-binding and oligomerization domain–like receptor, leucine-rich repeat and pyrin domain–containing 3 inflammasome.[14–16] A high-fat diet might contribute to airway disease even without causing obesity, as illustrated by studies both in mouse models and in humans. Mice fed a high-fat compared with normal chow diet for only 2 weeks developed increased airway reactivity, and higher levels of interleukin-1β (IL-1β) in lung tissue, although this is not associated with overt pulmonary inflammation.[17] In humans, a single high-fat diet meal challenged increased airway neutrophilic inflammation and decreased response to bronchodilator.[18]

Targeting Dietary Components to Treat Asthma

Studies of dietary and lifestyle interventions in asthma could transform the approach to patients with asthma. As of yet, there is a paucity of controlled trials in this field: lifestyle interventions are complex and implementation challenging, but there are some studies that suggest that targeting diet and lifestyle can improve asthma control. Wood and colleagues[19] compared a diet high in fruit and vegetables (2 servings of fruit and 5 of vegetables) with one low fruit and vegetables (1 serving of fruit, and up to 2 servings of vegetables): participants on the high fruit and vegetable intervention had reduced asthma exacerbations over the 16 weeks of the study. Some of the participants in the low fruit and vegetable arm received an antioxidant supplement, but this did not mitigate the increased risk of asthma exacerbations, suggesting that the whole food dietary component was more important than antioxidant supplementation. Ma and colleagues[20] performed a 6-month controlled study targeting improved dietary quality versus maintaining usual diet. In this pilot study with 90 participants, better dietary quality tended to improve asthma control and asthma quality of life. Sexton and colleagues[21] performed a small 12-week pilot study in 38 patients with asthma and found that implementing a Mediterranean diet might have some efficacy in asthma, although it did not achieve statistical significance in this small study.

Of note, it is not just obese patients who seem to benefit from improved dietary quality and exercise: Toennesen and colleagues[22] studied the effects of an 8-week intervention of high-intensity exercise versus diet (high protein, low glycemic index) versus a combination of both: 125 participants completed the study; only participants in the combined intervention experienced a significant benefit in terms of asthma control and quality of life. This combined diet and exercise intervention was not associated with significant changes in airway reactivity or inflammation.

Effects of Weight Loss on Asthma

Lifestyle interventions
Weight loss can be achieved with lifestyle interventions. There have been a few studies of this in children and adults with asthma (**Table 1**). These studies suggest that a weight loss of 5% to 10% may produce a significant improvement in asthma control.[16–19,30–32] Exercise may have an additional benefit on asthma control, but it is not clear whether this is attributable to a direct effect of exercise on asthma control, or whether it is related to greater weight loss.[23]

Weight loss surgery
There have now been several studies suggesting that bariatric surgery produces dramatic improvements in asthma control and lung function.[23–31] Bariatric surgery is an expensive, complex procedure, but it may have a significant public health impact: Hasegawa and colleagues[32] found approximately 22% of patients with asthma had an asthma exacerbation leading to an Emergency Department visit or hospitalization annually before bariatric surgery; this decreased to 11% annually after surgery. The mechanisms by which bariatric surgery improves asthma control likely include mechanical unloading of the respiratory system, reduced metabolic inflammation, and changes in dietary composition.[33]

Exercise
There are no published studies of the effects of exercise in obese animal models of asthma, although several reports in lean mouse models of asthma suggest favorable effects on a variety of parameters pertinent to allergic asthma; these include the following:

- Decreases chemokine responsive migration to lung: lean ovalbumin (OVA) mouse model[34]
- Enhanced Treg cell number and function in the lung: lean OVA mouse model[35]
- Decreased airway smooth muscle thickness: lean OVA mouse model[36]
- Decreased airway inflammation, airway reactivity, and remodeling: lean OVA mouse model[37–39]
- Decreased airway inflammation, increased epithelial modeling: lean OVA guinea pig model[40]

The effects of exercise on asthma in people have been studied in the context of both obese and nonobese asthma. In contrast to animal studies, these reports have not shown effects on airway inflammation, perhaps because they have included multiple phenotypes of asthma, but in general do seem to improve symptoms and asthma control, especially when combined with a dietary intervention, even in those nonobese patients with asthma (**Table 2**).[22,23,27,41–45]

METABOLISM
Metabolic Syndrome

Metabolic syndrome (MetS), a condition defined by a grouping of clinical factors, including abdominal obesity, poor glycemic control, dyslipidemias (elevated triglycerides and/or reduced high-density lipoprotein cholesterol levels), and hypertension, is present in about two-thirds of the obese population.[46,47] Although not a specific disease per se, MetS increases the risk for diabetes, cardiovascular diseases, hepatic steatosis, and cancer, to name a few. Given obese subjects that concomitantly have this condition have a greater propensity for developing chronic diseases in multiple organs, it is reasonable to speculate that MetS can also affect the lungs, and to some extent, potentially explain why obesity is associated with asthma. The question of whether in fact MetS is independently associated with

Table 1
Studies of the effect of diet-induced weight loss on asthma control

Author	Intervention	n	Weight Change in Intervention Group	Effect on Asthma
Freitas et al,[23] 2017	Diet and sham vs diet and exercise	55	Diet alone: ↓ 3.1% Diet and exercise: ↓ 6.8%	Significantly greater improvement in asthma control and quality of life with addition of exercise
Pakhale et al,[24] 2015	Liquid meal replacement	22	↓ 19%	Significant improvement in airway reactivity and asthma control
Ma et al,[25] 2015	Diet and exercise	330	↓ 4.1% (vs ↓ 2.1% in enhanced care)	Improved asthma control in those who lost ≥5% weight
Dias-Junior et al,[26] 2014	Diet and weight loss medication (controlled study)	22 adults	↓ 7.5%	Improved asthma control
Scott et al,[27] 2013	Diet and exercise (controlled study)	28 adults	↓ 8.5%	Improved asthma control
Jensen et al,[28] 2013	Dietary intervention vs wait list control	32 children	↓5.7% vs ↑ 1.8%	Improved asthma control in intervention group
Hernández Romero et al,[29] 2008	Diet including meal replacements Diet	96 adults	↓ 10.6% (diet + meal replacement) ↓ 6.1% (diet)	Improved symptoms, decreased medication
Johnson et al,[30] 2007	Diet (single arm)	10 adults	↓ 8%	Improved asthma control
Stenius-Aarniala et al,[31] 2000	Diet (controlled study)	19 adults	↓ 14.5%	Improved lung function and symptoms

changes in lung function or asthma diagnosis and morbidity has been evaluated in several epidemiologic studies (**Table 3**). In large cross-sectional studies of adults and children, MetS diagnosis was associated with reduced forced expiratory volume in 1 second (FEV_1) and forced vital capacity (FVC)[54–56] and increased respiratory symptoms after adjusting for potential confounders. Longitudinally, it is associated with steeper loss of lung function over time and increased risk for asthma diagnosis; however, it remains unclear how much of this incidence is confounded by BMI.[49] Individual MetS components are also associated with asthma in adult and children, particularly poor glycemic control, dyslipidemias, and abdominal girth.[48]

The mechanisms by which MetS relates to asthma are likely multifactorial and involve several pathways.[57] Poor glycemic control, associated with insulin resistance and hyperinsulinemia, could explain deficits in lung function and greater respiratory symptoms. Insulin may induce hypercontractility in airway smooth muscle via phosphoinositide 3-kinase and Rho-kinase-dependent pathways, and through vagally mediated bronchoconstriction with loss of inhibitory muscarinic receptor 2 functionality on parasympathetic nerves.[58–60] Epidemiologic and clinical data support a role for insulin by showing an inverse association between insulin resistance and lung function decrements and by the fact that subjects inhaling human insulin (now discontinued Exubera) exhibited more respiratory symptoms, including cough and mild dyspnea, along with reductions in FEV_1 and diffusing capacity of the lung for carbon monoxide.[61]

Oxidative Stress

Compared with their leaner counterparts, obese asthmatics have increased levels of airway and systemic biomarkers of oxidative stress, which are associated with increased asthma morbidity and reduced response to inhaled

Table 2
Studies of the efficacy of exercise intervention for asthma

Author	Intervention	n	Duration	Main Findings
Turk et al,[41] 2017	Outpatient pulmonary rehabilitation	53 obese, 85 nonobese	12 wk	Improved 6-min walk distance and asthma control score
Freitas et al,[23] 2017	Weight loss vs exercise and weight loss	55 obese	12 wk	More significant improvement in asthma control in the diet and exercise group (also lost more weight)
Toennesen et al,[22] 2018	Improved dietary quality, exercise and diet, exercise or control	125 nonobese	8 wk	Participants randomized to improved dietary quality and exercise had most significant improvement in asthma control and quality of life, no effect on airway inflammation or airway reactivity
França-Pinto et al,[42] 2015	Exercise vs control	58 (obese and nonobese)	12 wk	Exercise group experienced improved asthma control and decreased airway reactivity
Scott et al,[27] 2013	Exercise vs diet vs exercise and diet	46 obese	10 wk	Exercise not as effective as inducing either weight loss or improved asthma control as diet and diet plus exercise intervention
Boyd et al,[43] 2012	Usual care or walking program	19 (obese and nonobese)	12 wk	Showed feasibility of intervention, likely underpowered to see effects on clinical outcomes
Turner et al,[44] 2011	Exercise vs control	35 older adults	3 mo	Improved symptoms and quality of life in the exercise intervention group
Mendes et al,[45] 2010	Usual care or exercise	101 nonobese	3 mo	Improved aerobic capacity and asthma symptom-free days in the exercise group

corticosteroids.[62–64] Oxidative stress is a complex process involving a fine balance between many potential oxidative sources and the function of antioxidant mechanisms. Although MetS has been widely associated with greater systemic oxidative stress and inflammation,[65] it is unclear if it has similar effects in the airways of asthmatics. However, animal models and epidemiologic studies suggest that altered L-arginine and NO metabolism as a potential pathway by which obesity, MetS, and airway oxidative stress are linked. Compared with mice fed regular chow, those taking high-fat or high-fructose diet for 18 weeks developed MetS and had increased inducible nitric oxide synthase (iNOS) protein and nitrotyrosine lung levels (a marker for oxonitrative stress), whereas having lower NO in the absence of increased airway inflammation.[66]

The unexpected lack of NO increase while iNOS is upregulated suggests an NO redox imbalance, which was explained by the fact that diet-induced MetS reduced the lung L-arginine/asymmetric dimethyl arginine (ADMA, a methylated product of L-arginine catabolism) ratio levels. When this imbalance occurs, iNOS becomes uncoupled, producing anion superoxide at the expense of NO production.[67] These results have been replicated in primary human airway epithelial cells of asthmatics treated with ADMA. Interestingly, the clinical relevance of these results were recently validated in a cross-sectional study of participants from the Severe Asthma Research Program, which showed that obese subjects had lower L-arginine/ADMA ratios, which were associated with lesser exhaled NO levels, reduced lung function, and more frequent respiratory

Table 3
Epidemiologic studies linking metabolic syndrome with lung function or asthma diagnosis and morbidity

Author	Exposure	Study Design	Population	Outcomes
Brumpton et al,[48] 2013	MetS	Prospective	23,191 Nord-Trondelag Health Study participants from 1995-2008, ages 19–55 y	MetS is associated with higher risk for incident asthma; not BMI adjusted
Assad et al,[49] 2013	MetS	Prospective	4619 eligible participants in the Coronary Artery Risk Development in Young Adults cohort followed over 25 y	MetS predicted incident asthma among women but not men; this association was confounded by BMI
Kuschnir et al,[50] 2018	MetS	Cross-sectional, multicenter school survey	MetS and asthma	MetS was associated with severe asthma
Forno et al,[51] 2015	MetS, insulin resistance	Cross-sectional	1429 adolescents aged 12–17 y in the 2007–2010 National Health and Nutrition Examination Survey	Insulin resistance and MetS are associated with worsened lung function in overweight/obese adolescents
Lee et al,[52] 2009	MetS	Cross-sectional	9942 individuals (4716 men and 5226 women) participating in The Korean Health and Genome Study	MetS was associated with asthma-related respiratory symptoms. Those with symptoms had lower lung function
Cardet et al,[53] 2016	Obesity and insulin resistance	Cross-sectional	12,421 adults, ages 18–85 y from the National Health and Nutrition Examination Survey 2003–2012	The relationship between obesity and current asthma was stronger with increasing insulin resistance levels

symptoms.[68] Having greater ADMA levels in obesity and MetS coupled with increased levels of allergic inflammatory mediators, such as IL-4, can have synergistic effects in producing mitochondrial dysfunction, which is a common feature of these conditions and also associated with asthma.[69]

Dyslipidemias Immunometabolism

Elevated triglycerides and/or reduced high-density lipoprotein (HDL) are MetS factors, which have independently been associated with greater asthma prevalence, respiratory morbidity, and reduced lung function in children and adults.[70,71] These dyslipidemias are not only indicative of adipose metabolic dysfunction but also related to immune changes that may explain the underlying mechanism supporting these associations.[72] Obesity is a low-grade inflammatory state in which adipocytes secrete cytokines activating and recruiting macrophages that play pivotal roles in systemic inflammatory responses, including activation of T helper (Th) cells, in particular Th1 polarization, which has been described in obese asthmatic children.[73] A large cross-sectional study of obese and normal weight adolescents with and without asthma showed that having reduced HDL was significantly associated with increased Th1/Th2 (Th1 [CD4$^+$IFNγ(interferon γ)$^+$]/Th2 [CD4$^+$IL4$^+$] cells) cell responses to phytohemagglutinin, and inversely associated with percent patrolling monocytes but directly associated with CCR2 expression on patrolling and resident monocytes. These associations suggested a role for obesity-mediated dyslipidemia in monocyte activation among obese subjects with asthma and may explain why these lipid disorders are associated with asthma in the context of MetS and obesity.[71] The immunologic consequences of metabolic dysregulation in obesity have far reaching consequences beyond Th1 polarization. For example, obese subjects, independently of asthma, have increased odds for developing H1N1 influenza, and when they do, it can be of greater severity.[74] This phenomenon may be partly explained by the fact that 12 months after vaccination, greater BMI is associated with a steeper decline in influenza antibody titers.[75] Furthermore, peripheral blood monocytes cells from obese individuals challenged ex vivo with vaccine strain virus show decreased CD8 T-cell activation and decreased expression of functional proteins compared with healthy weight individuals.[76] In addition, obese individuals also have dysfunctional natural killer cells and a greater degree of B-cell immune activation, which is associated with a suboptimal humoral response to vaccines.[77]

In summary, metabolic dysregulation associated with obesity is linked to changes in oxidative stress, airway function, and immunologic changes, which increase asthma morbidity as well as risk for viral respiratory infections and pneumonia that can indirectly also worsen asthma.

SUMMARY

Obesity is a complex disorder associated with altered exposures and behaviors (diet, lifestyle, and physical activity). Excess adipose tissue contributes to immunometabolic disarray, increased oxidative stress, and decreased bioavailability of NO. All these factors combine to alter the pattern of established airway disease, and to produce de novo airway disease. Obesity is producing an epidemic of airway disease poorly responsive to conventional therapies, therapies developed for treatment of disease in lean patients. Understanding the interactions between altered exposures, MetS, and airway disease will yield fundamental insights into the relationship between respiration and metabolism, and to new and better treatments for patients with obesity and asthma.

REFERENCES

1. Hales CM, Fryar CD, Carroll MD, et al. Trends in obesity and severe obesity prevalence in US youth and adults by sex and age, 2007-2008 to 2015-2016. JAMA 2018;319(16):1723–5.
2. Dixon AE, Poynter ME. Mechanisms of asthma in obesity. Pleiotropic aspects of obesity produce distinct asthma phenotypes. Am J Respir Cell Mol Biol 2016;54(5):601–8.
3. Peters U, Suratt BT, Bates JHT, et al. Beyond BMI: obesity and lung disease. Chest 2018;153(3):702–9.
4. Brigham EP, Steffen LM, London SJ, et al. Diet pattern and respiratory morbidity in the atherosclerosis risk in communities study. Ann Am Thorac Soc 2018;15(6):675–82.
5. Han YY, Forno E, Shivappa N, et al. The dietary inflammatory index and current wheeze among children and adults in the United States. J Allergy Clin Immunol Pract 2018;6(3):834–41.e2.
6. Gerard P. Gut microbiota and obesity. Cell Mol Life Sci 2016;73(1):147–62.
7. Trompette A, Gollwitzer ES, Yadava K, et al. Gut microbiota metabolism of dietary fiber influences allergic airway disease and hematopoiesis. Nat Med 2014;20(2):159–66.
8. Thorburn AN, McKenzie CI, Shen S, et al. Evidence that asthma is a developmental origin disease influenced by maternal diet and bacterial metabolites. Nat Commun 2015;6:7320.

9. Halnes I, Baines KJ, Berthon BS, et al. Soluble fibre meal challenge reduces airway inflammation and expression of GPR43 and GPR41 in asthma. Nutrients 2017;9(1) [pii:E57].

10. Shore SA. Obesity and asthma: lessons from animal models. J Appl Physiol (1985) 2007;102(2):516–28.

11. Calixto MC, Lintomen L, Schenka A, et al. Obesity enhances eosinophilic inflammation in a murine model of allergic asthma. Br J Pharmacol 2010; 159(3):617–25.

12. Johnston RA, Zhu M, Rivera-Sanchez YM, et al. Allergic airway responses in obese mice. Am J Respir Crit Care Med 2007;176(7):650–8.

13. Dahm PH, Richards JB, Karmouty-Quintana H, et al. Effect of antigen sensitization and challenge on oscillatory mechanics of the lung and pulmonary inflammation in obese carboxypeptidase E-deficient mice. Am J Physiol Regul Integr Comp Physiol 2014; 307(6):R621–33.

14. Kien CL, Bunn JY, Fukagawa NK, et al. Lipidomic evidence that lowering the typical dietary palmitate to oleate ratio in humans decreases the leukocyte production of proinflammatory cytokines and muscle expression of redox-sensitive genes. J Nutr Biochem 2015;26(12):1599–606.

15. Deopurkar R, Ghanim H, Friedman J, et al. Differential effects of cream, glucose, and orange juice on inflammation, endotoxin, and the expression of Toll-like receptor-4 and suppressor of cytokine signaling-3. Diabetes Care 2010;33(5):991–7.

16. Ralston JC, Lyons CL, Kennedy EB, et al. Fatty acids and NLRP3 inflammasome-mediated inflammation in metabolic tissues. Annu Rev Nutr 2017;37: 77–102.

17. Fricke K, Vieira M, Younas H, et al. High fat diet induces airway hyperresponsiveness in mice. Sci Rep 2018;8(1):6404.

18. Wood LG, Garg ML, Gibson PG. A high-fat challenge increases airway inflammation and impairs bronchodilator recovery in asthma. J Allergy Clin Immunol 2011;127(5):1133–40.

19. Wood LG, Garg ML, Smart JM, et al. Manipulating antioxidant intake in asthma: a randomized controlled trial. Am J Clin Nutr 2012;96(3): 534–43.

20. Ma J, Strub P, Lv N, et al. Pilot randomised trial of a healthy eating behavioural intervention in uncontrolled asthma. Eur Respir J 2016;47(1):122–32.

21. Sexton P, Black P, Metcalf P, et al. Influence of mediterranean diet on asthma symptoms, lung function, and systemic inflammation: a randomized controlled trial. J Asthma 2013;50(1):75–81.

22. Toennesen LL, Meteran H, Hostrup M, et al. Effects of exercise and diet in nonobese asthma patients-a randomized controlled trial. J Allergy Clin Immunol Pract 2018;6(3):803–11.

23. Freitas PD, Ferreira PG, Silva AG, et al. The role of exercise in a weight-loss program on clinical control in obese adults with asthma. A randomized controlled trial. Am J Respir Crit Care Med 2017; 195(1):32–42.

24. Pakhale S, Baron J, Dent R, et al. Effects of weight loss on airway responsiveness in obese adults with asthma: does weight loss lead to reversibility of asthma? Chest 2015;147(6):1582–90.

25. Ma J, Strub P, Xiao L, et al. Behavioral weight loss and physical activity intervention in obese adults with asthma. A randomized trial. Ann Am Thorac Soc 2015;12(1):1–11.

26. Dias-Junior SA, Reis M, de Carvalho-Pinto RM, et al. Effects of weight loss on asthma control in obese patients with severe asthma. Eur Respir J 2014;43(5): 1368–77.

27. Scott HA, Gibson PG, Garg ML, et al. Dietary restriction and exercise improve airway inflammation and clinical outcomes in overweight and obese asthma: a randomized trial. Clin Exp Allergy 2013;43(1):36–49.

28. Jensen ME, Gibson PG, Collins CE, et al. Diet-induced weight loss in obese children with asthma: a randomized controlled trial. Clin Exp Allergy 2013;43(7):775–84.

29. Hernández Romero A, Matta Campos J, Mora Nieto A, et al. Clinical symptom relief in obese patients with persistent moderate asthma secondary to decreased obesity. Rev Alerg Mex 2008;55(3): 103–11 [in Spanish].

30. Johnson JB, Summer W, Cutler RG, et al. Alternate day calorie restriction improves clinical findings and reduces markers of oxidative stress and inflammation in overweight adults with moderate asthma. Free Radic Biol Med 2007;42(5):665–74.

31. Stenius-Aarniala B, Poussa T, Kvarnstrom J, et al. Immediate and long term effects of weight reduction in obese people with asthma: randomised controlled study. BMJ 2000;320(7238):827–32.

32. Hasegawa K, Tsugawa Y, Chang Y, et al. Risk of an asthma exacerbation after bariatric surgery in adults. J Allergy Clin Immunol 2015;136(2):288–94.e8.

33. Dixon AE, Pratley RE, Forgione PM, et al. Effects of obesity and bariatric surgery on airway hyperresponsiveness, asthma control, and inflammation. J Allergy Clin Immunol 2011;128(3):508–15.e1-2.

34. Dugger KJ, Chrisman T, Jones B, et al. Moderate aerobic exercise alters migration patterns of antigen specific T helper cells within an asthmatic lung. Brain Behav Immun 2013;34:67–78.

35. Lowder T, Dugger K, Deshane J, et al. Repeated bouts of aerobic exercise enhance regulatory T cell responses in a murine asthma model. Brain Behav Immun 2010;24(1):153–9.

36. Hewitt M, Estell K, Davis IC, et al. Repeated bouts of moderate-intensity aerobic exercise reduce airway

reactivity in a murine asthma model. Am J Respir Cell Mol Biol 2010;42(2):243–9.

37. Vieira RP, Claudino RC, Duarte AC, et al. Aerobic exercise decreases chronic allergic lung inflammation and airway remodeling in mice. Am J Respir Crit Care Med 2007;176(9):871–7.

38. Silva RA, Vieira RP, Duarte AC, et al. Aerobic training reverses airway inflammation and remodelling in an asthma murine model. Eur Respir J 2010;35(5): 994 1002.

39. Silva RA, Almeida FM, Olivo CR, et al. Airway remodeling is reversed by aerobic training in a murine model of chronic asthma. Scand J Med Sci Sports 2015;25(3):e258–66.

40. Olivo CR, Vieira RP, Arantes-Costa FM, et al. Effects of aerobic exercise on chronic allergic airway inflammation and remodeling in Guinea pigs. Respir Physiol Neurobiol 2012;182(2–3):81–7.

41. Turk Y, van Huisstede A, Franssen FME, et al. Effect of an outpatient pulmonary rehabilitation program on exercise tolerance and asthma control in obese asthma patients. J Cardiopulm Rehabil Prev 2017; 37(3):214–22.

42. França-Pinto A, Mendes FA, de Carvalho-Pinto RM, et al. Aerobic training decreases bronchial hyperresponsiveness and systemic inflammation in patients with moderate or severe asthma: a randomised controlled trial. Thorax 2015;70(8): 732–9.

43. Boyd A, Yang CT, Estell K, et al. Feasibility of exercising adults with asthma: a randomized pilot study. Allergy Asthma Clin Immunol 2012;8(1):13.

44. Turner S, Eastwood P, Cook A, et al. Improvements in symptoms and quality of life following exercise training in older adults with moderate/severe persistent asthma. Respiration 2011;81(4):302–10.

45. Mendes FA, Goncalves RC, Nunes MP, et al. Effects of aerobic training on psychosocial morbidity and symptoms in patients with asthma: a randomized clinical trial. Chest 2010;138(2):331–7.

46. Beltran-Sanchez H, Harhay MO, Harhay MM, et al. Prevalence and trends of metabolic syndrome in the adult U.S. population, 1999-2010. J Am Coll Cardiol 2013;62(8):697–703.

47. Cameron AJ, Shaw JE, Zimmet PZ. The metabolic syndrome: prevalence in worldwide populations. Endocrinol Metab Clin North Am 2004;33(2):351–75. table of contents.

48. Brumpton BM, Camargo CA Jr, Romundstad PR, et al. Metabolic syndrome and incidence of asthma in adults: the HUNT study. Eur Respir J 2013;42(6): 1495–502.

49. Assad N, Qualls C, Smith LJ, et al. Body mass index is a stronger predictor than the metabolic syndrome for future asthma in women. The longitudinal CARDIA study. Am J Respir Crit Care Med 2013; 188(3):319–26.

50. Kuschnir FC, Felix MMR, Caetano Kuschnir MC, et al. Severe asthma is associated with metabolic syndrome in Brazilian adolescents. J Allergy Clin Immunol 2018;141(5):1947–9.e4.

51. Forno E, Han YY, Muzumdar RH, et al. Insulin resistance, metabolic syndrome, and lung function in US adolescents with and without asthma. J Allergy Clin Immunol 2015;136(2):304–11.e8.

52. Lee EJ, In KH, Ha ES, et al. Asthma-like symptoms are increased in the metabolic syndrome. J Asthma 2009;46(4):339–42.

53. Cardet JC, Ash S, Kusa T, et al. Insulin resistance modifies the association between obesity and current asthma in adults. Eur Respir J 2016;48(2): 403–10.

54. Kim SK, Bae JC, Baek JH, et al. Decline in lung function rather than baseline lung function is associated with the development of metabolic syndrome: a six-year longitudinal study. PLoS One 2017;12(3): e0174228.

55. Leone N, Courbon D, Thomas F, et al. Lung function impairment and metabolic syndrome: the critical role of abdominal obesity. Am J Respir Crit Care Med 2009;179(6):509–16.

56. Lim SY, Rhee EJ, Sung KC. Metabolic syndrome, insulin resistance and systemic inflammation as risk factors for reduced lung function in Korean nonsmoking males. J Korean Med Sci 2010;25(10): 1480–6.

57. Agrawal A, Mabalirajan U, Ahmad T, et al. Emerging interface between metabolic syndrome and asthma. Am J Respir Cell Mol Biol 2011;44(3):270–5.

58. Dekkers BG, Schaafsma D, Tran T, et al. Insulin-induced laminin expression promotes a hypercontractile airway smooth muscle phenotype. Am J Respir Cell Mol Biol 2009;41(4):494–504.

59. Lee H, Kim SR, Oh Y, et al. Targeting insulin-like growth factor-I and insulin-like growth factor-binding protein-3 signaling pathways. A novel therapeutic approach for asthma. Am J Respir Cell Mol Biol 2014;50(4):667–77.

60. Nie Z, Jacoby DB, Fryer AD. Hyperinsulinemia potentiates airway responsiveness to parasympathetic nerve stimulation in obese rats. Am J Respir Cell Mol Biol 2014;51(2):251–61.

61. Rosenstock J, Cefalu WT, Hollander PA, et al. Safety and efficacy of inhaled human insulin (exubera) during discontinuation and readministration of therapy in adults with type 2 diabetes: a 3-year randomized controlled trial. Diabetes Technol Ther 2009;11(11): 697–705.

62. Lugogo NL, Bappanad D, Kraft M. Obesity, metabolic dysregulation and oxidative stress in asthma. Biochim Biophys Acta 2011;1810(11):1120–6.

63. Holguin F, Fitzpatrick A. Obesity, asthma, and oxidative stress. J Appl Physiol (1985) 2010; 108(3):754–9.

64. Anderson WJ, Lipworth BJ. Does body mass index influence responsiveness to inhaled corticosteroids in persistent asthma? Ann Allergy Asthma Immunol 2012;108(4):237–42.

65. Carrier A. Metabolic syndrome and oxidative stress: a complex relationship. Antioxid Redox Signal 2017; 26(9):429–31.

66. Singh VP, Aggarwal R, Singh S, et al. Metabolic syndrome is associated with increased oxo-nitrative stress and asthma-like changes in lungs. PLoS One 2015;10(6):e0129850.

67. Winnica D, Que LG, Baffi C, et al. l-citrulline prevents asymmetric dimethylarginine-mediated reductions in nitric oxide and nitrosative stress in primary human airway epithelial cells. Clin Exp Allergy 2017; 47(2):190–9.

68. Holguin F, Comhair SA, Hazen SL, et al. An association between L-arginine/asymmetric dimethyl arginine balance, obesity, and the age of asthma onset phenotype. Am J Respir Crit Care Med 2013;187(2):153–9.

69. Pattnaik B, Bodas M, Bhatraju NK, et al. IL-4 promotes asymmetric dimethylarginine accumulation, oxo-nitrative stress, and hypoxic response-induced mitochondrial loss in airway epithelial cells. J Allergy Clin Immunol 2016;138(1):130–41.e9.

70. Cottrell L, Neal WA, Ice C, et al. Metabolic abnormalities in children with asthma. Am J Respir Crit Care Med 2011;183(4):441–8.

71. Rastogi D, Fraser S, Oh J, et al. Inflammation, metabolic dysregulation, and pulmonary function among obese urban adolescents with asthma. Am J Respir Crit Care Med 2015;191(2):149–60.

72. Rastogi D, Holguin F. Metabolic dysregulation, systemic inflammation, and pediatric obesity-related asthma. Ann Am Thorac Soc 2017;14(Supplement_5):S363–7.

73. Rastogi D, Nico J, Johnston AD, et al. CDC42-related genes are upregulated in helper T cells from obese asthmatic children. J Allergy Clin Immunol 2018;141(2):539–48.e7.

74. Zhou Y, Cowling BJ, Wu P, et al. Adiposity and influenza-associated respiratory mortality: a cohort study. Clin Infect Dis 2015;60(10):e49–57.

75. Sheridan PA, Paich HA, Handy J, et al. Obesity is associated with impaired immune response to influenza vaccination in humans. Int J Obes (Lond) 2012;36(8):1072–7.

76. Frasca D, Ferracci F, Diaz A, et al. Obesity decreases B cell responses in young and elderly individuals. Obesity (Silver Spring) 2016;24(3):615–25.

77. Bahr I, Jahn J, Zipprich A, et al. Impaired natural killer cell subset phenotypes in human obesity. Immunol Res 2018;66(2):234–44.

The Exposome and Asthma

Ahila Subramanian, MD, MPH, Sumita B. Khatri, MD, MA*

KEYWORDS

- Asthma • Exposome • Allergen • Air pollution • Climate change

KEY POINTS

- The environment to which the individual is exposed (exposome) is continually influencing the pathobiology of asthma.
- Indoor and outdoor environments play a role in pathogenesis via levels and duration of exposure, with genetic susceptibility as a crucial factor that alters the initiation and trajectory of common conditions such as allergies and asthma.
- Knowledge of environmental exposures globally and changes that are occurring is necessary to function effectively as medical professionals and health advocates.

INTRODUCTION

Asthma is a common condition that can affect up to 339 million people, and the prevalence is rising.[1] Despite having common features, individuals diagnosed with asthma may have a unique etiology, symptomatology, and response to therapies, resulting in varying levels of asthma control. Intrinsic and genetic factors play a significant role, as demonstrated by a familial link. In addition, the environment to which the individual is exposed (exposome) is continually influencing the pathobiology of asthma.[2–5] This complex interaction of factors can often make the evolution and pathophysiology of asthma difficult to ascertain and comprehend. Among medical providers, there continues to be an enhanced awareness of environmental factors and how they have an impact on asthma pathogenesis, evolution, symptoms, and long-term morbidity. The exposome concept considers all exposures of an individual in a lifetime and how those exposures relate to health (**Fig. 1**).[6–8] In this context, there are known associations, associations that are not fully established, and exposures that demonstrate more distinctive effects based upon age, chronicity of exposure, and genetic predispositions.[9–11] It is through ongoing research and discourse that one will be able to determine precise treatments for individuals and have a better understanding of environment and exposure (exposome) impacts upon the health of individuals and larger at-risk populations.

This article focuses on the interaction of patients and their environments in various parts of their growth, development, and stages of life. It will discuss exposures from indoor and outdoor environments, consider many possible and probable exposures associated with asthma through a lifetime, and inform the reader how human impact on the environment locally and globally relates to public health, specifically respiratory health.

These topics are presented through the broader intent to support the role of medical professionals as educators and health advocates. Being knowledgeable of environmental exposures globally and changes that are occurring over time is necessary to function effectively in that realm. Ongoing research is revealing specific risks, means to mitigate human impact, and strategies to adapt to environmental changes. Such research and clinical expertise offer opportunities to influence public policy in this regard.[12,13]

Respiratory Institute, Cleveland Clinic, Cleveland Clinic Lerner College of Medicine, CWRU School of Medicine, 9500 Euclid Avenue/A90, Cleveland, OH 4419, USA
* Corresponding author.
E-mail address: khatris@ccf.org

Clin Chest Med 40 (2019) 107–123
https://doi.org/10.1016/j.ccm.2018.10.017

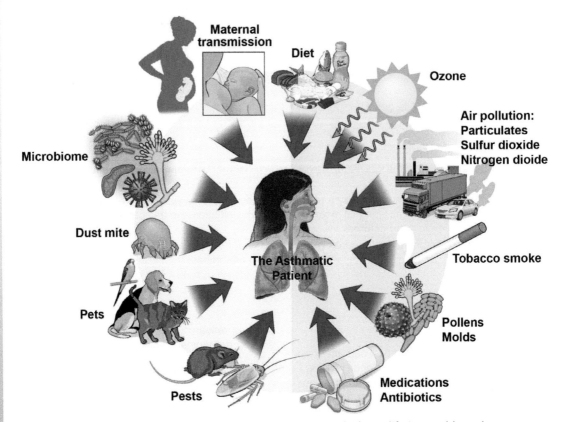

Fig. 1. The exposome concept considers all exposures of an individual in a lifetime and how those exposures relate to health.

PRENATAL AND POSTNATAL
Microbiome – Effect on Prenatal and Early Life Contributing to the Inception of Asthma

External exposures comprising the exposome contribute to the development of asthma, making it a potentially preventable disease process through environmental modifications. Allergic sensitization and respiratory infections with wheezing are independent and synergistic risk factors in the development of asthma. These factors are influenced in early life by the microbiome, which is a potential modifiable exposure in the natural history of asthma. Early microbial exposure and bacterial diversity within the human microbiome have been noted to be crucial elements in the development of innate immunity.[14] Factors associated with urbanization, improved sanitation, and vaccinations have led to decreased microbial exposure in early life and loss of biodiversity in the human microbiome over time. These changes in turn have been associated with increased susceptibility to the development of allergic sensitization and asthma.

Formation of the microbiome begins in utero largely through maternal transmission.[15] Differences in the gut microbiota during infancy with respect to diversity of strains and colonization of specific bacteria are linked with the likelihood of developing atopy. A comparison of diversity in stool flora at age 1 month showed that decreased diversity was predictive of allergic sensitization at age 6 years.[16] Another study revealed that risk of atopic sensitization was inversely related to diversity of infant gut microbiota.[17] Also, in contrast to colonization with *Bacteroides* and *Lactobacillus* species, which have been associated with decreased risk of allergy, specific colonization in the gut with *Clostridia* species was related to wheezing and allergic sensitization.[18]

Microbial colonization of the airways in early life has also been shown to play a role in risk of asthma development. One study showed that colonization with *Streptococcus* species in early life (age 2 months) was associated with chronic wheezing at age 5 years.[19] Another analysis of airway bacterial colonization in asymptomatic neonates at 1 month of age revealed that early colonization with *S pneumoniae*, *Haemophilus influenza*, and/or *Mycobacterium catarrhalis* was associated with recurrent wheeze by age 5 years.[20] Antibiotic use in infancy was associated with decreased abundance of *Bifidobacterium* and *Bacteroides* species.[21]

Given the compelling role of the microbiome in early life and development of asthma, it is important to understand the factors that can affect bacterial colonization and formation of the microbiome. Nutrition, medication use, environment (ie, farm exposures) and mode of delivery have all been demonstrated to have influences on the early life microbiome. Breastfeeding has been shown to alter the airway microbiome toward a more protective profile[22] and greater bacterial diversity.[3] Frequency of maternal urinary tract infections (use of maternal antibiotics) and infant antibiotic use in the first year of life were associated with increased risk of childhood asthma in a dose-dependent proportion.[23]

The benefit of bacterial diversity exposure in early life has been demonstrated through several human studies comparing children living in farm environments versus children living in urban environments. Children who lived on farms had increased indoor microbial exposure as well as more diversity within the microbial environment. These children also had less asthma and atopy compared with peers not living on farms.[14] Increased microbial diversity in the farm environment has been shown to be inversely associated with risk of asthma.[24] In a study comparing children of similar genetic ancestry living in traditional farming environment versus industrial farming, the prevalence of asthma was noted to be 4 to 6 times lower in the children living in the traditional farming environment (Amish community).[25] A proposed mechanism is the protective role of endotoxin, a component of gram-negative bacterial cell walls and a marker of microbial exposure. Amish homes contained higher levels of endotoxin in house dust. This finding is supported by a separate study where higher levels of endotoxin in child mattresses were associated with reduced risk of allergic sensitization and atopic asthma.[26]

Household/Indoor Exposures of Allergens

Indoor particulate matter (PM), including allergens and chemical pollutants, is a major factor in the propagation of asthma worldwide. The specific culprits of reduced indoor air quality vary greatly across countries, with differences influenced by climate, urbanization, and socioeconomic level. Developing countries bear a larger burden from indoor PM pollution because of the use of biomass fuel combustion. Geographic influences can be seen in colder climates where more time may be spent indoors. In the United States, the Environmental Protection Agency estimates most individuals spend approximately 93% of their time indoors.[27]

The relevant allergens in the indoor environment include house dust mites, cockroaches, molds, rodents, and pets. Sensitization in early life (before age 3 years) and multiple allergen sensitization are risk factors for the development of asthma that can persist through adulthood.[28] Perennial allergen sensitization has been linked with increased severity of asthma. Sensitization and exposure to these indoor allergens has been shown to contribute to asthma morbidity as measured by number of asthma exacerbations, days lost from school and work, hospital/emergency room visits, severity of asthma, and medication use.[29,30] In modern society, the efforts to make more energy-efficient homes and desire for comfort indoors (ie, increased indoor temperature, increased humidity, use of carpeting) all contribute to escalating the risk of poor indoor air quality by encouraging proliferation of allergens.

The most effective interventions in modifying indoor allergen exposure have used a multifaceted approach involving patient education, targeted remediation (ie, pest control, impermeable bed covers), and in-home visits/assessments.[31,32] As health care models shift toward value-based care, the use of effective environmental interventions may be increasingly desirable for decreasing asthma morbidity. Using environmental interventions to reduce allergen/irritant exposures can lessen reliance on medications and health care utilization, which will ultimately result in cost-effective and sustainable changes.

House dust mites

House dust mites (HDMs) are ubiquitous microscopic organisms found inside dwellings year-round. HDM sensitization is noted worldwide, with a higher prevalence among individuals with asthma compared with the general population. Asthmatics with HDM sensitization have increased risk for asthma morbidity as measured by health care utilization and increased medication use.[33]

The allergenic proteins of HDM are found in the gut and feces of the organism which contribute to both sensitization and clinical symptoms of the respiratory tract with ongoing exposure. HDMs thrive indoors with increased humidity and elevated temperatures. They feed off human skin cells and are found in high concentrations in bedding (pillows, mattress), carpeting, rugs, stuffed animals, and any item with padding. Interventions to reduce exposure to dust mites are geared toward removal as well as creating barriers: encasing any padded items in impermeable covers, removing likely reservoirs, frequent vacuuming, washing and drying bedding in high heat weekly, maintaining humidity less than 50%, and avoiding carpeted flooring, stuffed animals, and upholstered furniture. Studies evaluating the clinical effect of avoidance measures have shown varying degrees of improvement. The greatest impact is seen in children, where a single intervention of using mite-impermeable bed encasings correlated with reduced rate of hospital visits for asthma exacerbations.[34]

Another potential route of sensitization that has been proposed is oral sensitization to dust mite allergen through breastmilk. A study found the presence of dust mite allergen in breast milk correlating with risk of atopy and asthma at 5 years of age.[35] There was a higher risk in mothers with asthma and allergy themselves, suggesting that a combination of environmental factors and genetics plays a role in the development of asthma.[35] Further studies are needed to investigate the correlation with oral sensitization, as the implications could help shape guidelines for environmental avoidance measures in prenatal and early life.

Pets

Keeping domestic animals, typically cats and dogs, in the home is a common practice in many countries. It is estimated that in the United States over 50% of families are pet owners.[36] Cats are generally more allergenic than dogs; however, both can cause allergy from proteins found in the dander, saliva, and urine. The major allergenic protein of cats (Fel d 1) is small in size, lending this allergen to stay airborne and also easily stick to surfaces and clothing. Indoor exposure to animal allergen occurs inside homes as well as indoor commercial spaces, schools, and work places. This is highlighted by the fact that cat and dog allergenic proteins have been found in house dust from places where there are no animals.[37] The rate of sensitization to domestic animals appears to be rising in the United States and European countries.[38] Exposure to animal allergen in asthmatics who are sensitized is associated with significant asthma morbidity and increased health care utilization.[39]

The most effective remediation for animal allergens is removing pets from the home; yet studies show it can take up to 6 months to eliminate detectable allergen in the home after animal removal.[40] Eliminating animal allergen in the home has been shown to improve asthma symptoms for individuals in the home. Studies evaluating other mitigating measures including a combination of washing the cat weekly, reducing furnishings, vacuum cleaning, and air filtration have shown variable impact on control of asthma symptoms.

The relationship between early exposure to animal allergen and development of sensitization and asthma is more complicated. Some studies have shown early exposure to dogs having a protective effect against allergies. It is postulated that this may be in part caused by the effect of dogs on the home microbiome and in turn microbial exposure in early life. The relationship of sensitization with early exposure to cat on the other hand has not shown consistent patterns, and in some studies has noted an increased risk for sensitization. The link between allergen exposure and sensitization in early life seems to be influenced by timing, environmental factors, and epigenetics. This is an area in which further research may be helpful in elucidating clear guidelines on whether modifying animal exposure in the home can change risk of asthma development.

Mold

Mold spores are ubiquitous in indoor and outdoor environments. There are more than 100,000 known mold species, of which at least 80 have been identified in indoor dwellings.[41] Spores can be small, and, in some cases, microscopic, allowing them to enter deep into the airways. Mold spores thrive in high levels of humidity and are found indoors as result of excessive moisture from water intrusion, inadequate ventilation, defective plumbing, or other structural problems. Indoor mold exposure can be a potential asthma trigger in homes as well as public indoor environments such as schools and places of work. There is a well-established link between sensitization to mold and presence of asthma in adults and children, and early exposure to mold or dampness in infancy has been associated with increased risk of asthma.[42–44] Mold sensitization and exposure are associated with asthma morbidity. Indoor dampness, linked with mold exposure, has been shown to increase the risk of poor asthma control, asthma exacerbations, and increased health care utilization.[45,46]

Indoor exposure to mold may be more prevalent among lower socioeconomic levels because of the higher costs associated with remediation. There is some evidence that mold remediation interventions (eg, removal of visible mold, decreasing humidity in damp basements, repairing leaks, and removal of water-damaged materials) can have impact on individuals with asthma with reduction in emergency room visits and hospitalizations due to asthma. However, some studies have shown no effect; therefore further study with larger sample sizes may be helpful in clarifying benefit of mold remediation efforts.

Cockroach

Cockroaches are a significant source of indoor allergen exposure; infestation is more common in urban environments with dense populations and linked with low socioeconomic status. The allergenic proteins are found in saliva, secretions, debris, and fecal material. Sensitization to cockroach varies across communities and has been found to be has high as 60% to 80% of children in low-income urban environments.[29,30] Cockroach sensitization and exposure have been associated with increases in asthma morbidity, severe asthma, and health care utilization, particularly in low-income inner-city populations.[47]

Interventions to eliminate cockroaches have been effective in reducing cockroach exposure and asthma symptoms. Integrated approaches appear most effective and include professional extermination using insecticide, use of roach traps, putting all food in sealed containers, plugging holes, keeping kitchens clean, promptly washing dishes, frequent disposal of garbage, and directed education on these avoidance measures.

The role of cockroach allergen sensitization in development of asthma is not clear. However, the known association with asthma morbidity and disproportionate burden of exposure in children of lower socioeconomic status have implications of impacting health care utilization well into adult hood.

Rodents

Rodents, including mice, rats, and guinea pigs, are a common source of indoor allergens in inner-city and urban dwellings. These are relevant allergens in homes, public buildings such as schools, and occupational exposure in laboratory facilities using mice for research. The exposure in homes varies greatly depending on geography and urban/rural setting. In certain locations, rodents have been found to be nearly ubiquitous, with mouse protein noted in house dust of the majority of homes in a community. The allergenic protein can be found in urine, skin cells, and hair follicles. Sensitization to mouse and allergen exposure is associated with asthma morbidity and appears to be dose-dependent.[48,49]

Risk factors for higher concentration of mouse allergen in a home include presence of holes or cracks in the wall or doors, reports of mouse sightings, and presence of cockroaches.

Integrated pest management is a remediation approach that has been shown to effectively reduce allergen level in the home. It is a multifaceted plan including vacuuming, using low-toxicity pesticides, placing traps, and sealing holes.[50] This has been shown to reduce allergen levels and in some studies improve health outcomes, reduce health care utilization, and reduce missed days of school for individuals with asthma.[51,52]

Environmental tobacco smoke

Environmental tobacco smoke (ETS) is smoke released into the air from burning cigarette, cigar, or pipes. This contaminates indoor air in homes and common spaces, causing increased asthma morbidity.[53] Exposure to ETS in utero and in early life has been linked with development of asthma and atopy.[54,55] Residue from tobacco smoke, referred to as thirdhand smoke (THS), can persist for weeks to months by sticking to surfaces and dust after smoke is gone. The residue is comprised of chemicals that can react to other air pollutants, creating toxic particles. Young children who are crawling are at risk for exposure by ingesting particles residing on surfaces such as floors, walls, and furniture. A large study of a well-characterized cohort demonstrated that THS exposure was associated with poor asthma control, decreased quality of life, and lower lung function. Often the level of asthma severity was dependent solely on exposure to THS, converting nonsevere asthma to severe asthma. The relation also appeared to be related to genetic antioxidant capability.[56]

Although smoking cessation is the ideal remediation strategy, this has not been shown to be an effective intervention as it as depends on the cooperation of the smoking household members. The use of HEPA air purifiers can be helpful in reducing airborne particles and reducing asthma morbidity as measured by health care utilization in individuals with asthma who cannot avoid ETS.[57] Smoking outside the home may not be an effective mitigating strategy in young children because of the risk of thirdhand smoke (THS).[58]

Indoor chemical pollutants

Nitrogen dioxide Nitrogen dioxide is an important component of indoor air pollutants. It is produced from high-temperature combustion and accumulates in the indoor atmosphere with unvented combustion processes most commonly from gas stoves, kerosene heaters, and poorly vented furnaces and fireplaces. Elevated nitrogen dioxide levels in homes, even below the EPA outdoor standard (53 ppb) has been associated with increased symptoms and use of rescue medications in children with asthma.[59] Interventions such as replacing existing gas stoves with electric stoves, installing ventilation hoods over existing gas stoves, and using air purifiers with HEPA and carbon filters have been shown to be effective in reducing indoor nitric oxide levels. Indoor air quality is also significantly related not only to smoking and cleaning products, but also from using a fireplace or cooking. Cooking may actually increase particulate matter concentration by 1.5- to 27-fold.[60]

Volatile organic compounds Volatile organic compounds (VOCs) are often from human/anthropogenic sources including construction materials, formaldehyde in particle board, oil-based paints, printer toner, fragrant decorations, and indoor plants.[61]

Endotoxin

Endotoxin is a component of the outer membrane of gram-negative bacteria. It is associated with the presence of dampness, mold, pets, or rodents in homes. Endotoxin has been implicated in a variety of toxic effects including airway inflammation and airflow obstruction and therefore an interesting target for indoor air quality improvements. Elevated levels of endotoxin are relevant in the home, school, and workplace for certain occupations. Endotoxin exposure in an inner-city community was positively associated with wheeze at 2 years of age, and personal endotoxin exposure has been associated with increased asthma symptoms and decreased forced expiratory volume in 1 second (FEV_1).[28,62] Occupations in agricultural industry and farming have higher exposure to endotoxin through work, which has been associated with acute and chronic respiratory disease.[63,64] Further study is needed to elucidate the effect of endotoxin exposure on asthma and utility of remediation measures to reduce endotoxin levels.

As described previously, there are a multitude of sources and types of indoor air pollution that affect asthma. In the next sections, relationships of indoor-to-outdoor and primarily global outdoor pollutants will be discussed.

RELATION OF INDOOR AND OUTDOOR AIR QUALITY

Poor or suboptimal indoor air quality is influenced by many sources (eg, mold, pets, dust mites, and chemicals) and can have an adverse effect upon respiratory conditions. This is notable, because most people spend more than 90% of their time indoors.[27] However, indoor environments are not an isolated environment system, and outdoor air quality affects indoor spaces.[65] These correlations vary based upon ventilation, circulation of air indoors, pollution levels outside the housing envelope, and meterological conditions.[27,66] Air exchange rates of 0.35 per hour are recommended in order for the actual amount of air changed to be 63.2% in 1 hour. However, these guidelines may need to be modified based on factors such as outdoor air pollution and number of people occupying the home (eg, more than 15 cubic feet per meter per person).[65,67]

Various factors affect this relationship.[68] Particulate matter levels depend on baseline indoor particulate matter, and are increased by cooking (grilling or frying), exhaust from burners, tobacco smoking, and increased foot traffic. Air circulation and ventilation of the indoor-outdoor environment affect total levels. Particulate matter levels indoors depend largely upon velocity of air movement. Some pollutant such as nitrogen dioxide and other byproducts of VOCs linger until they become diluted or dissociate into radicals and nitrogen dioxide. In addition to air conditioning, appropriate exchange rates, smoke-free homes, maintaining allergen protective measures, and removing or wiping shoes at entrances can reduce indoor particulate matter levels.[68]

Three mechanisms allow outdoor air to enter and affect indoor environments, including mechanical ventilation (via intake for air conditioning and HVAC systems), natural ventilation from outdoor airflow, and infiltration through poorly sealed areas of the housing envelope.[69] Importantly, as changes in the outdoor environment occur, indoor exposures will also change. For example, more than 75% of daily indoor variations of particle and black smoke can be explained by daily outdoor variations.[70] Indoor to outdoor ratios of nitrogen oxides (NOx) vary from 0.5 to 1 with little effect on building permeability while ratios of ozone vary from 0 to 0.5 with building permeability being a significant factor.[71,72] Therefore, the indoor-outdoor relationship of air quality depends upon sources in either compartment, the exchange factors, and attempts to control the sources in each sector.

OUTDOOR EXPOSURES
Pollen

Windborne pollen is a major contributor to allergic asthma. Pollen grains from trees, grass, and weeds are transmitted by the wind and can cause upper and lower respiratory symptoms through immunoglobulin E (IgE)-mediated hypersensitivity reactions on mucosal surfaces. The degree of clinical reaction to pollen depends on the amount of pollen dispersed by a plant, the duration of exposure, and the allergenicity of the pollen. Certain plants may be more influential due to these factors, such as the ragweed plant, which is known to produce over 1 billion pollen grains in 1 allergy season.[73]

The effect of pollen allergy is seen worldwide and most prominent in temperate regions. Depending upon the geographic location, there may be distinct seasons for different types of pollen. For example, in North America, tree pollen exposure is in the spring, grass pollen in the summer, and weeds and ragweed in the fall. Exposure to airborne pollen is linked to increased asthma morbidity, as a study New York showed emergency room visits for asthma attacks, particularly in children, were associated with peaks in tree pollen levels.[74]

Outdoor Air Pollution

Air pollution is a varied mix of components dependent upon industrial and traffic-related emissions and geographic factors such as mountains and valleys. In addition, weather factors such as rainfall, wind speed, and temperature play a role. Mechanisms of air pollution-related compromise to lung health occur via increased permeability of bronchial epithelia, affecting clearance and protection of the airway from allergens and irritants. Environment can also affect respiratory health via epigenetic processes, including by regulation of chromatin, which is one's gene expression profile. DNA methylation and histone modifications are dynamic processes that have been shown to be altered by the external environment. Genes may also be modulated by changes in microRNA expression.[4,7,75] These epigenetic phenomena in which genes may respond to environmental influences explain the gene and environment interactions for disease occurrence and amplification.[4,7]

Air pollution is often related to combustion processes, which also contribute to greenhouse gas emissions.[13] This perpetuates the cyclical issue of air pollution. Methods to evaluate modes of air quality-related lung health have been varied. These include large national health databases, prospective cohort studies, panel studies, and more recently cohort studies in collaboration with more specific air quality monitoring and respiratory-related health markers.[76–79] Outdoor pollutants such as ozone, particulate matter, sulfur dioxide, and nitrogen dioxide are well known to trigger asthma exacerbations and have been associated with reductions in the rate of lung development.[80] Sources include motor vehicle traffic, industrial sources such as petrochemical plants, or coal-fired power plants.[81–83] Another factor that affects the health associations with air quality is the various sources (steel mills), species (organic or inorganic), and components (diesel with adherent pollen grains) of air pollution.[84–86]

Ozone

In contrast to stratospheric ozone levels that protect the earth's atmosphere from 6 to 30 miles above the earth's surface, ambient ozone is present at the respirable ground level closer to the earth's surface. This ambient ozone poses health risks, particularly for those with chronic pulmonary conditions. Ozone is comprised of 3 molecules of oxygen O_3 formed from an oxidative reaction in the presence of pollutants in the atmosphere (eg, VOCs and NOx), heat, and sunlight. Substrate chemicals are released from sources such as burning of fossil fuels, motor vehicle exhaust, and emissions from industrial facilities where molecular oxygen has added oxygen radical, and O_3 is formed. Ozone is therefore a seasonal pollutant that builds up over the course of the day, and in North America, high ozone season occurs from May to September.[87]

Effects of ozone on respiratory conditions include worsening susceptibility to allergens. Summer ozone levels affect respiratory allergy and hay fever symptoms, even when stratified by urban versus rural status.[88–91] Ozone effects are higher after a lag period 24 to 48 hours after exposures, as there is a priming effect to enhance the inflammatory effect of allergen exposures. This lag effect may account for people's inability to perceive the association. Exposure to higher ambient ozone levels has been related to eosinophilia in airways, reducing in small airway airflows FEF25 to 75.[78] Further, ambient ozone levels have been shown not only to worsen existing disease but also with incidence of asthma.[92] The Children's Health study found that children playing 3 or more sports during high ozone days were more likely to have newly diagnosed asthma. Children are particularly sensitive/susceptible to ozone and experience more asthma symptoms, emergency department visits, and intensive care unit admissions.[75,93,94] Children may be also more predisposed because of lungs that are in growth phase, have higher minute ventilation, and more time spent outdoors during summer.

The pathophysiology of these associations may be caused by inflammation, oxidative stress including from increased NADPH oxidase activity, or enhanced allergenic stimulation/eosinophilia.[95] Higher ambient ozone exposures have been temporally associated with higher IgE levels and peripheral eosinophilia[82,96,97] and present oxidant stress to the airways.[98] Exhaled nitric oxide has been shown to correlate with higher ozone levels, indicating increased allergic airway inflammation in patients with asthma.[78,91] Molecular mechanisms may be varied; however, there is evidence of cells' ability to change their behaviors due to environmental exposures (also called plasticity) in cell phenotypes.[75]

Particulate Matter

Particle matter is a year-round pollutant, comprised of a mixture of suspended solids and liquids in the air categorized based upon size.

The particles are produced from industrial, traffic, and geological sources (dust from roads or via chemical reactions in the atmosphere caused by released chemicals from motor vehicles or industrial sources). PM is not visible. Coarse particles (PM10) are 2.5 to 10 um in diameter and fine particles (PM 2.5) are 2.5 um in diameter or less and released from combustion. Although PM is formed in the presence of incomplete combustion of fossil fuels, it can further combine with organic material such as pollen, endotoxins, and fungal spores, creating the immunomodulating and inflammatory responses related to asthma.[27] PM size is related to its potential health effects, as transit in the airways, and absorption/inflammation, are related to particle size and the efficiency of airway defense mechanisms. Inhalable particulate matter that can reach the lower airways includes PM10, PM2.5, and ultrafine (<1 um) particulate matter. PM 2.5, because of its smaller size, is thought to possess a greater health risk due to being able to be inhaled more deeply into the lungs. PM larger than 5 um and less than 10 um may only reach the proximal airways and be expelled by mucociliary clearance. Fine PM is able to transit to the alveolar level and cause inflammatory responses through mediator release more systemically, predisposing to respiratory and cardiac diseases.[99–101]

PM has been associated with the exacerbation of respiratory illnesses. Proximity of homes to major roadways and highways is associated with increased asthma symptoms, emergency department visits, and hospitalizations.[77,100,101] Children who lived within 150 meters of nearest freeway had more deficits in lung function, which been associated with NOx pollutants.[100] Morbidity from chronic asthma and chronic obstructive pulmonary disease (COPD) had consistent associations with PM pollution.[102] These associations are likely caused by the increased inflammatory processes from inhalation with irritation of airways, oxidative stress with formation of inflammatory markers, and mitochondrial dysfunction.[103,104] By promoting release of specific cytokines, chemokines, immunoglobulins, and oxidants in the upper and lower airway, symptoms appear from inflammatory cascade, resulting in increased mucus secretion and bronchial hyperresponsiveness.[103] As demonstrated in the Hyde Park study, which compared exposure to high traffic pollution (Oxford Street) to lower pollution (Hyde Park), airway acidification and sputum myeloperoxidase concentration at 24 hours was higher after exposure on Oxford Street. These inflammatory markers are higher even in instances with relatively modest reductions in lung function, demonstrating the mechanisms by which traffic-related air pollution may affect individuals with asthma.[79] Particles are inhaled, and, depending upon the size and components from the region adherent to molecule (allergens or LPS from bacterial cell walls), airway inflammation may then occur.[89,105]

Diesel exhaust particles (DEPs) and their components such as polycyclic aromatic hydrocarbons make up the majority of particulate matter pollution in urban areas. PM sizes are fine and ultrafine; however, they can coalesce and have other particles adhere to the vehicle provided. The hydrophobic nature of DEPs allow deposition onto the mucosa and not only causes immediate irritant effects but also more chronic symptoms over time such as cough, production of sputum, and diminished lung function. DEPs can enhance the allergenicity of aeroallergens, rendering atopic subjects more susceptible through synergistic expression of allergen-specific IgE and Th2 cytokines.[106,107] In addition, modifications of genetic signaling have been thought to be a mechanism of gene-environment interplay with air pollution and asthma pathogenesis.[75]

Traffic-related air pollution (also known as TRAP), a combination of particulate matter, nitrogen dioxide, and suspended road dust, has been consistent as a trigger for patients with asthma.[80] Traffic-related air pollution affects not only asthma but also COPD, suggesting an even longer-term effect.[108] TRAP and PM in general also affect other chronic conditions. Cardiovascular diseases are also increased and have increased mortality and morbidity from PM.[13]

Nitrogen Dioxide

Nitrogen dioxide is a precursor of ozone, which is formed with additive presence of heat and sunlight. The predominant source of nitrogen dioxide is automobile exhaust, followed by power plants and other industries that burn fossil fuels.[27] However, there are some studies that demonstrate that acute exposure to nitrogen dioxide is associated with asthma and rhinitis and decrement in lung function in individuals with asthma part of TRAP, as in conjunction with black carbon and particulate matter, is the mixture related to TRAP. Growth of lung function is impaired in children with chronic exposure to traffic-related pollutants such as nitrogen dioxide.[109,110]

Sulfur Dioxide

Sulfur dioxide can be a pulmonary irritant and results in increased bronchial responsiveness and bronchomotor tone in patients with asthma.[111,112] Formed from industrial pollutants, sulfur dioxide is a year-round substance in the air formed with the burning of fossil fuels that contain sulfur. In contrast to ozone, where there are more lingering and lag effects of asthma-related symptoms, sulfur dioxide-related symptoms are more short term, during periods of exercise and high ventilatory rates, and may be related to cholinergic-mediated neural mechanisms.[13] However, sulfur dioxide is felt to be more deleterious in combination with other pollutants than as a single agent of concern. These associations were noted during the Beijing Olympics. When industrial pollutant sources were curbed around the times of the games and resulted in lower sulfur dioxide levels, public health metrics related to exacerbations of asthma were reduced.[113,114]

How climate affects air pollutants and environmental triggers for asthma

Greenhouse gas emissions and carbon pollution contribute to increases in temperature in the atmosphere.[13] Climate change is caused by increases in global surface temperatures from greenhouse gases in the troposphere that reflect back infrared radiation to the earth's surface.[12] These greenhouse gases include predominantly carbon dioxide and also methane, nitrous oxide, black carbon, ozone, and various hydrofluorocarbons in the atmosphere. The heat-trapping nature of carbon dioxide is what provides the greenhouse effect and promotes enhanced warming of the earth's surface.[115] Approximately half of total carbon dioxide increase in the earth's atmosphere has occurred in the last 40 years; this phenomenon was recognized as early as the 1800s.[116]

During the American Thoracic Society International Conference in 2010, clinical researchers and scientists authored a consensus statement on climate change and health.[12] There was agreement that the most serious health risks include heat-related illness from heat waves and increased air pollution, but also from desertification, which poses particular risks to pulmonary health (asthma and COPD) from increases in air pollution and particulate matter exposure.

Heat Illnesses/Extreme Temperatures

Heat waves are defined as daily maximum temperature of more than 5 consecutive days exceeding the average max temp by 5°, compared with reference normal period between 1960 and 1990 from (World Meterological Organization).[117] Health is affected by climate change in direct and indirect ways. Directly, changes in temperature produce sources of stress for chronic diseases. Indirectly, with heat as a precursor of many pollutants (particulate matter and ozone), higher levels of air pollutants potentiate the inherent risk of air pollutants

and airway inflammation in asthma. Increased desertification and dust storms create increased inflammation in airways.[86,115,118] With respect to ozone and climate, more warm days with higher surface temperatures and continued burning of fossil fuels allow buildup of VOCs as a substrate in the natural chemical reaction to produce more ground level ozone. This occurs without increased substrate; thus higher temperatures alone prolong peak episodes of ambient ozone.

Air Pollution

Various air quality simulations demonstrate that climate-induced increases in ozone lead to adverse health impacts, suggesting that 50% to 90% of the United States will be exposed to increased levels of ozone exposure.[119] However, in combination with other pollutants such as particulate matter and TRAP, the estimated ozone-related health effects will likely be amplified.[120] With particulate matter, traffic in colder climates, and stagnation with weather patterns, it has been suggested that the global population-weighted PM 2.5 exposure has already increased by 11.2% since 1990.[6,13,117] Estimated projections of the future suggest that 130 million people (half of the global population) will have allergic disease by 2050.[13] Certain patterns have already been noted. Areas with lower temperatures and pollen counts have lower prevalence of allergy, while extreme dry environments with sunlight combining with high pollen counts result in higher prevalence of allergy.[121,122] With changes in climate, earlier flowering has been seen from ragweed pollen as well as from birch, oak, and olive trees. Longer seasons are likely also supplemented by the enhanced allergen content of pollen caused by the altered ecosystem. However, it should be noted that this molecular aerobiology evidence is still in its infancy.[11]

Pollen

The gradual temperature warming associated with climate change has had a major impact on air quality with respect to pollen through its influence on the length of pollen seasons, amount of pollen produced, and the allergenicity and distribution of pollen spores. These influences are seen in emerging patterns, where regions with lower temperature and pollen counts have relatively lower prevalence of allergy, and areas with warmer temperature and dryer environments, conducive to spread of windborne pollen, have higher prevalence of allergy.[121]

Rising temperatures have been associated with longer pollen seasons, with the greatest impact seen in higher latitudes. In North America for example, since 1995 the ragweed season has lengthened from 13 to 27 days.[123] With longer pollen seasons, allergenic plants such as ragweed can grow bigger and produce more pollen over time, leading to increased seasonal asthma morbidity.

In laboratory studies, the size of a ragweed plant and amount of pollen produced were shown to increase with higher levels of carbon dioxide exposure; this showed that as a product of fossil fuel combustion, carbon dioxide is a powerful food for allergenic plants.[124] This has also been demonstrated with timothy grass pollen, where exposure to higher levels of carbon dioxide show approximately doubling of pollen production.[125] Examining this relationship in a natural environment showed a similar association; ragweed plants planted in an urban Baltimore grew faster, flowered earlier, and produced more pollen than plants grown outside the city.[126] Living in proximity to heavy traffic areas is associated with increased pollen-induced respiratory symptoms.[86]

Urbanization is associated with higher traffic patterns and industrial emissions. creating a significant difference in air quality and PM compared with rural environments. The prevalence of paved and dark surface roads, buildings, and open lots increases heat absorption and leads to higher temperatures in the urban environment.[127] This has been referred to as the urban heat island effect, which subsequently leads to acceleration in pollen production and air pollution.

The rise in carbon dioxide levels associated with climate change has driven an increase in air pollutants, which in turn interact with pollen to increase allergen particles and allergenicity. Several mechanisms have been identified, including direct damage of pollen cell wall facilitating allergen release, stimulation of specific allergen production in pollen grains, and acting as an adjuvant by carrying small allergen particles through the airways. The mechanism of increasing allergen protein within the pollen has not been well studied.

Strategies for pollen avoidance can help reduce exposure, but it is difficult to achieve complete avoidance. Use of air conditioning is an effective intervention that can filter out pollen from indoor spaces. Avoiding prolonged outdoor exposure during high pollen counts and bathing/changing clothes after pollen exposure can also be helpful.

The role of climate change and allergies is a broader issue, ultimately highlighting the need to curb fossil fuel combustion and invest in clean energy. Some studies have shown that increasing green spaces within urban environments can help reduce allergy and asthma symptoms.[128]

However, some studies have shown increased association with green space and allergen sensitization.[129] Further studies are needed to clarify how to develop interventions that will lead to a positive impact on the health of communities.

Outdoor Mold

Outdoor mold spore counts are increased with warmer temperatures and humidity. The effects of climate change can lead to increased exposure to mold outdoors (through weather change) and indoors as a result of extreme weather events such hurricanes and flooding, leading to more opportunity for indoor dampness. Warmer weather associated with climate change is contributing to rising sea levels worldwide, which in turn play a role in extreme weather events such as flooding. Outdoor mold exposure has been linked to asthma morbidity. In an Australian study, outdoor mold exposure was associated with child asthma hospitalizations.[124]

Mitigating exposure to outdoor mold spores can be challenging similar to pollen avoidance strategies. However, knowledge of individual mold sensitization may help with risk stratification among individuals with asthma and help guide who may benefit most from strict outdoor avoidance during high mold spore counts and associated weather conditions. Remediation of indoor mold is expensive, and the projected likely increase in prevalence of indoor dampness related to climate change will pose another challenge in optimizing avoidance measures to reduce asthma morbidity. This will likely have a disproportionately larger impact on communities with older homes, restricted access to maintenance capabilities, and rental properties, thus adding to the health disparities in urban environments and communities of lower socioeconomic status.

OTHER ITEMS COMPRISING EXPOSOME
Antibiotics

As previously mentioned in the microbiome section of this article, exposures to consider both prenatally and postnatally that may contribute to asthma as part of the exposome include medications such as antibiotics. In the United States, more than 12% of clinic visits result in a prescription for an antibiotic, and 30% of those prescriptions may be unnecessary.[130,131] Antibiotic exposure during infancy has been shown to be a risk factor for the diagnosis of asthma, as shown in a study in Canada evaluating 213, 661 mother-child dyads, which found that 36.8% of children were prenatally exposed to antibiotics, and 10.1% developed asthma. This antibiotic exposure was associated with increased risk of asthma (hazard ratio 1.23 [1.20–1.27]). A relation to number of antibiotic courses with increased risk of asthma was also found.[131]

Studies have demonstrated an increased association of asthma in children with the prescribing and dispensation of antibiotics to mothers during pregnancy. However, there also appears to be an effect before pregnancy or after birth when mothers are lactating or afterward. These associations of antibiotic use and development of asthma (with odds ratio [OR] of at least 1.23), although present in larger cohort studies, may have a causal role or may be related to other confounding factors that increase the propensity of a child having asthma. Confounders are obvious, such that the mother may have a predisposition to asthma, may have a trend for multiple infections warranting treatment and thus are already compromised, and/or that alteration of the mother's microbiome may lead to an intrinsic predisposition toward asthma. However, in many cases, even with such predispositions, analyses still demonstrate that antibiotic exposure has been a risk factor.[132–134]

Although causal association with alteration of immune function may be part of this association, familial factors such as genetic predisposition (examined by sibling controls), family propensity for infection, and other individual factors such as nutrition (vitamin D), environmental, or genetics are likely at play.[135,136] Finally, health care utilization patterns may be influencing these associations.[136] In summary, although the precise mechanism of these associations is not fully clear, judicious use of antibiotics during this period, as in other times, appears to be warranted.

Related factors of the exposome, such as diet/nutrition and exposures related to occupation and hobbies, have been indirectly or briefly touched upon in this article. These factors should be explored and taken into consideration during the evaluation and management of such patients. **Table 1** lists occupations that need to be considered as potential risks for initiating or enhancing asthma.

MEDICAL COMMUNITY CALL TO ACTION

The implications of the science of exposome, environment, and asthma are immense. The World Health Organization (WHO) and Health Effects Institute (HEI) and Lancet report on climate change estimate that by 2016, approximately 125 million additional vulnerable adults will be exposed to heat waves, putting them at risk for additional disease and premature death.[13] Societies are evaluating the evidence, valuing the science, and

| Table 1 Occupations at high risk for influencing respiratory health ||
Occupation	Trigger
Painters, roofers, insulators	Isocyanates
Famers, agricultural workers	Animal proteins, plants, fungicides
Cleaners	Amines
Bakers	Flours and cereals
Laboratory workers	Animal proteins, chemical exposure (eg, formaldehyde or glutaraldehyde)
Factory workers (manufacturing facilities of paint, plastics, epoxy resins)	Anhydrides
Carpenters	Wood dust
Welders and metal workers	Metals
Hair dressers	Chemicals in hair products, dyes
Health professionals	Latex, biocides, acrylates

speaking up to have a concerted effort to address these threats.[137,138] Ambient air pollution caused 3 million premature deaths from overlapping effects of increased greenhouse gas emissions and air pollution. This is particularly relevant to respiratory health, as future projections estimate 130 million people (half of the global population) will have allergic disease by 2050.[139] There have been more accelerated changes in climate in the last 40 years, and it has been suggested that a feasible goal, that of limiting the temperature rise to 2° above preindustrial times, would prevent the accelerated consequences on ecology, human access to food, and health.[139]

Professional Medical Societies Are Recognizing This to Be a Problem

Although there is a growing awareness among the health care community, environmental factors and climate change have been slow to become part of the partnerships between patients and health care providers. However, professional societies and public health advocates have become more vocal and proactive with statements that highlight the known epidemiologic and pathophysiologic rationale and mechanisms of air quality/environment and health.

Experts agree upon the need to increase public recognition and awareness of this issue as well as educate regarding early warning signs to mitigate the effects on vulnerable populations. To do this, coordinated efforts are necessary among communities of clinicians to engage in, advocate, and influence public policy. Development and funding of climate change research centers are essential.[12,13]

Populations at disproportionate risk for air pollution-related asthma morbidity

It is well established that these effects target people who are young, older, and with chronic medical problems. Studies globally have demonstrated that the population older than 65 years has a greater risk of death.[99,101] Meanwhile in many instances, children appear to be at higher susceptibility compared with adults for emergency department visits for asthma.[11,84] These effects also disproportionately affect those in minority and impoverished communities. Heat waves affect certain populations preferentially, include older individuals, children, laborers, certain ethnic or racial groups, and individuals of low socioeconomic status. These are additive risk factors to air pollution, high humidity, and lack of air conditioning.[9]

There are different levels of risk of mortality and morbidity from air pollution depending on baseline chronic conditions and other factors. The elderly population worldwide is at risk, varying from groups greater than 65 or greater than 75 years old, with higher rates of death in association with particulate matter in the United States (6 cities), South America, and Europe.[99] Ozone and total suspended particles were also associated with mortality in the Netherlands.[140] These associations with mortality remain temporally associated, as rates decrease when air pollution levels become lower again.[141] Children are at risk with exposures to particulate matter, sulfur and nitrogen dioxides, and diesel. These pollutants have been associated with reduced lung function parameters, asthma, and respiratory symptoms. Ozone, nitrogen dioxide, particulate matter, and sulfur dioxide are associated with asthma attacks.[80] Therefore, health effects from short- and longer-term air pollution exposures likely are derived from oxidative stress and immune dysfunction. Those of lower socioeconomic status are at heightened risk because of other usual additional risk factors, home environment/geographic conditions, living in areas of higher pollution, access to care, and related health factors such as malnutrition and smoking.[142]

Importantly, it should be noted that as the exact mechanisms, pace of change, and effects on human respiratory health are debated, regardless of which scientific and mathematical models are used, having policies that address and mitigate climate change consistently indicates that a large number of deaths would be avoided as compared to a scenario where no policy is implemented at all.[143]

SUMMARY

Knowledge of intrinsic and extrinsic factors that predispose people to develop asthma is growing. It is also clear that there is a unique interplay of endosome and exposome in the pathophysiology of respiratory diseases from allergies and asthma. Both indoor and outdoor environments play a role in pathogenesis via levels and duration of exposure, with genetic susceptibility as a crucial factor that alters the initiation and trajectory of a common conditions. The scientific evidence is clear with these known associations. To some degree these exposures can be reduced via a collaborative multinational and global intent to do so. Members of the medical community must understand these factors to better care for patients and potentially prevent future disease from occurring or guard patients with means to mitigate their risks for worsening asthma.

REFERENCES

1. Network GA. The global asthma report 2018. Auckland (New Zealand): 2018.
2. Joubert BR, Reif DM, Edwards SW, et al. Evaluation of genetic susceptibility to childhood allergy and asthma in an African American urban population. BMC Med Genet 2011;12:25.
3. Schwartz S, Friedberg I, Ivanov IV, et al. A metagenomic study of diet-dependent interaction between gut microbiota and host in infants reveals differences in immune response. Genome Biol 2012;13(4):r32.
4. Yang IV, Lozupone CA, Schwartz DA. The environment, epigenome, and asthma. J Allergy Clin Immunol 2017;140(1):14–23.
5. Zhang Y, Salam MT, Berhane K, et al. Genetic and epigenetic susceptibility of airway inflammation to PM2.5 in school children: new insights from quantile regression. Environ Health 2017;16(1):88.
6. Burbank AJ, Sood AK, Kesic MJ, et al. Environmental determinants of allergy and asthma in early life. J Allergy Clin Immunol 2017;140(1):1–12.
7. Cecchi L, D'Amato G, Annesi-Maesano I. External exposome and allergic respiratory and skin diseases. J Allergy Clin Immunol 2018;141(3):846–57.
8. Renz H, Holt PG, Inouye M, et al. An exposome perspective: early-life events and immune development in a changing world. J Allergy Clin Immunol 2017;140(1):24–40.

9. Kravchenko J, Abernethy AP, Fawzy M, et al. Minimization of heatwave morbidity and mortality. Am J Prev Med 2013;44(3):274–82.

10. Pope CA 3rd, Hansen ML, Long RW, et al. Ambient particulate air pollution, heart rate variability, and blood markers of inflammation in a panel of elderly subjects. Environ Health Perspect 2004;112(3): 339–45.

11. Sun J, Fu JS, Huang K, et al. Estimation of future PM2.5- and ozone-related mortality over the continental United States in a changing climate: an application of high-resolution dynamical downscaling technique. J Air Waste Manag Assoc 2015;65(5):611–23.

12. Pinkerton KE, Rom WN, Akpinar-Elci M, et al. An official American Thoracic Society workshop report: climate change and human health. Proc Am Thorac Soc 2012;9(1):3–8.

13. Watts N, Amann M, Ayeb-Karlsson S, et al. The Lancet Countdown on health and climate change: from 25 years of inaction to a global transformation for public health. Lancet 2018; 391(10120):581–630.

14. Illi S, von Mutius E, Lau S, et al. Perennial allergen sensitisation early in life and chronic asthma in children: a birth cohort study. Lancet 2006;368(9537): 763–70.

15. Jimenez E, Fernandez L, Marin ML, et al. Isolation of commensal bacteria from umbilical cord blood of healthy neonates born by cesarean section. Curr Microbiol 2005;51(4):270–4.

16. Abrahamsson TR, Jakobsson HE, Andersson AF, et al. Low diversity of the gut microbiota in infants with atopic eczema. J Allergy Clin Immunol 2012; 129(2):434–40, 440.e1-2.

17. Boyce JA, Bochner B, Finkelman FD, et al. Advances in mechanisms of asthma, allergy, and immunology in 2011. J Allergy Clin Immunol 2012;129(2):335–41.

18. van Nimwegen FA, Penders J, Stobberingh EE, et al. Mode and place of delivery, gastrointestinal microbiota, and their influence on asthma and atopy. J Allergy Clin Immunol 2011;128(5):948–55.e1-3.

19. Teo SM, Mok D, Pham K, et al. The infant nasopharyngeal microbiome impacts severity of lower respiratory infection and risk of asthma development. Cell Host Microbe 2015;17(5):704–15.

20. Bisgaard H, Hermansen MN, Buchvald F, et al. Childhood asthma after bacterial colonization of the airway in neonates. N Engl J Med 2007; 357(15):1487–95.

21. Penders J, Gerhold K, Stobberingh EE, et al. Establishment of the intestinal microbiota and its role for atopic dermatitis in early childhood. J Allergy Clin Immunol 2013;132(3):601–7.e8.

22. Biesbroek G, Bosch AA, Wang X, et al. The impact of breastfeeding on nasopharyngeal microbial communities in infants. Am J Respir Crit Care Med 2014;190(3):298–308.

23. Wu P, Feldman AS, Rosas-Salazar C, et al. Relative importance and additive effects of maternal and infant risk factors on childhood asthma. PLoS One 2016;11(3):e0151705.

24. Wlasiuk G, Vercelli D. The farm effect, or: when, what and how a farming environment protects from asthma and allergic disease. Curr Opin Allergy Clin Immunol 2012;12(5):461–6.

25. Stein MM, Hrusch CL, Gozdz J, et al. Innate immunity and asthma risk in Amish and Hutterite farm children. N Engl J Med 2016;375(5):411–21.

26. von Mutius E, Braun-Fahrländer C, Schierl R, et al. Exposure to endotoxin or other bacterial components might protect against the development of atopy. Clin Exp Allergy 2000;30(9):1230–4.

27. Agency UEP. 2018. Available at: https://www.epa.gov/indoor-air-quality-iaq. Accessed September 16, 2018.

28. Perzanowski MS, Miller RL, Thorne PS, et al. Endotoxin in inner-city homes: associations with wheeze and eczema in early childhood. J Allergy Clin Immunol 2006;117(5):1082–9.

29. Gruchalla RS, Pongracic J, Plaut M, et al. Inner City Asthma Study: relationships among sensitivity, allergen exposure, and asthma morbidity. J Allergy Clin Immunol 2005;115(3):478–85.

30. Gruchalla RS, Sampson HA. Peanut consumption in infants at risk for peanut allergy. N Engl J Med 2015;372(22):2165–6.

31. Crocker DD, Kinyota S, Dumitru GG, et al. Effectiveness of home-based, multi-trigger, multicomponent interventions with an environmental focus for reducing asthma morbidity: a community guide systematic review. Am J Prev Med 2011;41(2 Suppl 1):S5–32.

32. Dixon SL, Fowler C, Harris J, et al. An examination of interventions to reduce respiratory health and injury hazards in homes of low-income families. Environ Res 2009;109(1):123–30.

33. Wang J, Visness CM, Calatroni A, et al. Effect of environmental allergen sensitization on asthma morbidity in inner-city asthmatic children. Clin Exp Allergy 2009;39(9):1381–9.

34. Murray CS, Foden P, Sumner H, et al. Preventing severe asthma exacerbations in children. a randomized trial of mite-impermeable bedcovers. Am J Respir Crit Care Med 2017;196(2):150–8.

35. Baiz N, Macchiaverni P, Tulic MK, et al. Early oral exposure to house dust mite allergen through breast milk: a potential risk factor for allergic sensitization and respiratory allergies in children. J Allergy Clin Immunol 2017;139(1):369–72.e10.

36. Arbes SJ Jr, Cohn RD, Yin M, et al. Dog allergen (Can f 1) and cat allergen (Fel d 1) in US homes: results from the National Survey of Lead and

Allergens in Housing. J Allergy Clin Immunol 2004; 114(1):111–7.

37. Munir AKM, Bjorksten B, Einarsson R, et al. Cat (Fel d I), dog (Can f I), and cockroach allergens in homes of asthmatic children from three climatic zones in Sweden. Allergy 1994;49(7):508–16.

38. Asher MI, Montefort S, Bjorksten B, et al. Worldwide time trends in the prevalence of symptoms of asthma, allergic rhinoconjunctivitis, and eczema in childhood: ISAAC Phases One and Three repeat multicountry cross-sectional surveys. Lancet 2006; 368(9537):733–43.

39. Gergen PJ, Mitchell HE, Calatroni A, et al. Sensitization and exposure to pets: the effect on asthma morbidity in the US Population. J Allergy Clin Immunol Pract 2018;6(1):101–7.e2.

40. Wood RA, Chapman MD, Adkinson NF Jr, et al. The effect of cat removal on allergen content in household-dust samples. J Allergy Clin Immunol 1989;83(4):730–4.

41. Gautier C, Charpin D. Environmental triggers and avoidance in the management of asthma. J Asthma Allergy 2017;10:47–56.

42. O'Driscoll BR, Hopkinson LC, Denning DW. Mold sensitization is common amongst patients with severe asthma requiring multiple hospital admissions. BMC Pulm Med 2005;5:4.

43. Reponen T, Vesper S, Levin L, et al. High environmental relative moldiness index during infancy as a predictor of asthma at 7 years of age. Ann Allergy Asthma Immunol 2011;107(2):120–6.

44. Thacher JD, Gruzieva O, Pershagen G, et al. Mold and dampness exposure and allergic outcomes from birth to adolescence: data from the BAMSE cohort. Allergy 2017;72(6):967–74.

45. Jaakkola MS, Nordman H, Piipar R, et al. Indoor dampness and molds and development of adult-onset asthma: a population-based incident case-control study. Environ Health Perspect 2002;110(5):543–7.

46. Jaakkola JJK, Hwang B-F, Jaakkola N. Home dampness and molds, parental atopy, and asthma in childhood: a six-year population-based cohort study. Environ Health Perspect 2004;113:357–61.

47. Rosenstreich DL, Eggleston P, Kattan M, et al. The role of cockroach allergy and exposure to cockroach allergen in causing morbidity among inner-city children with asthma. N Engl J Med 1997; 336(19):1356–63.

48. Ahluwalia SK, Peng RD, Breysse PN, et al. Mouse allergen is the major allergen of public health relevance in Baltimore City. J Allergy Clin Immunol 2013;132(4):830–5.e1-2.

49. Torjusen EN, Diette GB, Breysse PN, et al. Dose-response relationships between mouse allergen exposure and asthma morbidity among urban children and adolescents. Indoor Air 2013;23(4): 268–74.

50. Phipatanakul W, Cronin B, Wood RA, et al. Effect of environmental intervention on mouse allergen levels in homes of inner-city Boston children with asthma. Ann Allergy Asthma Immunol 2004;92(4):420–5.

51. Kattan M, Stearns SC, Crain EF, et al. Cost-effectiveness of a home-based environmental intervention for inner-city children with asthma. J Allergy Clin Immunol 2005;116(5):1058–63.

52. Pongracic JA, Visness CM, Gruchalla RS, et al. Effect of mouse allergen and rodent environmental intervention on asthma in inner-city children. Ann Allergy Asthma Immunol 2008;101(1):35–41.

53. Morkjaroenpong V, Rand CS, Butz AM, et al. Environmental tobacco smoke exposure and nocturnal symptoms among inner-city children with asthma. J Allergy Clin Immunol 2002;110(1):147–53.

54. Hu FB, Persky V, Flay BR, et al. Prevalence of asthma and wheezing in public schoolchildren: association with maternal smoking during pregnancy. Ann Allergy Asthma Immunol 1997;79(1):80–4.

55. Lannero E, Wickman M, Pershagen G, et al. Maternal smoking during pregnancy increases the risk of recurrent wheezing during the first years of life (BAMSE). Respir Res 2006;7:3.

56. Comhair SA, Gaston BM, Ricci KS, et al. Detrimental effects of environmental tobacco smoke in relation to asthma severity. PLoS One 2011;6(5): e18574.

57. Lanphear BP, Hornung RW, Khoury J, et al. Effects of HEPA air cleaners on unscheduled asthma visits and asthma symptoms for children exposed to secondhand tobacco smoke. Pediatrics 2011; 127(1):93–101.

58. Ferrante G, Simoni M, Cibella F, et al. Third-hand smoke exposure and health hazards in children. Monaldi Arch Chest Dis 2013;79(1):38–43.

59. Belanger E, Kielb C, Lin S. Asthma hospitalization rates among children, and school building conditions, by New York State school districts, 1991-2001. J Sch Health 2006;76(8):408–13.

60. He C, Morawska L, Hitchings J, et al. Contribution from indoor sources to particle number and mass concentration in residential houses. Atmos Environ 2004;38:3405–15.

61. Weschler CJ, Shields HC. Indoor ozone/terpene reactions as a source of indoor particles. Atmos Environ 1999;33:2301–12.

62. Rabinovitch N, Liu AH, Zhang L, et al. Importance of the personal endotoxin cloud in school-age children with asthma. J Allergy Clin Immunol 2005; 116(5):1053–7.

63. Bolund AC, Miller MR, Basinas I, et al. The effect of occupational farming on lung function development in young adults: a 15-year follow-up study. Occup Environ Med 2015;72(10):707–13.

64. Schlunssen V, Basinas I, Zahradnik E, et al. Exposure levels, determinants and IgE mediated

sensitization to bovine allergens among Danish farmers and non-farmers. Int J Hyg Environ Health 2015;218(2):265–72.

65. Lai AC, Thatcher TL, Nazaroff WW. Inhalation transfer factors for air pollution health risk assessment. J Air Waste Manag Assoc 2000;50(9):1688–99.

66. Medicine Io. Clearing the air: asthma and indoor air exposures. Washington, DC: The National Academies Press; 2000.

67. Mudarri DH. Building coes and indoor air quality-EPA. Arlington (VA): 2010.

68. Thompson CR, Hensel EG, Kats G. Outdoor-indoor levels of six air pollutants. J Air Pollut Control Assoc 1973;23(10):881–6.

69. Johnson T, Myers J, Kelly T, et al. A pilot study using scripted ventilation conditions to identify key factors affecting indoor pollutant concentration and air exchange rate in a residence. J Expo Anal Environ Epidemiol 2004;14:1–22.

70. Cyrys J, Pitz M, Bischof W, et al. Relationship between indoor and outdoor levels of fine particle mass, particle number concentrations and black smoke under different ventilation conditions. J Expo Anal Environ Epidemiol 2004;14:275–83.

71. Blondeau P, Lordache V, Poupard O, et al. Relationship between outdoor and indoor air quality in eight French Schools. Indoor Air 2005;15:2–12.

72. Leung DY. Outdoor-indoor air pollution in urban environment: challenges and opportunity. Front Environ Sci 2015;2:1–6.

73. Rees AM. 2nd edition. Consumer health USA: essential information from the federal health network, vol. 2. Westwood (CT): Greenwood; 1997.

74. Ito K, Weinberger KR, Robinson GS, et al. The associations between daily spring pollen counts, over-the-counter allergy medication sales, and asthma syndrome emergency department visits in New York City, 2002-2012. Environ Health 2015;14:71.

75. Feinberg AP. Phenotypic plasticity and the epigenetics of human disease. Nature 2007;447(7143):433–40.

76. Bowatte G, Lodge CJ, Knibbs LD, et al. Traffic-related air pollution exposure is associated with allergic sensitization, asthma, and poor lung function in middle age. J Allergy Clin Immunol 2017;139(1):122–9.e1.

77. Gauderman WJ, Avol E, Lurmann F, et al. Childhood asthma and exposure to traffic and nitrogen dioxide. Epidemiology 2005;16(6):737–43.

78. Khatri SB, Holguin FC, Ryan PB, et al. Association of ambient ozone exposure with airway inflammation and allergy in adults with asthma. J Asthma 2009;46(8):777–85.

79. McCreanor J, Cullinan P, Nieuwenhuijsen MJ, et al. Respiratory effects of exposure to diesel traffic in persons with asthma. N Engl J Med 2007;357(23):2348–58.

80. Delfino RJ, Chang J, Wu J, et al. Repeated hospital encounters for asthma in children and exposure to traffic-related air pollution near the home. Ann Allergy Asthma Immunol 2009;102(2):138–44.

81. Peled R. Air pollution exposure: who is at high risk? Atmos Environ 2011;45(10):1781–5.

82. Peled R, Friger M, Bolotin A, et al. Fine particles and meteorological conditions are associated with lung function in children with asthma living near two power plants. Public Health 2005;119(5):418–25

83. Wickman M, Lupinek C, Andersson N, et al. Detection of IgE reactivity to a handful of allergen molecules in early childhood predicts respiratory allergy in adolescence. EBioMedicine 2017;26:91–9.

84. Khatri SB, Newman C, Rose J, et al. Associations of air quality with asthma during the Cleveland Multiple Air Pollutant Study (CMAPS). Am J Respir Crit Care Med 2010;181:A6827.

85. Norris G, Larson T, Koenig J, et al. Asthma aggravation, combustion, and stagnant air. Thorax 2000;55(6):466–70.

86. D'Amato G, Cecchi L, D'Amato M, et al. Urban air pollution and climate change as environmental risk factors of respiratory allergy: an update. J Investig Allergol Clin Immunol 2010;20(2):95–102 [quiz following: 102].

87. Schultz AA, Schauer JJ, Malecki KM. Allergic disease associations with regional and localized estimates of air pollution. Environ Res 2017;155:77–85.

88. Parker JD, Akinbami LJ, Woodruff TJ. Air pollution and childhood respiratory allergies in the United States. Environ Health Perspect 2009;117(1):140–7.

89. D'Amato G, Liccardi G, D'Amato M, et al. Environmental risk factors and allergic bronchial asthma. Clin Exp Allergy 2005;35(9):1113–24.

90. D'Amato G. Urban air pollution and plant-derived respiratory allergy. Clin Exp Allergy 2000;30(5):628–36.

91. D'Amato G, Liccardi G, D'Amato M. Environmental risk factors (outdoor air pollution and climatic changes) and increased trend of respiratory allergy. J Investig Allergol Clin Immunol 2000;10(3):123–8.

92. McConnell R, Berhane K, Gilliland F, et al. Asthma in exercising children exposed to ozone: a cohort study. Lancet 2002;359(9304):386–91.

93. Ege MJ, Mayer M, Normand AC, et al. Exposure to environmental microorganisms and childhood asthma. N Engl J Med 2011;364(8):701–9.

94. Pakarinen J, Hyvarinen A, Salkinoja-Salonen M, et al. Predominance of gram-positive bacteria in house dust in the low-allergy risk Russian Karelia. Environ Microbiol 2008;10(12):3317–25.

95. Kanter U, Heller W, Durner J, et al. Molecular and immunological characterization of ragweed

(Ambrosia artemisiifolia L.) pollen after exposure of the plants to elevated ozone over a whole growing season. PLoS One 2013;8:e61518.

96. Peled R, Pilpel D, Bolotin A, et al. Young infants' morbidity and exposure to fine particles in a region with two power plants. Arch Environ Health 2004; 59(11):611–6.

97. Rage E, Jacquemin B, Nadif R, et al. Total serum IgE levels are associated with ambient ozone concentration in asthmatic adults. Allergy 2009;64(1): 40–6.

98. Khatri SB, Peabody J, Burwell L, et al. Systemic antioxidants and lung function in asthmatics during high ozone season: a closer look at albumin, glutathione, and associations with lung function. Clin Transl Sci 2014;7(4):314–8.

99. Dockery DW, Stone PH. Cardiovascular risks from fine particulate air pollution. N Engl J Med 2007; 356(5):511–3.

100. Gauderman WJ, Avol E, Gilliland F, et al. The effect of air pollution on lung development from 10 to 18 years of age. N Engl J Med 2004;351(11):1057–67.

101. Schwartz J. Air pollution and blood markers of cardiovascular risk. Environ Health Perspect 2001; 109(Suppl 3):405–9.

102. Halonen JI, Lanki T, Yli-Tuomi T, et al. Particulate air pollution and acute cardiorespiratory hospital admissions and mortality among the elderly. Epidemiology 2009;20(1):143–53.

103. Pandya RJ, Solomon G, Kinner A, et al. Diesel exhaust and asthma: hypotheses and molecular mechanisms of action. Environ Health Perspect 2002;110(Suppl 1):103–12.

104. Salo PM, Xia J, Johnson CA, et al. Indoor allergens, asthma, and asthma-related symptoms among adolescents in Wuhan, China. Ann Epidemiol 2004; 14(8):543–50.

105. Nordenhall C, Pourazar J, Blomberg A, et al. Airway inflammation following exposure to diesel exhaust: a study of time kinetics using induced sputum. Eur Respir J 2000;15:1046–51.

106. Diaz-Sanchez D, Riedl M. Diesel effects on human health: a question of stress? Am J Physiol Lung Cell Mol Physiol 2005;289(5):L722–3.

107. Riedl M, Diaz-Sanchez D. Biology of diesel exhaust effects on respiratory function. J Allergy Clin Immunol 2005;115(2):221–8 [quiz: 229].

108. Lindgren A, Stroh E, Montnemery P, et al. Traffic-related air pollution associated with prevalence of asthma and COPD/chronic bronchitis. A cross-sectional study in Southern Sweden. Int J Health Geogr 2009;8:2.

109. Gauderman WJ, Urman R, Avol E, et al. Association of improved air quality with lung development in children. N Engl J Med 2015;372(10):905–13.

110. Gauderman WJ, Zhang P, Morrison JL, et al. Finding novel genes by testing G x E interactions in a genome-wide association study. Genet Epidemiol 2013;37(6):603–13.

111. Sheppard D, Eschenbacher WL, Boushey HA, et al. Magnitude of the interaction between the bronchomotor effects of sulfur dioxide and those of dry (cold) air. Am Rev Respir Dis 1984;130(1):52–5.

112. Balmes JR, Fine JM, Sheppard D. Symptomatic bronchoconstriction after short-term inhalation of sulfur dioxide. Am Rev Respir Dis 1987;136(5): 1117–21.

113. Rich DQ, Kipen HM, Zhang J, et al. Triggering of transmural infarctions, but not nontransmural infarctions, by ambient fine particles. Environ Health Perspect 2010;118(9):1229–34.

114. Corrigan AE, Becker MM, Neas LM, et al. Fine particulate matters: the impact of air quality standards on cardiovascular mortality. Environ Res 2018;161: 364–9.

115. National Academies of Sciences Engineering and Medicine (U.S.). Committee on extreme weather events and climate change attribution. Attribution of extreme weather events in the context of climate change. Washington, DC: The National Academies Press; 2016. Available at: https://www.nap.edu/catalog/21852/attribution-of-extreme-weather-events-in-the-context-of-climate-change Electronic version. Unrestricted access.

116. Swaminathan MS, Kesavan PC. Agricultural research in an era of climate change. Agricultural Research 2012;1(1):3–11.

117. Upperman CR, Parker JD, Akinbami LJ, et al. Exposure to extreme heat events is associated with increased hay fever prevalence among nationally representative sample of US adults: 1997-2013. J Allergy Clin Immunol Pract 2017;5(2): 435–41.e2.

118. Pollock J, Shi L, Gimbel RW. Outdoor environment and pediatric asthma: an update on the evidence from North America. Can Respir J 2017;2017: 8921917.

119. Post ES, Grambsch A, Weaver C, et al. Variation in estimated ozone-related health impacts of climate change due to modeling choices and assumptions. Environ Health Perspect 2012;120(11):1559–64.

120. Tagaris E, Manomaiphiboon K, Liao K-J, et al. Impacts of global climate change and emissions on regional ozone and fine particulate matter concentrations over the United States. J Geophys Res Atmos 2007;112:D14312.

121. Silverberg JI, Braunstein M, Lee-Wong M. Association between climate factors, pollen counts, and childhood hay fever prevalence in the United States. J Allergy Clin Immunol 2015;135(2):463–9.

122. Stinson KA, Albertine JM, Hancock MS, et al. Northern ragweed ecotypes flower earlier and longer in response to elevated CO2: what are you sneezing at? Oecologia 2016;182(2):587–94.

123. Ziska L, Knowlton K, Rogers C, et al. Recent warming by latitude associated with increased length of ragweed pollen season in central North America. Proc Natl Acad Sci U S A 2011;108(10):4248–51.

124. Tham R, Vicendese D, Dharmage SC, et al. Associations between outdoor fungal spores and childhood and adolescent asthma hospitalizations. J Allergy Clin Immunol 2017;139(4):1140–7.e4.

125. Albertine JM, Manning WJ, DaCosta M, et al. Projected carbon dioxide to increase grass pollen and allergen exposure despite higher ozone levels. PLoS One 2014;9(11):e111712.

126. Ziska LH, Gebhard DE, Frenz DA, et al. Cities as harbingers of climate change: common ragweed, urbanization, and public health. J Allergy Clin Immunol 2003;111(2):290–5.

127. Schmidt CW. Environmental crimes: profiting at the earth's expense. Environ Health Perspect 2004; 112(2):A96–103.

128. Ruokolainen L, von Hertzen L, Fyhrquist N, et al. Green areas around homes reduce atopic sensitization in children. Allergy 2015;70(2):195–202.

129. Andrusaityte S, Grazuleviciene R, Kudzyte J, et al. Associations between neighbourhood greenness and asthma in preschool children in Kaunas, Lithuania: a case-control study. BMJ Open 2016; 6(4):e010341.

130. Fleming-Dutra KE, Hersh AL, Shapiro DJ, et al. Prevalence of inappropriate antibiotic prescriptions among US ambulatory care visits, 2010-2011. JAMA 2016;315(17):1864–73.

131. Loewen K, Monchka B, Mahmud SM, et al. Prenatal antibiotic exposure and childhood asthma: a population-based study. Eur Respir J 2018;52(1) [pii:1702070].

132. Hoskin-Parr L, Teyhan A, Blocker A, et al. Antibiotic exposure in the first two years of life and development of asthma and other allergic diseases by 7.5 yr: a dose-dependent relationship. Pediatr Allergy Immunol 2013;24(8):762–71.

133. Penders J, Kummeling I, Thijs C. Infant antibiotic use and wheeze and asthma risk: a systematic review and meta-analysis. Eur Respir J 2011; 38(2):295–302.

134. Kuo CH, Kuo HF, Huang CH, et al. Early life exposure to antibiotics and the risk of childhood allergic diseases: an update from the perspective of the hygiene hypothesis. J Microbiol Immunol Infect 2013;46(5):320–9.

135. Metsala J, Kilkkinen A, Kaila M, et al. Perinatal factors and the risk of asthma in childhood—a population-based register study in Finland. Am J Epidemiol 2008;168(2):170–8.

136. Stokholm J, Chawes BL, Vissing NH, et al. Azithromycin for episodes with asthma-like symptoms in young children aged 1–3 years: a randomised, double-blind, placebo-controlled trial. Lancet 2016;4(1):19–26.

137. Bayram H, Bauer AK, Abdalati W, et al. Environment, global climate change, and cardiopulmonary health. Am J Respir Crit Care Med 2017;195(6): 718–24.

138. Hopkinson NS, Hart N, Jenkins G, et al. Climate change and lung health: the challenge for a new president. Thorax 2017;72(4):295–6.

139. Asher K, Pearce N. Global burden of asthma among children. Int J Tuberc Lung Dis 2014; 21(1):59–63.

140. Hoek G, Schwartz JD, Groot B, et al. Effects of ambient particulate matter and ozone on daily mortality in Rotterdam, The Netherlands. Arch Environ Health 1997;52(6):455–63.

141. Maddison D. Dose response functions and the harvesting effect. Resour Energy Econ 2006;28(4): 299–368.

142. O'Noill MS, Jerrett M, Kawachi I, et al. Health, wealth, and air pollution: advancing theory and methods. Environ Health Perspect 2003;111(16): 1861–70.

143. Garcia-Menendez F, Saari RK, Monier E, et al. U.S. air quality and health benefits from avoided climate change under greenhouse gas mitigation. Environ Sci Technol 2015;49(13):7580–8.

Life Cycle of Childhood Asthma
Prenatal, Infancy and Preschool, Childhood, and Adolescence

Kristie R. Ross, MD, MS[a],*, W. Gerald Teague, MD[b],
Benjamin M. Gaston, MD[c]

KEYWORDS

- Asthma • Wheezing • Preschool • Prenatal • Childhood • Adolescence • Puberty

KEY POINTS

- Wheezing episodes are common in young children, and a substantial minority will go on to develop asthma.
- Childhood asthma is a heterogeneous condition, but atopy is the most important risk factor.
- Adolescence is a time of remission of symptoms with persistent lung function deficits.

INTRODUCTION AND OBJECTIVES

Episodic wheezing and other lower respiratory tract symptoms are common in infancy and during the preschool years. Although most of these children will see their symptoms resolve by school age, a substantial minority will develop asthma. Allergic sensitization early in life is the strongest risk factor for the development of asthma in childhood, although there are important interactions with prenatal and early life exposures and genotic background. Severe childhood asthma, characterized by significant symptoms or exacerbations despite treatment with high-dose inhaled corticosteroids (ICS) and additional therapies, is a heterogeneous collection of conditions with a broad range of underlying endotypes. It is present in a minority of children with asthma but accounts for a substantial proportion of the burden of childhood asthma on families, the health care system, and public health. Adolescence is a time of remission of symptoms in many children with asthma, although important lung function deficits may remain. Most adults with asthma report the onset of their symptoms or disease during childhood, but given the complexity and heterogeneity of the pathobiology of asthma in adulthood, important questions remain about the transition from childhood to adult asthma. In this review, the

Disclosures: Dr K.R. Ross reports grant funding from NIH, the Ohio Department of Jobs and Family Services, and nonfinancial support from Boehringer Ingelheim, TEVA Respiratory, Glaxo Smith Kline, and Merck. Dr W.G. Teague reports salary support from the Ivy Foundation, grant support from NIH, Panera Bread, TEVA Respiratory, the American Lung Association, AstraZeneca, Sanofi/Regeneron, advisory board participation with Sanofi/Regeneron, TEVA Respiratory, GlaxoSmithKline, Genentech, Aviragen, and serves on speaker bureaus for Genentech/Novartis and TEVA Respiratory.
[a] Division of Pediatric Pulmonology, Allergy, Immunology and Sleep Medicine, Case Western Reserve University School of Medicine, 11100 Euclid Avenue, Cleveland, OH 44106, USA; [b] Pediatric Asthma Center of Excellence, Department of Pediatrics, University of Virginia School of Medicine, 409 Lane Road, Building MR4, Room 2112, PO Box 801349, Charlottesville, VA 22908, USA; [c] Division of Pediatric Pulmonology, Allergy, Immunology and Sleep Medicine, Rainbow Babies and Children's Hospital, Case Western Reserve University School of Medicine, Children's Lung Foundation, 2109 Adelbert Road, BRB 827, Cleveland, OH 44106, USA
* Corresponding author.
E-mail address: Kristie.ross@uhhospitals.org

Clin Chest Med 40 (2019) 125–147
https://doi.org/10.1016/j.ccm.2018.10.008
0272-5231/19/© 2018 Elsevier Inc. All rights reserved.

authors describe current understanding of the epidemiology and risk factors for the asthma throughout childhood, describe the pathobiology underlying the phenotypes of wheezing and asthma in childhood, and highlight important unanswered questions.

INFANCY AND THE PRESCHOOL YEARS
Epidemiology

Up to 50% of children experience at least one episode of wheezing before the age of 6 years.[1] Although most adults with asthma report the onset of wheezing in childhood,[2,3] most young children with wheezing do not develop persistent asthma.[1,4–6] The ideal classification system of young children with asthmalike symptoms would use clinical, immunologic, and/or physiologic characteristics during one of the first episodes of wheezing to classify the child into an endotype that predicted her response to therapy and prognosis for persistence or remittance of disease. The ideal classification system would address questions important to parents: *"Why is my child wheezing?," "How can I prevent/manage these episodes?," "Does this mean my child has asthma?,"* and help direct health care resources. Longitudinal birth cohorts have provided some understanding of the risk factors for the emergence of wheezing in this age group and its persistence into later childhood, although accurate prediction of response to therapy and prognosis for an individual child remains challenging.

Birth Cohorts and Phenotypes of Early Wheezing

Table 1 shows a selection of the more than 30 studies[7] that include longitudinal follow-up from birth or early infancy through at least the third year of life, focusing on those discussed further in later discussion. The earliest large longitudinal study was the Tucson Children's Respiratory Study (TCRS), which enrolled more than 1200 healthy newborns from a health maintenance organization primary care ambulatory practice between 1980 and 1984, with remarkable success in long-term follow-up of the population during which they characterized respiratory and atopic symptoms.[8] At the age of 6, children in the study were described by 4 clinical phenotypes: (1) never wheezing (51.5%); (2) transient early wheezing (19.9%); (3) persistent wheezing (13.7%); and (4) late-onset (after age 3) wheezing (15%).[1]

Unsupervised analyses of more recent birth cohorts have suggested that there may be additional phenotypes to those described in the Tucson cohort.[4,6] In contrast to hypothesis-driven

analyses, unsupervised analyses use statistical methods to allow the data to aggregate into categories without prespecified restrictions, based on the supposition that a priori restrictions may impose bias that could prevent the identification of novel patterns or categories. In the population-based Avon Longitudinal Study of Parents and Children (ALSPAC) study, investigators used latent class analysis (LCA) to identify phenotypes.[4] Although there were reassuring similarities to broadly accepted classifications including the TCRS phenotypes, this analytical technique identified additional subsets that may be helpful to consider in clinical practice and for future research studies. Prolonged early wheeze and intermediate (18–42 months) onset wheeze were found in addition to 4 phenotypes similar to those described in the Tucson cohort. Clinical features at ages 8 to 9 years were compared among the phenotypes, and the children in the phenotypes in which wheezing began after the age of 18 months (intermediate onset and late onset) had the strongest associations with atopy and bronchodilator reversibility at school age. Bias may have resulted from attrition, because nearly half of the children in the original cohort had incomplete data and were not included in this analysis. Children lost to follow-up were more likely to be from a socially deprived background; given findings in a separate analysis of this cohort that suggesting that socioeconomic exposures can influence asthma phenotypes,[9] this is an important limitation.

The relevance of the intermediate and later onset wheezing phenotype was confirmed in a separate LCA of the Prevention and Incidence of Asthma and Mite Allergy (PIAMA) study.[6,10] Similar to the ALSPAC cohort, children in the PIAMA cohort with intermediate onset wheeze, late onset wheeze, and persistent wheeze had the strongest associations with allergic sensitization, bronchial hyperreactivity, and clinical diagnosis of asthma at the age of 8 years. Other evidence that transient early wheezing with viral infections is a distinct phenotype from later onset wheezing includes the findings that daycare attendance or exposure to multiple older siblings increases the risk for wheezing episodes before age 3 but reduces the risk of asthma in later childhood.[11] Taken together, these findings support the concept that precision in terms of the age at the onset of wheeze, the persistence of symptoms, and the presence of atopy may be helpful considerations in evaluating the preschool child with wheezing. However, although the classification systems derived from these birth cohort studies are helpful from a population health construct, phenotypes that are defined by course over time retrospectively cannot

Table 1
Selected asthma birth cohorts

Cohort Name	Selection Criteria and Study Design	Population Included	Baseline and Serial Measures	Outcome Measure Description
Tucson Children's Respiratory Study (TCRS)[1]	Healthy unselected newborns Longitudinal cohort study No intervention	1246 infants enrolled in Tucson, AZ 1980–1984 826 had complete data aged 3 and 6 y 401 had at least one episode of wheezing	Cord serum IgE, infant lung function measurements before illnesses, serum IgE at 9 mo, questionnaires at age 1, assessments during lower respiratory tract illnesses through age 3 y	Age 6: Clinical examination Wheezing questionnaires Serum IgE Spirometry Skin testing
Avon Longitudinal Study of Parents and Children (ALSPAC)[4]	Healthy unselected newborns Longitudinal cohort study No intervention	14,026 infants enrolled in the UK in 1991–1992 11,678 reported wheeze at ≥2 time points of which 6265 had complete data	Parent completed wheezing questionnaires approximately yearly beginning at age 6 mo	Skin prick testing age 7–8 y Lung function age 8–9 y Parent reported physician diagnosis of asthma at age 7.5 y
Prevention and Incidence of Asthma and Mite Allergy (PIAMA)[10]	Infants born to allergic (n = 855) and nonallergic (n = 3291) mothers Allergic mothers only enrolled in randomized trial using dust mite covers	4146 infants enrolled in The Netherlands 1996–1997 2810 had complete data 2067 had no or infrequent reports of wheezing	Parent completed questionnaires approximately yearly beginning at age 3 mo	Clinical examination with specific IgE (4 and 8 y) Lung function (8 y) Measures made in all children born to allergic mothers and subset of children born to nonallergic mothers

(continued on next page)

Table 1
(continued)

Cohort Name	Selection Criteria and Study Design	Population Included	Baseline and Serial Measures	Outcome Measure Description
The Copenhagen Prospective Study on Asthma in Childhood (COPSAC)[76]	Mothers with asthma enrolled	411 infants enrolled in 1998–2001 384 participated through 2 y of age Longitudinal cohort study with nested interventional study using budesonide	Symptom questionnaires, microbiology, inflammatory markers, diet, air quality, allergen exposures and sensitization, genetics, lifestyle measures, lung function measures assessed at 1 m, 6 m, then yearly through age 6 y	Outcomes assessed include preasthma, asthma, atopic dermatitis, allergic rhinitis, allergy, lung function and bronchial responsiveness, subjective and objective testing and clinical examinations at various time points through age 6 y
Childhood Origins of Asthma (COAST)[58]	At least one parent had positive skin testing and/or physician-diagnosed asthma Longitudinal cohort study with no intervention	289 newborns enrolled in 1998–2000 240 had at least one moderate to severe respiratory illness in year 1 76 children had at least one wheezing episode during the third year of life	Questionnaires about symptoms and exposures (frequently in infancy, then yearly ages 1–3 y), nasal lavage samples during scheduled visits in infancy and acute illnesses with and without wheezing, allergen-specific IgE (1 y)	Wheezing during the third year of life

be applied prospectively to the young child with wheezing in your office. The authors discuss prediction models in more detail later in this review.

Risk Factors and Pathobiology of Wheezing in the Preschool Years: "Why Is My Child Wheezing?"

Risk factors for wheezing in early childhood examined in longitudinal cohorts include infections, allergen exposure and sensitization, diet and nutritional factors, stress and adverse life events, obesity, prematurity, irritant and oxidant exposure including smoke exposure and air pollution, and genetic factors. As highlighted by a more detailed discussion of some of these factors in later discussion, when evaluating these studies one must consider the timing of the exposure, interactions between exposures and host factors, and the outcome assessment timing and method. The recent explosion in the ability to measure risk factors with precision, exemplified best by the advances in genetic technology in the last 10 years but also relevant to many other risk factors, and the concurrent advances in complex statistical techniques used to handle these rapid advancements, has resulted in more complex analyses attempting to account for interactions between risk factors. Advancements in the science of analysis techniques may allow one to reconcile some of the conflicting studies surrounding risk factors for wheezing and asthma.

Overview of the Pathobiology of the Inception of Asthma

Asthma susceptibility is determined by a family of genes modified by prenatal and early life environmental factors. Meta-analyses of published reports identify 23 candidate genes associated with asthma risk.[12] Asthma likely is established in the first 3 years of life in children with genetic susceptibility during a critical inception phase of lung development. Among environmental determinants, prenatal factors related to placental function are important, and after birth, exposure to respiratory viruses, bacteria, and allergens likely have a fundamental role.[5,13,14] This gene by environment interaction results in an altered inflammatory airway milieu at or before birth that adversely influences airway function. For example, the authors have shown that the lower airways of young children with treatment-refractory wheeze display a dominant T-helper 1 (Th1) signature and atypical Th1, Th2, and Th17 cytokine profiles.[15]

Environmental exposures at a critical time in lung development normally upregulate T-cell function and promote innate immune responses to lower respiratory infections. However, the absence of certain environmental stimuli results in aberrant T-cell responses in a way that promotes lung inflammation and wheeze with viral infections. Children raised in Amish communities exposed to high levels of endotoxin, known to drive Th1 immune responses, have less asthma and allergen sensitization.[16] An intact respiratory epithelial Th1 immune response to viral infections is required to direct epigenetic changes in airway epithelial cell chromatin that enhances the airway cells' ability to resist infection.[17] Thus, a broad paradigm of the pathobiology of asthma is based on the concept that children born with an array of susceptibility genes acquire dysfunctional innate immune responses to respiratory infections that promote epigenetic changes that subsequently modify the function of the developing airways.

Prenatal Exposures

Prenatal exposures that are associated with the development of wheezing and asthma in childhood are listed in **Table 2**. Epidemiologic associations between exposures and outcomes may be explained by direct effects of the exposure, or by unmasking of an intrinsic tendency. Prenatal and perinatal exposures have been postulated to influence the development of asthma and atopy through a variety of mechanisms, including direct effects on the growth and/or mechanics of developing fetal lungs/airways, modulation of the developing immune system through multiple mechanisms, including effects on the maternal and infant microbiome, and epigenetic modifications. For most exposures, there are likely complex interactions between the child's genetic background, the timing of the exposure, and individual exposures. The high level of complexity of these interactions, as well as the heterogeneity of early childhood wheezing, likely contributes to the heterogeneity of effects seen across studies.

Tobacco Exposure

Active smoking during pregnancy adversely affects lung function in all children,[18] with stronger effects in children with asthma.[19] Active and passive maternal smoking increases the risk of wheezing in early childhood and the development of asthma later in childhood.[19–21] Tobacco affects a variety of genes involved in airway function, oxidative stress, and immune function.[22–26] The finding that prenatal tobacco exposure is more important than postnatal exposure on the child's subsequent respiratory health may be explained by the finding that prenatal tobacco exposure is

Table 2
Prenatal exposures associated with childhood respiratory outcomes

Exposure	Outcome	Comments
Active smoking during pregnancy	Associated with: Reduced lung function[18,19] Increased risk (~40%) for early wheezing[20,21] Increased risk (~20%) for asthma[20]	May have direct effects on airway growth Associated with lifelong epigenetic changes that influence immune and airway development[27,28] Interactions with genetic background[22–26]
Air pollution	Some pollutants associated with generally small but significant (generally <10%) increased risk for early wheezing and asthma[31]	Possible stronger effects in boys and when mothers have high stress[32,177] Animal models suggest epigenetic changes important mechanism[33,34]
Maternal stress	Increased risk (~50%) for early wheezing and asthma[36]	Gender differences[37] Interactions with timing of stress exposure and genetic background[38] Proposed to affect immune programming, airway and lung development[35]
Vitamin D deficiency	Associated with early wheezing and other troublesome lung symptoms in some[178] but not all[179] studies	Postulated to affect immune programming, including reduced antiviral immunity in the infants
Maternal obesity	Increased risk for asthma[180] Increased risk for ever wheezing[180]	Significant heterogeneity in studies
Maternal diet	Limited evidence in most studies that maternal diet is associated with childhood asthma and atopy[41]	Most studies have significant methodological limitations, including recall bias and difficulty accounting for confounders
Vitamin D supplementation	Nonsignificant reduction in wheezing through age 3 OR (0.8, 95% CI 0.6–1.0)[42] OR 0.76 (0.52–1.12)[43]	Subsequent analysis combining the 2 studies showed a protective effect (OR 0.74 [0.57–0.96]) with the strongest effect in women who were vitamin D deficient[44]
Fatty acid supplementation	Fatty acid supplements derived from fish oil during mid gestation reduced persistent wheezing by 30% in a well-designed trial[45]	Single-center study in Denmark; effect was strongest in women with low fatty acid levels at randomization
Folic acid supplements	Increased risk for transient early wheezing[47] No effect on long-term asthma risk in a meta-analysis[46]	A study describing an association between folic acid and allergic airway disease in a mouse model was subsequently retracted[181]
Maternal infections	Prenatal urinary tract infections[50] and chorioamnionitis[54] have been associated with increased childhood wheezing Meta-analysis pooled OR 1.55 (95% CI 1.24–1.92)[51]	Limitations to studies in this area include retrospective nature of most studies, difficulties controlling for confounding, limited duration of follow-up into childhood
Maternal antibiotics	Two meta-analyses of antibiotic use showed increase risk of childhood wheeze or asthma OR 1.2 (95% CI 1.13–1.27)[52] OR 1.24 (95% CI 1.02–1.5)[53]	Confounding by indication is challenging to address
Farming environments	Protective effect on allergic disease[48,49]	Prenatal effect appears to be independent of postnatal exposure to farming environment

associated with lifelong changes in the epigenome[27,28] during a critical window of susceptibility.[29,30] The concepts that there may be a critical window of exposure and that exposures interact with genes are nicely highlighted by the literature on tobacco exposure and asthma, but are also relevant in other exposures.

Air Quality

Studies of the role prenatal exposure to outdoor air pollution has on the risk of wheezing or asthma in childhood have mixed results. Challenges in undertaking these studies include isolating prenatal from postnatal exposures, challenges in measurement and modeling of pollution exposures, and controlling for interactions with other exposures and risk factors. In a recent meta-analysis that included 18 studies, significant associations were found between exposure and childhood wheezing or asthma for nitrogen dioxide and particulate matter of 10 micrometers or less in diameter (PM_{10}).[31] Several studies have shown that timing of exposure,[22] interactions with other exposures,[32] or interaction with sex[22,32] impact the relationship between prenatal air pollution and asthma outcomes. Animal models suggest that prenatal air pollution exposure may affect the development of asthma through immune modulation, increased transcription of genes related to oxidative stress in the absence of ongoing exposure,[33] and via effects on airway hyperreactivity,[34] but the mechanisms in humans have yet to be determined.

Stress

Maternal stress has been linked to multiple physical and mental health outcomes in children and has been postulated to affect the developing respiratory system through inflammation directly affecting fetal airways, disruption in the fetal neuroendocrine system, and alterations in the autonomic nervous system.[35] In a meta-analysis that includes 10 studies with a low level of heterogeneity, children born to mothers exposed to prenatal stress were 1.56 (95% confidence interval [CI] 1.36–1.80) more likely to have wheezing or asthma.[36] Boys born to mothers reporting higher frequencies of negative life events during pregnancy may be more vulnerable to poor respiratory outcomes than girls.[37] Others have found that the timing of events and genetic background are important confounders, with negative life events during the second half of gestation in mothers without a personal history of asthma linked to higher risk of asthma in adolescents.[38]

Nutritional Factors

Maternal nutrition is critical for fetal development and has been postulated to specifically affect the risk of wheezing and asthma through effects on the developing immune system. Although there are many biologically plausible mechanisms that might explain how maternal intake of specific nutrients with immunomodulatory properties could influence the respiratory outcome of offspring,[39] and there are substantial data from animal models supporting this concept,[40] most human studies have been disappointing. A recent meta-analysis of 29 cohorts found that among 16 nutritional components assessed, only maternal intake of vitamin E, zinc, and vitamin D was protective against the development of wheezing, asthma, and other atopic diseases.[41] Limitations to many of these studies include lack of assessment for interactions between nutrients and other risk factors, imprecise assessments of timing and dose of exposures, recall bias, and difficulties controlling for confounding.

Although studies of macronutrients and general diets have been disappointing, there are some data to support the effect of specific vitamins or supplements on respiratory outcomes in the preschool period. When data from 2 randomized controlled trials[42,43] were pooled, vitamin D supplementation during pregnancy was associated with a reduction in asthma or recurrent wheezing at the age of 3 (odds ratio [OR] 0.74, 95% CI 0.57–0.96).[44] Supplementation with fish oil during the last trimester of pregnancy was associated with a lower prevalence of recurrent wheeze or asthma through age 5 in the Copenhagen Prospective Study on Asthma in Childhood (COPSAC) cohort (OR 0.68, 95% CI 0.47–0.98).[45] Maternal use of folic acid supplements has also been studied, with associations found only between use and a small transient increase in risk of wheeze during first year of life not sustained later in childhood.[46,47]

Infections, Bacteria in the Environment, and Antibiotics

Given the interest in the role of the microbiome in the developing immune system, the association between childhood respiratory outcomes and prenatal infections and antibiotic use has also been studied extensively. Prenatal exposure to the high endotoxin burden found in farming environments appears to be protective,[48,49] whereas prenatal infections and antibiotic use increase the risk for early wheezing and asthma.[50–54]

Early Childhood Exposures

Viral infections and the interaction with allergic sensitization

Lower respiratory tract infections are common in early childhood, with more than 30% of participants in the TCRS experiencing a lower respiratory tract infection associated with wheezing in the first year of life, most commonly due to respiratory syncytial virus (RSV).[55] Maternal smoking and low lung function before the onset of symptoms and lack of early allergic sensitization were the strongest risk factors for early but transient wheezing, suggesting this phenotype is driven by substantially different pathobiology than asthma. Cord-serum immunoglobulin E (IgE) was not related to any of the wheezing phenotypes described in the TCRS. In contrast, children with persistent wheezing had higher IgE levels at age 9 months and lower lung function at age 6 years but not at birth.[1] Wheezing with RSV infections in early childhood appears more strongly associated with nonatopic wheeze later in childhood rather than persistent allergic asthma,[56] although there are some contradictory findings.[57]

As the technology to detect a wider variety of microorganisms has advanced, later cohorts established the importance of pathogens other than RSV. In the Childhood Origins of Asthma Study (COAST), in a birth cohort of infants at increased risk for developing asthma due to family history, nasal lavage samples were collected during all acute illnesses and tested for respiratory viruses using polymerase chain reaction (PCR) technology, which was relatively new at the time.[58] The strongest risk factor for wheezing in the third year of life was having a wheezing illness associated with human rhinovirus (HRV) during infancy, although wheezing illnesses with RSV, moderate to severe lower respiratory tract infections without wheezing with any virus, passive smoke exposure, older siblings, and sensitization to foods were all also associated with wheezing in the third year. In a subsequent analysis of the COAST cohort at the age of 6, investigators found that sensitization to aeroallergens increased the risk for subsequent wheezing with HRV, but not RSV.[13] Wheezing with either virus early in life did not increase the risk for allergic sensitization. Adding to the complexity, there are interactions between risk variants in the 17q21 gene locus and wheezing illnesses with HRV with subsequent development of asthma.[59,60] These and other studies highlight the complexities in understanding how the timing of exposures, interactions between exposures, and interactions with host factors including genetic background influence the development of wheezing in the preschool years and childhood asthma.

Bacteria

Culture-based methodology used in the COPSAC study provided evidence that early life colonization with respiratory pathogens (*Streptococcus pneumoniae*, *Haemophilus infuenzae*, or *Moraxella catarrhalis*) is associated with increased risk for recurrent wheezing, doctor-diagnosed asthma, and increased airway resistance responsive to beta-agonists at the age of 5.[5] In contrast, colonization of the oropharynx with *Staphylococcus aureus* was not associated with these respiratory outcomes, nor was colonization with any of the respiratory pathogens at the age of 1 year. Investigators later showed that immune response to the respiratory pathogens at the age of 6 months was different in children who subsequently developed asthma compared with those who did not, characterized by increased interleukin-5 (IL-5) and IL-13 levels with no differences in the activation of T cells or the composition of peripheral T-cell compartments.[61] As methodology to detect microorganisms grew to culture-independent molecular methods, the authors learned that there is a complex symbiotic relationship between humans and microorganisms. The composition, quantity, and diversity of bacteria and other organisms comprising the gut and airway microbiomes likely influence the development and severity of childhood asthma (reviewed in Ref.[62]).

Predictive Models: "Does This Mean My Child Has Asthma?"

Although there has been extensive work to develop prediction models (**Table 3**), early identification of young children with wheezing episodes who are at high risk for progression to established asthma at school age remains an important unmet need. Improvements in the available prediction models would allow directed diagnostic testing, monitoring, and treatment that could deploy resources appropriately while improving quality of life in children and their families by preventing both undertreatment and overtreatment. Accurate prediction of those at highest risk could also advance research in the primary and secondary prevention of asthma. The Asthma Predictive Index (API), developed using the TCRS,[63] and its modified version[64] are the most widely used and cited models. The API and 11 other prediction models developed using birth cohorts and other prospective studies were recently examined in a systematic review.[65] All models included in the review used predictors obtained before the age of 4 years and outcomes obtained between 6 and

Table 3
Models to predict the development of asthma in preschool children with wheezing

Name of Model or Study	Components, Age at Assessment	Outcome, Age at Assessment	PPV	NPV	Validation Studies and Other Comments
Asthma Predictive Index (API)[63] and modified API[64,75] Derived from unselected birth cohort, TCRS	Positive API for children with: 3 or more wheezing episodes before age 3 AND one of: • Parental doctor-diagnosed asthma • Doctor-diagnosed eczema in child (age 2 or 3 y) OR at least 2 of: • Doctor-diagnosed allergic rhinitis (age 2 or 3 y) • Wheezing apart from colds • Eosinophilia (>4%) at age 10 mo	Active asthma by clinical assessment at ages 6, 8, 11, 13 y PPV and NPV are for asthma diagnosis during at least one assessment	77	68	Most widely cited predictive model (>130 citations in PubMed) The mAPI was used in the PEAK study as entry criteria[75] and validated in another cohort[64], added allergic sensitization to at least 1 aeroallergen by age 3 to major criteria and substituted allergic sensitization to milk, egg, or peanut for allergic rhinitis diagnosis
Clinical Asthma Predictive Index (CAPS)[67] Longitudinal cohort study of children ages 1–5 y presenting to primary care provider in The Netherlands for symptoms	Continuous score calculated using: Age at presentation (0–4 points) Family history of asthma/ allergy (0 or 1) Sleep disturbance due to wheezing (0 or 2) Wheezing outside viral infections (0 or 2) Positive specific IgE to cat, dog, OR dust mite (0 or 2) Range 0–11 ≥7 positive score <3 negative score	Symptoms with medication use plus bronchodilator reversibility at age 6 y	74	78	Older age at presentation with first symptoms resulted in higher points Continuous score allows for separate negative and positive cut offs No validation studies reported

(continued on next page)

Table 3
(continued)

Name of Model or Study	Components, Age at Assessment	Outcome, Age at Assessment	PPV	NPV	Validation Studies and Other Comments
From a population-based study in Leicestershire, UK, 1226 children seeing a primary care provider for symptoms were included (n = 1226)[69]	Continuous score with 10 predictors: Sex (1 point for boys) Age at onset (0 points for age 1, 1 point for 2–3 y) Wheezing without colds (0 or 1 points); more than 3 episodes in the last year (2 points) Degree of interference with activities (0–2 points) Degree of dyspnea with symptoms (0, 2, 3 points) Triggered by exercise, play, crying, laughing (0 or 1 point), triggered by exposure to grass, dust, pets (0 or 1 point) Atopic dermatitis (0 or 1 point) Parent family history of wheezing/asthma (1 point for each parent) Range 0–15 ≥5 positive score	Asthma defined as current wheezing + use of asthma medications at 6–8 y	49	86	Used only noninvasive predictors that can be assessed in primary care setting Validated in population based Multicentre Allergy Study, a birth cohort of 1314 German children of whom 140 had cough and wheeze at age 3 and were followed until age 20[182] with similar performance to original study

Study	Score	Outcome	Sensitivity (%)	Specificity (%)	Comments
PIAMA risk score[71]	Continuous score: Male sex (4.6 points), Postterm birth (>42 wk) (0 or 7.3 points), Parental education (medium/low) (0 or 4.2 points), Parental use of inhaled medications (0 or 7 7 points), Wheezing episode frequency per year (0 or 4.2 or 9.1 points), Wheezing apart from colds (0 or 7.1 points), Doctor diagnosis of eczema (0 or 8.2 points), Range 0–55 points, >20 positive score	Age 7 and 8 y, in the last 12 mo: Doctor diagnosis of asthma OR use of ICS OR wheezing episode	23	94	Simplified scoring in validation study[66]. Male sex (2 points), Parental education (medium/low) (0 or 1 point), Parental asthma (0 or 4 points), Wheezing episode frequency per year (0, 4, or 7 points), Wheezing apart from colds (0 or 2 points), Eczema (0 or 6 points), Changed postterm delivery to preterm birth (1 point), Range 0–23 points, ≥8 positive score with PPV 12.4%, NPV 97%, No differences in discriminative ability by ethnic, SE subgroup analyses
Isle of Wight study 1536 children born between 1989 and 1990	Continuous score with one point each for: Recurrent chest infections at age 2 (viral or bacterial), Family history of asthma, Skin test positive at age 4, Absence of chronic nasal symptoms at age 1, Range 0–4 points, ≥3 positive score	Wheezing at age 10	68	74	Very simple scoring system, although skin testing not done in primary care setting in general. Variability in timing of assessments of risk factors, may be challenging to use in real time
10-y follow-up of Environment and Childhood Asthma Study in Oslo, birth cohort study.[72] Nested case control study of 233 children with recurrent or persistent wheezing at age 2 (doctor confirmed) and 216 children without those without any symptoms	Severity of obstructive symptoms was scored: 0–6 points for no. of episodes or months with persistent symptoms; 2 points for each hospitalization (maximum 6 points), Range 0–12, >5 positive score	Symptoms requiring medication and/or positive exercise challenge test at age 10 y	54	87	Applied API to their population with similar performance. Subsequent analysis of inclusion of sIgE (Phadiotop Infant) improved model[70]

Abbreviations: mAPI, modified asthma predictive index; NPV, negative predictive value; PPV, positive predictive value.; SE, socioeconomic; sIgE, serum immunoglobulin E.

12 years, but there was substantial variability in how predictors and outcomes were obtained and defined. A minority of studies (4 out of 12) included physiologic or clinical tests as part of the outcome measure definition of asthma. As might be expected with longitudinal studies, all models had moderate to high risk of bias due to attrition or study flow. Positive predictive values ranged from 12.4%[66] to 74.3%,[67] and negative predictive values ranged from 75.9%[68] to 97.2%.[66] Wheezing in the later preschool years was more strongly associated with asthma in childhood than wheezing in the first 1 to 2 years of life across several studies.[67,69] Some models include diagnostic testing for allergies or atopy,[63,64,67,70] but several models use clinical data obtained noninvasively in the primary care setting.[69,71,72] Authors of the systematic review suggested that these models could form a platform for improvement using advance data techniques; validation and comparison of the available models in a large diverse population may allow integration of components of these models to create an ideal model with better performance.[65] The study of novel biomarkers and more physiologic testing was also suggested as a method to improve performance.

Response to Therapy

Treatment recommendations for preschool children with recurrent wheezing vary from use of anti-inflammatory medications (eg, ICS) in a minority of these children[73] to more liberal use based on symptoms and exacerbations[74] similar to constructs used in older children. In terms of the ability of predictive models to direct symptom management, preschool-aged children with a positive API have been shown to have improved control while treated with low-dose ICS,[75] whereas young children who were at high risk for asthma based on maternal history of asthma but who were otherwise unselected did not show benefit.[76] Preschool children with persistent asthma-type symptoms were also more likely to respond to low-dose ICS if they had evidence for both allergic sensitization and eosinophilia than if they had only one or none of these markers.[77] The recommendation to classify and treat young children based on trigger (viral vs multiple trigger) made in the 2008 European Respiratory Society (ERS) Task Force report[73] has been updated recently to account for the variability over time for individual children, and to shift the emphasis from trigger to the severity and frequency of both symptoms and exacerbations.[78] Many children in this age group have frequent flares of wheezing without day-to-day impairment, and in those children, use of

intermittent high-dose inhaled steroids resulted in similar clinical improvement to daily use with fewer adverse effects.[79] For those with more frequent symptoms between exacerbations, use of daily ICS reduces exacerbation frequency.[80]

Primary and Secondary Prevention

Given the increasing understanding of asthma as a developmental disorder characterized by interactions between prenatal and early life exposures with genetic susceptibility, with a particular focus on the interactions between viral infections and allergens in susceptible children, the development of strategies to intervene and prevent asthma is an exciting prospect. Although there is some evidence that a multifaceted approach to reduce exposure to allergens may prevent the development of asthma in high-risk populations,[81,82] larger studies of more generalizable and practical strategies that target single allergen exposure have not been able to prevent asthma development.[83–86] Trials of immunotherapy to prevent sensitization have also been disappointing.[87]

Strategies that prevent viral infection have also been studied. In a randomized controlled trial of RSV prophylaxis in healthy preterm infants, infants in the treatment group had 61% fewer wheezing days in the first year of life.[88] Longer-term follow-up will be needed to determine if this expensive strategy reduces the development of asthma later in life. The prevention of HRV infection is more complex, and although there is some evidence it is possible in select populations,[89] the paradox that early life daycare exposure, where HRV infection is high with prolonged viral shedding,[90] is associated with reduced asthma risk[11,91] highlights the need for further study in this area with careful attention to measuring exposures and outcomes and their interactions.

Strategies that might influence the developing immune system to boost antiviral response, reduce skew toward Th2 signaling, and enhance T-regulatory cells in a manner that replicates the protective effects of early life farm living[92] that have been shown to be effective in animal models include bacterial products[93–96] and probiotics.[97–99] Human studies of probiotics to prevent asthma have been largely disappointing,[100] and there are limited data on the use of bacterial extracts in children.[101]

Although ICS improve symptom control in young children with wheezing, they are not effective in secondary prevention, with multiple studies showing no impact on the natural history of early wheezing.[75,76,102] There are some epidemiologic data that secondary prevention of asthma using immunotherapy may be possible,[103] although confirmation in well-controlled trials is needed. Although there is interest in the use of monoclonal antibodies directed against Th2 inflammatory pathways as secondary prevention strategies,[104] concerns about long-term safety and expense must be considered.

SCHOOL-AGED CHILDREN
Epidemiology and Pathobiology of Established Asthma

Asthma progresses from an evolving phase during early development characterized by virus-associated wheeze to an established phase by 4 to 6 years of age.[1] Although virus-associated wheeze episodes are highly prevalent in preschool children, most children with this clinical pattern do not develop persistent asthma. Treatment with inhaled corticosteroids in this age group can reduce symptom burden and exacerbations in children at high risk for asthma development, but does not have a lasting effect on symptoms or exacerbations once treatment is discontinued.[75] Evidence of allergen sensitization to foods and inhalants, which starts during infancy and can progress during early maturation, is the most important determinant of persistent asthma by school age.[105] The phenotype of atopy, the pattern and timing of sensitization to aeroallergens, is an important determinant of asthma risk.[106,107] More than two-thirds of school-age and adolescent children with persistent asthma are allergen sensitized, regardless of asthma severity.[108]

Children who reach school age with ongoing episodic or persistent wheezing that is not caused by structural abnormalities or rare lung disease, particularly when reversible airway obstruction is demonstrated, generally meet epidemiologic and clinical criteria for a firm diagnosis of asthma.[74,109] Asthma prevalence estimates in this age group vary by sex and race, with a prevalence of 12.4% among boys and 8.8% among girls aged 5 to 14 years.[110] In addition to atopy, male sex,[2] maternal or paternal history of asthma,[111] preterm birth,[112] overweight/obesity,[113] minority race,[114,115] and socioeconomic and geographic factors[116] are all well established risk factors for childhood asthma. As previously discussed, each of these risk factors has important interactions with genetic background and other exposures in determining whether an individual child develops asthma.

Response to Treatment

The landmark Childhood Asthma Management Program (CAMP) showed that most, but not all, children with asthma will respond well to low-dose ICS with improved lung function and airway hyperreactivity and reduced symptoms and exacerbations.[117] Beneficial effects of ICS do not last once therapy is discontinued, whereas small but significant reductions in height are sustained, particularly in girls.[118] The CAMP investigators and others have shown that lack of response to ICS is predicted by prenatal smoke exposure,[119] lack of bronchodilator reversibility,[120,121] and overweight and obesity.[122] Atopy[123] and airway inflammation[124] may predict better response to ICS in children with mild to moderate asthma. Further work is needed to allow accurate and personalized approaches to choose the best option for an individual child among the several alternatives for step-up therapy in those not responding to low-dose ICS.[125,126]

Lung Function Trajectories

Early wheezing and childhood asthma are associated with lung function deficits, most of which are established by early school age. All children with a wheezing phenotype in the ALSPAC birth cohort had lung function deficits at school age,[4] whereas others have shown that there are stronger relationships between more persistent wheezing phenotypes in the preschool years and later lung function deficits.[127] Some studies have shown little progression of lung function abnormalities as children age, including the Melbourne Asthma Study,[128] the TCRS,[129] and the Dunedin Multidisciplinary Health and Development Study.[130] However, more recently published findings from the CAMP study suggest that three-quarters of young adults with childhood onset asthma have abnormal patterns of lung growth, including 11% who met guideline-defined chronic obstructive pulmonary disease.[131] Taken together, these studies suggest lung function deficits begin early in life and impact lifelong lung growth.

Asthma Exacerbations

Exacerbations of asthma result in missed school and work and health care utilization, important outcomes to children and their families and drivers of direct and indirect asthma-related costs. Longitudinal follow-up of participants in CAMP and other cohort studies of asthma in childhood, including the Severe Asthma Research Program (SARP) and The Epidemiology and Natural History of Asthma: Outcomes and Treatment Regimens (TENOR), suggest exacerbations are associated with uncontrolled or severe asthma, and that exacerbation-prone asthma in children may also be a distinct phenotype not fully explained by severity or control.[132–135] Infection with HRV, particularly by the A and C strains, is the most important trigger in children hospitalized for asthma.[136] As in preschool children, there are important interactions between atopy and response to viral infections. Children with HRV infection and demonstrable sensitivity to dust mite have a much higher probability of wheeze compared with nonsensitized children in a Costa Rica emergency room study.[14] Current evidence supports the concept that in children with problematic wheeze and asthma, infection with HRV amplifies smoldering Th2 inflammation to produce inflammatory cytokines, which are present during exacerbations of asthma. The fundamental importance of IgE responses as regulating HRV-associated exacerbations is illustrated by a study of inner city children with asthma wherein treatment with omalizumab, an anti-IgE biological therapy, completely ameliorated the expected spike in exacerbations expected during the fall viral respiratory season.[137]

Severe Asthma

Severe asthma, characterized by a significant symptom burden despite high-dose corticosteroid therapy,[138] is present in approximately 10% of children with asthma. Findings from the SARP and TENOR study confirm that severe asthma of childhood has heterogeneous clinical features and pathobiology.[139–141] There is no one dominant "phenotype" that is appropriate for severe asthma; instead, specific molecular "endotypes" are present that explain the heterogeneity of its clinical symptoms and treatment response. In ongoing studies, the authors have found that children with the most severe asthma and morbid clinical features have increased eosinophils and neutrophils in the airway's fluid accompanied by prevalent infection with HRV, blood eosinophilia, and a high degree of allergen sensitization (WG Teague, unpublished data, 2017). The inflammatory pattern appears to be relatively insensitive to high-dose corticosteroid therapy in these children. The heterogeneity in childhood severe asthma is narrower than that seen in adult severe asthma with more consistent findings of atopy and reversible airways obstruction.[142,143]

PUBERTY AND ADOLESCENCE
Epidemiology of Asthma in Adolescence

After a peak in school age, asthma prevalence appears to decrease between the beginning and end of adolescence.[108,110,144] The authors discuss the role of endogenous sex hormone changes in puberty on asthma in later discussion. In addition,

although developmental maturation of innate immune responses is probably important, one study has shown that persistent respiratory eosinophilia is a fundamental determinant of bronchial hyperresponsiveness and asthma remission.[145] With adult maturation, the pathobiology of asthma becomes increasingly complex with an array of inflammatory endotypes.[108] The epidemiology of asthma in adults is markedly different than children, transitioning from increased prevalence in boys compared with girls to increased prevalence in women compared with men.[110] It seems likely that severe asthma in adulthood includes those who had severe atopic asthma in childhood, with the addition of other later onset phenotypes.[146]

Notwithstanding the decline in prevalence during adolescence, there is a subpopulation of children with persistent asthma who had had childhood impairment of lung function and have subsequent lung function decline in adolescence. The persistent lung function decline suggests that early wheezing and obstruction increase risk for fixed airflow obstruction in adolescence and early adulthood.[131] Indeed, preadolescent children with persistent wheeze have, on follow-up, consistently lower lung function in adolescence and young adulthood.[130] Thus, although there is a tendency for many children to outgrow asthma symptoms, at least transiently, in adolescence, those who had persistent wheezing in childhood had lower lung function in adolescence. Wheezing and obstruction in children less than 3 years old, in particular, may predict persistent obstruction in adolescence and later in life.[1,129]

Of note, about half of children with severe asthma in early childhood no longer meet criteria for severe asthma as adolescents.[147] Severe asthma is defined by American Thoracic Society (ATS)/ERS criteria as asthma, managed by an asthma specialist, that requires treatment with high-dose ICS plus a second controller, and/or systemic corticosteroids, but remains symptomatic and exacerbation prone.[138] In general, severe asthma accounts for nearly half of the morbidity, mortality, and cost of asthma.[108,138,144] However, both asthma severity and hospitalizations start to decrease in late childhood and remain relatively low into young adulthood.[110,144,147] Cross-sectional data[144,147,148] suggest that severe asthma prevalence and asthma admissions are lower in late adolescence (14–18 years old) and early adulthood (19–30 years old) than in earlier childhood and in middle age. Longitudinal data from the SARP show a decrease in the proportion of subjects with qualifying factors for severe asthma, and a corresponding increase in the proportion of subjects who are well controlled without qualifying medications over 3 years.[147] Moreover, individual aspects of severe asthma improved longitudinally, including symptom scores, exacerbations, and controller medication requirements.[147]

Surprisingly, there were 3 important factors that were not associated with improvement in severe asthma.[147] First, lung function did not, overall, change among children with severe asthma followed into adolescence. Consistent with previous reports, there were some children with lower lung function and some with higher, likely determined early in childhood, but lung function did not decline during adolescence, nor was it a predictor or resolution of severe asthma. Second, body mass index (BMI) did not change in the population, nor was it a predictor of failure to resolve severe asthma in adolescence. Finally, the proportion of boys and girls with severe asthma in childhood improved equally during adolescence, despite dramatic gender-based differences in early childhood and adulthood (see later discussion).

Endocrine Effects on Asthma in Adolescence

Assessment of the stage of pubertal maturation is different in boys than in girls. In boys, surges in central and peripheral androgens are parallel, whereas in girls, the peripheral effects of androgens are not necessarily synchronized with centrally stimulated release of estradiol and breast bud development.[149,150] Surges in endogenous sex hormones across adolescence could affect asthma status. For example, dehydroepiandrosterone sulfate (DHEAS), a circulating androgen that increases with puberty, inhibits human airway smooth muscle and airway fibroblast proliferation[151,152] and may influence airway epithelial-to-mesenchymal transition.[153] Testosterone promotes airway smooth muscle relaxation[154] and has anti-inflammatory effects.[155] Androgen receptors are expressed in bronchial smooth muscle tissue, and testosterone relaxes airway smooth muscle, suggesting a beneficial effect of androgens on airway smooth muscle tone.[154] Note that, in children with asthma, studies of adrenarche may be affected by corticosteroid treatment.[156]

In women both with and without asthma, forced expiratory volume in 1 second (FEV_1) % peaks at the end of the luteal phase to the beginning of menstruation and then decreases when circulating estrogen and progesterone decrease.[157] Accordingly, the decrease in circulating estrogen and progesterone from the luteal to the follicular phase of the menstrual cycle is accompanied by a reduction in lymphocyte β_2 adrenoceptor density[158] and increased bronchial responsiveness in women

with asthma.[159] Recent studies of dysanapsis (differential growth of airway caliber and lung volume) in healthy subjects suggest that, by adulthood, women develop more small airways resistance than do men.[160] Taken together, these studies suggest that sex steroids can affect lung function and airway inflammation during puberty.

In the SARP, there were differences in phenotypic features according to sex and pubertal stage, taking all asthmatic children into account (both severe and nonsevere).[161] For boys 6 to 18 years old, lung function associated positively with log DHEAS values. The prebronchodilator FEV_1% ($\beta = 8.05$; $P = .01$), post-bronchodilator (BD) FEV_1% ($\beta = 8.82$, $P = .008$), and pre-BD forced vital capacity (FVC%) ($\beta = 8.33$, $P = .01$) had strongly positive β coefficients. In addition, boys with high DHEAS had fewer symptoms. The Asthma Control Questionnaire 6 (ACQ6) had a negative β coefficient with higher log DHEAS values ($\beta = -0.59$, $P = .007$). The model predicting ACQ6 included negative β coefficients for both log DHEAS and testosterone as well as the interaction of log DHEAS with testosterone. Circulating DHEAS levels in boys did not vary significantly when compared according to treatment with high-dose versus medium-dose ICS. Furthermore, treatment with high-dose corticosteroids did not suppress DHEAS levels in boys. Although the testosterone increase is orders of magnitude greater than that of DHEAS with puberty,[162,163] DHEAS levels in the authors' analysis were more strongly associated with better lung function and improved ACQ6 than was testosterone.

For girls 6 to 18 years of age, androgens associated positively, but estrogens negatively, with lung function. Free testosterone had a positive association with post-BD FEV_1% ($\beta = 3.99$, $P = .04$). In contrast, estradiol had negative β coefficients for pre-BD FEV_1% ($\beta = -0.47$, $P = .03$), post-BD FEV_1% ($\beta = -0.62$, $P = .0009$), pre-BD FVC% ($\beta = -0.36$, $P = .04$), and post-BD FVC% ($\beta = -0.33$, $P = .03$). For the ACQ6, only log DHEAS had a significant association; it varied positively ($\beta = 0.49$, $P = .05$), and the correlation was relatively weak. In girls, subtle but significant discordance between loss of lung function observed in association with late puberty assessed by breast staging relative to pubic hair staging suggests that estrogen, which drives breast development, may be the main factor affecting lung function.[161] Only girls have a surge of estrogen or progesterone during puberty, and breast development is exclusively associated with this surge. The authors also cannot exclude an adverse effect of progesterone. For example, the effects of pregnancy on lung function may be both estrogen and progesterone dependent, and both hormones have been hypothesized to play roles in the worsening of lung function.

What Are the Determinants of Change in Asthma Incidence and Severity During Adolescence?

As noted above, both asthma incidence and severity decrease, on the whole, during adolescence. Identifying the factors associated with this decrease could help "flatten the risk curve" as a function of age in asthma, as has been done for cardiovascular disease.[164,165] That is, if it is known why adolescents improve, that knowledge could possibly be applied to younger children and older adults in whom asthma risk remains higher.

First, adrenal androgens may help decrease asthma during adolescence. Production is increased during puberty in both boys and girls.[159,166] Higher DHEAS is associated with better lung function[161]; DHEA supplementation can improve pulmonary outcomes,[167] and DHEAS has beneficial airway effects in vitro. However, interpretation of androgen data can be confounded by corticosteroid use[156] and by additional endocrine factors,[168,169] and resolution of severe asthma occurred in both boys and girls Therefore, the authors suspect that additional factors are also at work.

Lung growth could be the principal reason for improvement in adolescence. Several longitudinal studies, such as the CAMP follow-up data, suggest that there is a subset of children with wheezing who have airflow limitation lasting into adulthood, measured by spirometry.[131,170] In this context, it is surprising that most younger children with severe asthma outgrow symptoms and medication requirements and can no longer be categorized as severe. Moreover, neither prealbuterol spirometry nor postalbuterol spirometry at enrollment predicted which children would outgrow severe asthma.[147] Obesity could also be a determinant of asthma severity, both affecting chest wall function[171,172] and, particularly through visceral fat, affecting non-Th2 inflammation (in part through IL-6).[172–174] However, the children who had severe asthma at the beginning of SARP III who were no longer severe after 3 years did not differ with regard to starting BMI, and BMI did not change with time. Furthermore, visceral fat increases in adolescence,[175] making it unlikely to be related to decreasing asthma severity. Importantly, adrenal androgens likely contribute to lung growth and improved chest wall strength, so increased androgen production and overall improved airway caliber/chest wall strength are not mutually exclusive.

Finally, it has been argued that chronic inflammation in asthmatic children could contribute to chronic long-term obstruction.[176] Mechanisms that could decrease inflammation might include moving to a residence with less antigenicity and/or improved medication adherence. However, neither of these are, overall, likely to occur during adolescence. Moreover, the SARP data suggest that Th2 markers are not decreased in children with severe asthma who go on to resolve; in fact, they tend to be increased.[147] Thus, it seems unlikely that a simple decrease in inflammation resulted in decreased asthma prevalence or severity.

SUMMARY

Wheezing in early childhood and childhood asthma are heterogeneous conditions, best conceptualized as developmental disorders arising from interactions between genetic susceptibility and exposures beginning in the prenatal period and continuing through childhood, resulting in modification of the immune and physiologic functioning of the developing airways. Prediction of which young children with wheezing will develop asthma remains challenging. Most school-aged children with asthma are atopic and respond well to low-dose ICS. Further work is needed to personalize care based on endotype for children with severe or difficult-to-treat asthma. Adolescence is a time of remission of symptoms but persistence of lung function deficits established in early life. The transition to asthma in adults is not well understood, because the pathobiology of asthma becomes increasingly complex as environmental influences, including smoking, air pollution exposure, and repeated infections, interact with obesity and hormonal changes to produce an array of inflammatory endotypes.

REFERENCES

1. Martinez FD, Wright AL, Taussig LM, et al. Asthma and wheezing in the first six years of life. N Engl J Med 1995;332(3):133–8.

2. Yunginger JW, Reed CE, O'Connell EJ, et al. A community-based study of the epidemiology of asthma: incidence rates, 1964–1983. Am Rev Respir Dis 1992;146(4):888–94.

3. Phelan PD, Robertson CF, Olinsky A. The Melbourne asthma study: 1964-1999. J Allergy Clin Immunol 2002;109:189–94.

4. Henderson J, Granell R, Heron J, et al. Associations of wheezing phenotypes in the first 6 years of life with atopy, lung function and airway responsiveness in mid-childhood. Thorax 2008;63(11): 974–80.

5. Bisgaard H, Hermansen MN, Buchvald F, et al. Childhood asthma after bacterial colonization of the airway in neonates. N Engl J Med 2007;357(15):1487–95.

6. Savenije OE, Granell R, Caudri D, et al. Comparison of childhood wheezing phenotypes in 2 birth cohorts: ALSPAC and PIAMA. J Allergy Clin Immunol 2011;127(6):1505–12.e14.

7. Bousquet J, Gern JE, Martinez FD, et al. Birth cohorts in asthma and allergic diseases: report of a NIAID/NHLBI/MeDALL joint workshop. J Allergy Clin Immunol 2014;133(6):1535–46.

8. Taussig LM, Wright AL, Morgan WJ, et al. The Tucson Children's Respiratory Study. I. Design and implementation of a prospective study of acute and chronic respiratory illness in children. Am J Epidemiol 1989;129(6):1219–31.

9. Galobardes B, Granell R, Sterne J, et al. Childhood wheezing, asthma, allergy, atopy, and lung function: different socioeconomic patterns for different phenotypes. Am J Epidemiol 2015;182(9):763–74.

10. Brunekreef B, Smit J, de Jongste J, et al. The prevention and incidence of asthma and mite allergy (PIAMA) birth cohort study: design and first results. Pediatr Allergy Immunol 2002;13(Suppl 15):55–60.

11. Ball TM, Castro-Rodriguez JA, Griffith KA, et al. Siblings, day-care attendance, and the risk of asthma and wheezing during childhood. N Engl J Med 2000;343(8):538–43.

12. Tizaoui K, Hamzaoui K, Hamzaoui A. Update on asthma genetics: results from meta-analyses of candidate gene association studies. Curr Mol Med 2017;17(10):647–67.

13. Jackson DJ, Evans MD, Gangnon RE, et al. Evidence for a causal relationship between allergic sensitization and rhinovirus wheezing in early life. Am J Respir Crit Care Med 2012;185(3):281–5.

14. Soto-Quiros M, Avila L, Platts-Mills TAE, et al. High titers of IgE antibody to dust mite allergen and risk for wheezing among asthmatic children infected with rhinovirus. J Allergy Clin Immunol 2012;129(6):1499–505.

15. Wisniewski JA, Muehling LM, Eccles JD, et al. TH1 signatures are present in the lower airways of children with severe asthma, regardless of allergic status. J Allergy Clin Immunol 2018;141(6):2048–60.e13.

16. Stein MM, Hrusch CL, Gozdz J, et al. Innate immunity and asthma risk in amish and hutterite farm children. N Engl J Med 2016;375(5):411–21.

17. Spalluto CM, Singhania A, Cellura D, et al. IFN-g influences epithelial antiviral responses via histone methylation of the RIG-I promoter. Am J Respir Cell Mol Biol 2017;57(4):428–38.

18. Gilliland FD, Berhane K, McConnell R, et al. Maternal smoking during pregnancy, environmental tobacco smoke exposure and childhood lung function. Thorax 2000;55(4):271–6.

19. Li Y-F, Gilliand FD, Berhane K, et al. Effects of in utero and environmental tobacco smoke exposure on lung function in boys and girls with and without asthma. Am J Respir Crit Care Med 2000;162(6):2097–104.

20. Burke H, Leonardi-Bee J, Hashim A, et al. Prenatal and passive smoke exposure and incidence of asthma and wheeze: systematic review and meta-analysis. Pediatrics 2012;129(4):735–44.

21. Vardavas CI, Hohmann C, Patelarou E, et al. The independent role of prenatal and postnatal exposure to active and passive smoking on the development of early wheeze in children. Eur Respir J 2016;48(1):115–24.

22. Wu C-C, Ou C-Y, Chang J-C, et al. Gender-dependent effect of GSTM1 genotype on childhood asthma associated with prenatal tobacco smoke exposure. Biomed Res Int 2014;2014:1–7.

23. Rogers AJ, Brasch-Andersen C, Ionita-Laza I, et al. The interaction of glutathione S-transferase M1-null variants with tobacco smoke exposure and the development of childhood asthma. Clin Exp Allergy 2009;39(11):1721–9.

24. Haley KJ, Lasky-Su J, Manoli SE, et al. RUNX transcription factors: association with pediatric asthma and modulated by maternal smoking. Am J Physiol Lung Cell Mol Physiol 2011;301(5):L693–701.

25. Ramadas RA, Sadeghnejad A, Karmaus W, et al. Interleukin-1R antagonist gene and pre-natal smoke exposure are associated with childhood asthma. Eur Respir J 2007;29(3):502–8.

26. Wang C, Salam MT, Islam T, et al. Effects of in utero and childhood tobacco smoke exposure and 2-adrenergic receptor genotype on childhood asthma and wheezing. Pediatrics 2008;122(1):e107–14.

27. Breton CV, Byun H-M, Wenten M, et al. Prenatal tobacco smoke exposure affects global and gene-specific DNA methylation. Am J Respir Crit Care Med 2009;180(5):462–7.

28. Breton CV, Siegmund KD, Joubert BR, et al. Prenatal tobacco smoke exposure is associated with childhood DNA CpG methylation. PLoS One 2014;9(6):e99716.

29. Guo H, Zhu P, Yan L, et al. The DNA methylation landscape of human early embryos. Nature 2014;511(7511):606–10.

30. Smith ZD, Chan MM, Humm KC, et al. DNA methylation dynamics of the human preimplantation embryo. Nature 2014;511(7511):611–5.

31. Hehua Z, Qing C, Shanyan G, et al. The impact of prenatal exposure to air pollution on childhood wheezing and asthma: a systematic review. Environ Res 2017;159:519–30.

32. Bose S, Chiu Y-HM, Hsu H-HL, et al. Prenatal nitrate exposure and childhood asthma. Influence

of maternal prenatal stress and fetal sex. Am J Respir Crit Care Med 2017;196(11):1396–403.

33. Manners S, Alam R, Schwartz DA, et al. A mouse model links asthma susceptibility to prenatal exposure to diesel exhaust. J Allergy Clin Immunol 2014;134(1):63–72.

34. Fedulov AV, Leme A, Yang Z, et al. Pulmonary exposure to particles during pregnancy causes increased neonatal asthma susceptibility. Am J Respir Cell Mol Biol 2008;38(1):57–67.

35. Wright RJ. Perinatal stress and early life programming of lung structure and function. Biol Psychol 2010;84(1):46–56.

36. van de Loo KFE, van Gelder MMHJ, Roukema J, et al. Prenatal maternal psychological stress and childhood asthma and wheezing: a meta-analysis. Eur Respir J 2016;47(1):133–46.

37. Lee A, Mathilda Chiu Y-H, Rosa MJ, et al. Prenatal and postnatal stress and asthma in children: temporal- and sex-specific associations. J Allergy Clin Immunol 2016;138(3):740–7.e3.

38. Hartwig IRV, Sly PD, Schmidt LA, et al. Prenatal adverse life events increase the risk for atopic diseases in children, which is enhanced in the absence of a maternal atopic predisposition. J Allergy Clin Immunol 2014;134(1):160–9.e7.

39. Prescott SL. Allergic disease: understanding how in utero events set the scene. Proc Nutr Soc 2010;69(03):366–72.

40. Thorburn AN, McKenzie CI, Shen S, et al. Evidence that asthma is a developmental origin disease influenced by maternal diet and bacterial metabolites. Nat Commun 2015;6(1):7320.

41. Beckhaus AA, Garcia-Marcos L, Forno E, et al. Maternal nutrition during pregnancy and risk of asthma, wheeze, and atopic diseases during childhood: a systematic review and meta-analysis. Allergy 2015;70(12):1588–604.

42. Litonjua AA, Carey VJ, Laranjo N, et al. Effect of prenatal supplementation with vitamin D on asthma or recurrent wheezing in offspring by age 3 years. JAMA 2016;315(4):362.

43. Chawes BL, Bønnelykke K, Stokholm J, et al. Effect of vitamin D 3 supplementation during pregnancy on risk of persistent wheeze in the offspring. JAMA 2016;315(4):353.

44. Wolsk HM, Chawes BL, Litonjua AA, et al. Prenatal vitamin D supplementation reduces risk of asthma/recurrent wheeze in early childhood: a combined analysis of two randomized controlled trials. PLoS One 2017;12(10):e0186657.

45. Bisgaard H, Stokholm J, Chawes BL, et al. Fish oil–derived fatty acids in pregnancy and wheeze and asthma in offspring. N Engl J Med 2016;375(26): 2530–9.

46. Brown SB, Reeves KW, Bertone-Johnson ER. Maternal folate exposure in pregnancy and childhood asthma and allergy: a systematic review. Nutr Rev 2014;72(1):55–64.

47. Bekkers MBM, Elstgeest LEM, Scholtens S, et al. Maternal use of folic acid supplements during pregnancy, and childhood respiratory health and atopy. Eur Respir J 2012;39(6):1468–74.

48. Ege MJ, Mayer M, Normand A-C, et al. Exposure to environmental microorganisms and childhood asthma. N Engl J Med 2011;364(8):701–9.

49. Douwes J, Cheng S, Travier N, et al. Farm exposure in utero may protect against asthma, hay fever and eczema. Eur Respir J 2008;32(3): 603–11.

50. Collier CH, Risnes K, Norwitz ER, et al. Maternal infection in pregnancy and risk of asthma in offspring. Matern Child Health J 2013;17(10): 1940–50.

51. Zhu T, Zhang L, Qu Y, et al. Meta-analysis of antenatal infection and risk of asthma and eczema. Medicine (Baltimore) 2016;95(35):e4671.

52. Zhao D, Su H, Cheng J, et al. Prenatal antibiotic use and risk of childhood wheeze/asthma: a meta-analysis. Pediatr Allergy Immunol 2015; 26(8):756–64.

53. Murk W, Risnes KR, Bracken MB. Prenatal or early-life exposure to antibiotics and risk of childhood asthma: a systematic review. Pediatrics 2011; 127(6):1125–38.

54. Getahun D, Strickland D, Zeiger RS, et al. Effect of chorioamnionitis on early childhood asthma. Arch Pediatr Adolesc Med 2010;164(2):187–92.

55. Wright AL, Taussig LM, Ray CG, et al. The tucson children's respiratory study. II. Lower respiratory tract illness in the first year of life. Am J Epidemiol 1989;129(6):1232–46.

56. Stein RT, Sherrill D, Morgan WJ, et al. Respiratory syncytial virus in early life and risk of wheeze and allergy by age 13 years. Lancet 1999;354(9178): 541–5.

57. Sigurs N, Gustafsson PM, Bjarnason R, et al. Severe respiratory syncytial virus bronchiolitis in infancy and asthma and allergy at age 13. Am J Respir Crit Care Med 2005;171(2):137–41.

58. Lemanske RF, Jackson DJ, Gangnon RE, et al. Rhinovirus illnesses during infancy predict subsequent childhood wheezing. J Allergy Clin Immunol 2005;116(3):571–7.

59. Çalışkan M, Bochkov YA, Kreiner-Møller E, et al. Rhinovirus wheezing illness and genetic risk of childhood-onset asthma. N Engl J Med 2013; 368(15):1398–407.

60. Smit LAM, Bouzigon E, Pin I, et al. 17q21 variants modify the association between early respiratory infections and asthma. Eur Respir J 2010;36(1): 57–64.

61. Larsen JM, Brix S, Thysen AH, et al. Children with asthma by school age display aberrant immune

responses to pathogenic airway bacteria as infants. J Allergy Clin Immunol 2014;133(4): 1008–13.e4.

62. Singanayagam A, Ritchie AI, Johnston SL. Role of microbiome in the pathophysiology and disease course of asthma. Curr Opin Pulm Med 2017; 23(1):41–7.

63. Castro-Rodriguez JA, Holberg CJ, Wright AL, et al. A clinical index to define risk of asthma in young children with recurrent wheezing. Am J Respir Crit Care Med 2000;162(4):1403–6.

64. Chang TS, Lemanske RF, Guilbert TW, et al. Evaluation of the modified asthma predictive index in high-risk preschool children. J Allergy Clin Immunol Pract 2013;1(2):152–6.

65. Smit HA, Pinart M, Antó JM, et al. Childhood asthma prediction models: a systematic review. Lancet Respir Med 2015;3(12):973–84.

66. Hafkamp-de Groen E, Lingsma HF, Caudri D, et al. Predicting asthma in preschool children with asthma-like symptoms: validating and updating the PIAMA risk score. J Allergy Clin Immunol 2013;132(6):1303–10.e6.

67. van der Mark LB, van Wonderen KE, Mohrs J, et al. Predicting asthma in preschool children at high risk presenting in primary care: development of a clinical asthma prediction score. Prim Care Respir J 2014;23(1):52–9.

68. Vial Dupuy A, Amat F, Pereira B, et al. A simple tool to identify infants at high risk of *mild* to *severe* childhood asthma: the *persistent* asthma predictive score. J Asthma 2011;48(10):1015–21.

69. Pescatore AM, Dogaru CM, Duembgen L, et al. A simple asthma prediction tool for preschool children with wheeze or cough. J Allergy Clin Immunol 2014;133(1):111–8.e13.

70. Lødrup Carlsen KC, Söderström L, Mowinckel P, et al. Asthma prediction in school children; the value of combined IgE-antibodies and obstructive airways disease severity score. Allergy 2010; 65(9):1134–40.

71. Caudri D, Wijga A, Schipper CM A, et al. Predicting the long-term prognosis of children with symptoms suggestive of asthma at preschool age. J Allergy Clin Immunol 2009;124(5):903–10.e7.

72. Devulapalli CS, Carlsen KCL, Haland G, et al. Severity of obstructive airways disease by age 2 years predicts asthma at 10 years of age. Thorax 2008;63(1):8–13.

73. Brand PLP, Baraldi E, Bisgaard H, et al. Definition, assessment and treatment of wheezing disorders in preschool children: an evidence-based approach. Eur Respir J 2008;32(4):1096–110.

74. Expert Panel Report-3. Guidelines for the Diagnosis and Management of Asthma, National Asthma Education and Prevention Program. National Institutes of Health. 2007. Available at: https://www.nhlbi.nih.gov/health-topics/guidelines-for-diagnosis-management-of-asthma.

75. Guilbert TW, Morgan WJ, Zeiger RS, et al. Long-term inhaled corticosteroids in preschool children at high risk for asthma. N Engl J Med 2006; 354(19):1985–97.

76. Bisgaard H, Hermansen MN, Loland L, et al. Intermittent inhaled corticosteroids in infants with episodic wheezing. N Engl J Med 2006;354(19): 1998–2005.

77. Fitzpatrick AM, Jackson DJ, Mauger DT, et al. Individualized therapy for persistent asthma in young children. J Allergy Clin Immunol 2016;138(6): 1608–18.e12.

78. Brand PLP, Caudri D, Eber E, et al. Classification and pharmacological treatment of preschool wheezing: changes since 2008. Eur Respir J 2014;43(4):1172–7.

79. Zeiger RS, Mauger D, Bacharier LB, et al. Daily or intermittent budesonide in preschool children with recurrent wheezing. N Engl J Med 2011;365(21): 1990–2001.

80. Kaiser SV, Huynh T, Bacharier LB, et al. Preventing exacerbations in preschoolers with recurrent wheeze: a meta-analysis. Pediatrics 2016;137(6) [pii:e20154496].

81. Chan-Yeung M, Ferguson A, Watson W, et al. The Canadian childhood asthma primary prevention study: outcomes at 7 years of age. J Allergy Clin Immunol 2005;116(1):49–55.

82. Arshad SH, Bateman B, Sadeghnejad A, et al. Prevention of allergic disease during childhood by allergen avoidance: the Isle of Wight prevention study. J Allergy Clin Immunol 2007;119(2): 307–13.

83. Woodcock A, Lowe LA, Murray CS, et al. Early life environmental control. Am J Respir Crit Care Med 2004;170(4):433–9.

84. Horak F, Matthews S, Ihorst G, et al. Effect of mite-impermeable mattress encasings and an educational package on the development of allergies in a multinational randomized, controlled birth-cohort study – 24 months results of the Study of Prevention of Allergy in Children in Europe. Clin Exp Allergy 2004;34(8):1220–5.

85. Corver K, Kerkhof M, Brussee JE, et al. House dust mite allergen reduction and allergy at 4 yr: follow up of the PIAMA-study. Pediatr Allergy Immunol 2006;17(5):329–36.

86. Toelle BG, Garden FL, Ng KKW, et al. Outcomes of the childhood asthma prevention study at 11.5 years. J Allergy Clin Immunol 2013;132(5):1220–2.e3.

87. Zolkipli Z, Roberts G, Cornelius V, et al. Randomized controlled trial of primary prevention of atopy using house dust mite allergen oral immunotherapy in early childhood. J Allergy Clin Immunol 2015; 136(6):1541–7.e11.

88. Blanken MO, Rovers MM, Molenaar JM, et al. Respiratory syncytial virus and recurrent wheeze in healthy preterm infants. N Engl J Med 2013; 368(19):1791–9.

89. Luoto R, Ruuskanen O, Waris M, et al. Prebiotic and probiotic supplementation prevents rhinovirus infections in preterm infants: a randomized, placebo-controlled trial. J Allergy Clin Immunol 2014;133(2):405–13.

90. Martin ET, Fairchok MP, Stednick ZJ, et al. Epidemiology of multiple respiratory viruses in childcare attendees. J Infect Dis 2013;207(6):982–9.

91. Nicolaou NC, Simpson A, Lowe LA, et al. Day-care attendance, position in sibship, and early childhood wheezing: a population-based birth cohort study. J Allergy Clin Immunol 2008;122(3):500–6.e5.

92. von Mutius E, Vercelli D. Farm living: effects on childhood asthma and allergy. Nat Rev Immunol 2010;10(12):861–8.

93. Johnson JL, Jones MB, Cobb BA. Bacterial capsular polysaccharide prevents the onset of asthma through T-cell activation. Glycobiology 2015;25(4):368–75.

94. Fu R, Li J, Zhong H, et al. Broncho-vaxom attenuates allergic airway inflammation by restoring GSK3β-related t regulatory cell insufficiency. PLoS One 2014;9(3):e92912.

95. Navarro S, Cossalter G, Chiavaroli C, et al. The oral administration of bacterial extracts prevents asthma via the recruitment of regulatory T cells to the airways. Mucosal Immunol 2011;4(1):53–65.

96. Strickland DH, Judd S, Thomas JA, et al. Boosting airway T-regulatory cells by gastrointestinal stimulation as a strategy for asthma control. Mucosal Immunol 2011;4(1):43–52.

97. Feleszko W, Jaworska J, Rha R-D, et al. Probiotic-induced suppression of allergic sensitization and airway inflammation is associated with an increase of T regulatory-dependent mechanisms in a murine model of asthma. Clin Exp Allergy 2007;37(4): 498–505.

98. Kim H-J, Kim Y-J, Lee S-H, et al. Effects of *Lactobacillus rhamnosus* on asthma with an adoptive transfer of dendritic cells in mice. J Appl Microbiol 2013; 115(3):872–9.

99. Kim H-J, Kim Y-J, Lee S-H, et al. Effects of Lactobacillus rhamnosus on allergic march model by suppressing Th2, Th17, and TSLP responses via CD4+CD25+Foxp3+ Tregs. Clin Immunol 2014; 153(1):178–86.

100. Azad MB, Coneys JG, Kozyrskyj AL, et al. Probiotic supplementation during pregnancy or infancy for the prevention of asthma and wheeze: systematic review and meta-analysis. BMJ 2013;347: f6471.

101. Razi CH, Harmancı K, Abacı A, et al. The immunostimulant OM-85 BV prevents wheezing attacks in preschool children. J Allergy Clin Immunol 2010; 126(4):763–9.

102. Murray CS, Woodcock A, Langley SJ, et al, IFWIN study team. Secondary prevention of asthma by the use of Inhaled Fluticasone propionate in Wheezy INfants (IFWIN): double-blind, randomised, controlled study. Lancet 2006;368(9537): 754–62.

103. Schmitt J, Schwarz K, Stadler E, et al. Allergy immunotherapy for allergic rhinitis effectively prevents asthma: results from a large retrospective cohort study. J Allergy Clin Immunol 2015;136(6): 1511–6.

104. Jackson DJ. Early-life viral infections and the development of asthma: a target for asthma prevention? Curr Opin Allergy Clin Immunol 2014;14(2):131–6.

105. Heymann PW, Carper HT, Murphy DD, et al. Viral infections in relation to age, atopy, and season of admission among children hospitalized for wheezing. J Allergy Clin Immunol 2004;114(2): 239–47.

106. Simpson A, Tan VYF, Winn J, et al. Beyond atopy: multiple patterns of sensitization in relation to asthma in a birth cohort study. Am J Respir Crit Care Med 2010;181(11):1200–6.

107. Hose AJ, Depner M, Illi S, et al. Latent class analysis reveals clinically relevant atopy phenotypes in 2 birth cohorts. J Allergy Clin Immunol 2017; 139(6):1935–45.e12.

108. Teague WG, Phillips BR, Fahy JV, et al. Baseline features of the Severe Asthma Research Program (SARP III) Cohort: differences with age. J Allergy Clin Immunol Pract 2018;6(2):545–54.e4.

109. Global Initiative for Asthma. Global strategy for Asthma Management and Prevention, 2016.

110. Centers for Disease Control and Prevention. National Center for Environmental Health, Division of Environmental Hazards and Health Effects, Centers for Disease Control and Prevention, Asthma Surveillance Data. Available at: www.cdc.gov/asthma/asthmadata.htm. Accessed April 30, 2018.

111. Lim RH, Kobzik L, Dahl M. Risk for asthma in offspring of asthmatic mothers versus fathers: a meta-analysis. PLoS One 2010;5(4):e10134.

112. Jaakkola J, Ahmed P, Ieromnimon A, et al. Preterm delivery and asthma: a systematic review and meta-analysis. J Allergy Clin Immunol 2006; 118(4):823–30.

113. Egan KB, Ettinger AS, Bracken MB. Childhood body mass index and subsequent physician-diagnosed asthma: a systematic review and meta-analysis of prospective cohort studies. BMC Pediatr 2013;13(1):121.

114. Gupta RS, Zhang X, Sharp LK, et al. Geographic variability in childhood asthma prevalence in Chicago. J Allergy Clin Immunol 2008;121(3):639–45.e1.

115. Forno E, Celedon JC. Asthma and ethnic minorities: socioeconomic status and beyond. Curr Opin Allergy Clin Immunol 2009;9(2):154–60.

116. Wright RJ, Subramanian SV. Advancing a multilevel framework for epidemiologic research on asthma disparities. Chest 2007;132(5):757S–69S.

117. Childhood Asthma Management Program Research Group, Szefler S, Weiss S, Tonascia J, et al. Long-term effects of budesonide or nedocromil in children with asthma. N Engl J Med 2000; 343(15):1054–63.

118. Strunk RC, Sternberg AL, Szefler SJ, et al. Long-term budesonide or nedocromil treatment, once discontinued, does not alter the course of mild to moderate asthma in children and adolescents. J Pediatr 2009;154(5):682–7.

119. Cohen RT, Raby BA, Van Steen K, et al. In Utero smoke exposure and impaired response to inhaled corticosteroids in children with asthma. J Allergy Clin Immunol 2010;126(3):491–7.

120. Zielen S, Christmann M, Kloska M, et al. Predicting short term response to anti-inflammatory therapy in young children with asthma. Curr Med Res Opin 2010;26(2):483–92.

121. Rogers AJ, Tantisira KG, Fuhlbrigge AL, et al. Predictors of poor response during asthma therapy differ with definition of outcome. Pharmacogenomics 2009;10(8):1231–42.

122. Forno E, Lescher R, Strunk R, et al. Decreased response to inhaled steroids in overweight and obese asthmatic children. J Allergy Clin Immunol 2011;127(3):741–9.

123. Gerald JK, Gerald LB, Vasquez MM, et al. Markers of differential response to inhaled corticosteroid treatment among children with mild persistent asthma. J Allergy Clin Immunol Pract 2015;3(4): 540–6.e3.

124. Knuffman JE, Sorkness CA, Lemanske RF, et al. Phenotypic predictors of long-term response to inhaled corticosteroid and leukotriene modifier therapies in pediatric asthma. J Allergy Clin Immunol 2009;123(2):411–6.

125. Lemanske RF, Mauger DT, Sorkness CA, et al. Step-up therapy for children with uncontrolled asthma receiving inhaled corticosteroids. N Engl J Med 2010;362(11):975–85.

126. Chang TS, Lemanske RF, Mauger DT, et al. Childhood asthma clusters and response to therapy in clinical trials. J Allergy Clin Immunol 2014;133(2): 363–9.e3.

127. Lodge CJ, Lowe AJ, Allen KJ, et al. Childhood wheeze phenotypes show less than expected growth in FEV$_1$ across adolescence. Am J Respir Crit Care Med 2014;189(11):1351–8.

128. Horak E, Lanigan A, Roberts M, et al. Longitudinal study of childhood wheezy bronchitis and asthma: outcome at age 42. BMJ 2003;326(7386):422–3.

129. Morgan WJ, Stern DA, Sherrill DL, et al. Outcome of asthma and wheezing in the first 6 years of life follow-up through adolescence. Am J Respir Crit Care Med 2005;172(10):1253–8.

130. Sears MR, Greene JM, Willan AR, et al. A Longitudinal, population-based, cohort study of childhood asthma followed to adulthood. N Engl J Med 2003;349(15):1414–22.

131. McGeachie MJ, Yates KP, Zhou X, et al. Patterns of growth and decline in lung function in persistent childhood asthma. N Engl J Med 2016;374(19): 1842–52.

132. Denlinger LC, Phillips BR, Ramratnam S, et al. Inflammatory and comorbid features of patients with severe asthma and frequent exacerbations. Am J Respir Crit Care Med 2017;195(3).

133. Haselkorn T, Zeiger RS, Chipps BE, et al. Recent asthma exacerbations predict future exacerbations in children with severe or difficult-to-treat asthma. J Allergy Clin Immunol 2009;124(5):921–7.

134. Wu AC, Tantisira K, Li L, et al. Predictors of symptoms are different from predictors of severe exacerbations from asthma in children. Chest 2011; 140(1):100–7.

135. Haselkorn T, Fish JE, Zeiger RS, et al. Consistently very poorly controlled asthma, as defined by the impairment domain of the Expert Panel Report 3 guidelines, increases risk for future severe asthma exacerbations in the Epidemiology and Natural History of Asthma: outcomes and Treatment Regimens (TENOR) study. J Allergy Clin Immunol 2009;124(5):895–902.e4.

136. Khetsuriani N, Lu X, Teague WG, et al. Novel human rhinoviruses and exacerbation of asthma in children. Emerg Infect Dis 2008;14(11):1793–6.

137. Busse WW, Morgan WJ, Gergen PJ, et al. Randomized trial of omalizumab (Anti-IgE) for asthma in inner-city children. N Engl J Med 2011;364(11): 1005–15.

138. Chung KF, Wenzel SE, Brozek JL, et al. International ERS/ATS guidelines on definition, evaluation and treatment of severe asthma. Eur Respir J 2014;43(2):343–73.

139. Fitzpatrick AM, Teague WG, Meyers DA, et al. Heterogeneity of severe asthma in childhood: confirmation by cluster analysis of children in the National Institutes of Health/National Heart, Lung, and Blood Institute Severe Asthma Research Program. J Allergy Clin Immunol 2011;127(2):382–9. e1-13.

140. Schatz M, Hsu J-WY, Zeiger RS, et al. Phenotypes determined by cluster analysis in severe or difficult-to-treat asthma. J Allergy Clin Immunol 2014; 133(6):1549–56.

141. Fitzpatrick AM, Gaston BM, Erzurum SC, et al, National Institutes of Health/National Heart, Lung, and Blood Institute Severe Asthma

Research Program. Features of severe asthma in school-age children: atopy and increased exhaled nitric oxide. J Allergy Clin Immunol 2006;118(6):1218–25.

142. Fitzpatrick AM, Teague WG. Severe asthma in children: insights from the National Heart, Lung, and Blood Institute's Severe Asthma Research Program. Pediatr Allergy Immunol Pulmonol 2010; 23(2):131–8.

143. Fleming L, Murray C, Bansal AT, et al. The burden of severe asthma in childhood and adolescence: results from the paediatric U-BIOPRED cohorts. Eur Respir J 2015;46(5):1322–33.

144. Zein JG, Udeh BL, Teague WG, et al. Impact of age and sex on outcomes and hospital cost of acute asthma in the United States, 2011-2012. PLoS One 2016;11(6):e0157301.

145. Broekema M, Timens W, Vonk JM, et al. Persisting remodeling and less airway wall eosinophil activation in complete remission of asthma. Am J Respir Crit Care Med 2011;183(3):310–6.

146. Moore WC, Meyers DA, Wenzel SE, et al. Identification of asthma phenotypes using cluster analysis in the severe asthma research program. Am J Respir Crit Care Med 2010;181(4):315–23.

147. Gupta R, Margevicius S, DeBoer M, et al. Children with severe asthma are LIkely to become less severe during adolescence: preliminary results of the SARP III pediatric longitudinal study. Am Thorac Soc Int Meet 2018;A7806.

148. Wu TJ, Wu CF, Lee YL, et al. Asthma incidence, remission, relapse and persistence: a population-based study in southern Taiwan. Respir Res 2014;15:135.

149. Marshall WA, Tanner JM. Variations in pattern of pubertal changes in girls. Arch Dis Child 1969; 44(235):291–303.

150. Marshall WA, Tanner JM. Variations in the pattern of pubertal changes in boys. Arch Dis Child 1970; 45(239):13–23.

151. Koziol-White CJ, Goncharova EA, Cao G, et al. DHEA-S inhibits human neutrophil and human airway smooth muscle migration. Biochim Biophys Acta 2012;1822(10):1638–42.

152. Mendoza-Milla C, Jiménez AV, Rangel C, et al. Dehydroepiandrosterone has strong antifibrotic effects and is decreased in idiopathic pulmonary fibrosis. Eur Respir J 2013;42(5):1309–21.

153. Xu L, Xiang X, Ji X, et al. Effects and mechanism of dehydroepiandrosterone on epithelial–mesenchymal transition in bronchial epithelial cells. Exp Lung Res 2014;40(5):211–21.

154. Kouloumenta V, Hatziefthimiou A, Paraskeva E, et al. Non-genomic effect of testosterone on airway smooth muscle. Br J Pharmacol 2006;149(8): 1083–91.

155. Cephus J-Y, Stier MT, Fuseini H, et al. Testosterone Attenuates Group 2 innate lymphoid cell-mediated airway inflammation. Cell Rep 2017;21(9):2487–99.

156. Dorsey MJ, Cohen LE, Phipatanakul W, et al. Assessment of adrenal suppression in children with asthma treated with inhaled corticosteroids: use of dehydroepiandrosterone sulfate as a screening test. Ann Allergy Asthma Immunol 2006;97(2):182–6.

157. Farha S, Asosingh K, Laskowski D, et al. Effects of the menstrual cycle on lung function variables in women with asthma. Am J Respir Crit Care Med 2009;180(4):304–10.

158. Wheeldon N, Newnham D, Coutie W, et al. Influence of sex-steroid hormones on the regulation of lymphocyte beta 2-adrenoceptors during the menstrual cycle. Br J Clin Pharmacol 1994;37(6):583–8.

159. Tan KS, McFarlane LC, Lipworth BJ. Loss of normal cyclical beta 2 adrenoceptor regulation and increased premenstrual responsiveness to adenosine monophosphate in stable female asthmatic patients. Thorax 1997;52(7):608–11.

160. Sheel AW, Dominelli PB, Molgat-Seon Y. Revisiting dysanapsis: sex-based differences in airways and the mechanics of breathing during exercise. Exp Physiol 2016;101(2):213–8.

161. DeBoer MD, Phillips BR, Mauger DT, et al. Effects of endogenous sex hormones on lung function and symptom control in adolescents with asthma. BMC Pulm Med 2018;18(1):58.

162. Mandhane PJ, Greene JM, Cowan JO, et al. Sex differences in factors associated with childhood- and adolescent-onset wheeze. Am J Respir Crit Care Med 2005;172(1):45–54.

163. Rosner W, Auchus RJ, Azziz R, et al. Position statement: Utility, limitations, and pitfalls in measuring testosterone: an endocrine society position statement. J Clin Endocrinol Metab 2007;92:405–13.

164. Alperovitch A, Kurth T, Bertrand M, et al. Primary prevention with lipid lowering drugs and long term risk of vascular events in older people: population based cohort study. BMJ 2015;350:h2335 (1756–1833 [Electronic]).

165. Ford I, Murray H, McCowan C, et al. Long-term safety and efficacy of lowering low-density lipoprotein cholesterol with statin therapy 20-year follow-up of west of Scotland coronary prevention study. Circulation 2016;133(11):1073–80.

166. Palmert MR, Dunkel L. Clinical practice. Delayed puberty. N Engl J Med 2012;366(5):443–53.

167. Wenzel SE, Robinson CB, Leonard JM, et al. Nebulized dehydroepiandrosterone-3-sulfate improves asthma control in the moderate-to-severe asthma results of a 6-week, randomized, double-blind, placebo-controlled study. Allergy Asthma Proc 2010; 31(6):461–71.

168. Orentreich N, Brind JL, Rizer RL, et al. Age changes and sex differences in serum dehydroepiandrosterone sulfate concentrations throughout adulthood. J Clin Endocrinol Metab 1984;59(3):551–5.

169. Phillips GB. Relationship between serum dehydroepiandrosterone sulfate, androstenedione, and sex hormones in men and women. Eur J Endocrinol 1996;134(2):201–6.

170. Berry CE, Billheimer D, Jenkins IC, et al. A distinct low lung function trajectory from childhood to the fourth decade of life. Am J Respir Crit Care Med 2016;194(5):607–12.

171. Forno E, Weiner DJ, Mullen J, et al. Obesity and airway dysanapsis in children with and without asthma. Am J Respir Crit Care Med 2017;195(3):314–23.

172. Holguin F, Comhair SAA, Hazen SL, et al. An association between l-arginine/asymmetric dimethyl arginine balance, obesity, and the age of asthma onset phenotype. Am J Respir Crit Care Med 2013;187(2):153–9.

173. Chen Y-C, Huang Y-L, Ho W-C, et al. Gender differences in effects of obesity and asthma on adolescent lung function: results from a population-based study. J Asthma 2017;54(3):279–85.

174. Dâmaso AR, De Piano A, Campos RMDS, et al. Multidisciplinary approach to the treatment of obese adolescents: effects on cardiovascular risk factors, inflammatory profile, and Neuroendocrine Regulation of Energy Balance. Int J Endocrinol 2013;2013:541032.

175. Huang TT, Johnson MS, Figueroa-Colon R, et al. Growth of visceral fat, subcutaneous abdominal fat, and total body fat in children. Obes Res 2001;9(5):283–9.

176. Sears MR. Consequences of long-term inflammation. The natural history of asthma. Clin Chest Med 2000;21(2):315–29.

177. Hsu H-HL, Chiu Y-HM, Coull BA, et al. Prenatal particulate air pollution and asthma onset in urban children. Identifying sensitive windows and sex differences. Am J Respir Crit Care Med 2015;192(9):1052–9.

178. Chawes BL, Bønnelykke K, Jensen PF, et al. Cord blood 25(OH)-vitamin D deficiency and childhood asthma, allergy and eczema: the COPSAC2000 birth cohort study. PLoS One 2014;9(6):e99856.

179. Wei Z, Zhang J, Yu X. Maternal vitamin D status and childhood asthma, wheeze, and eczema: a systematic review and meta-analysis. Pediatr Allergy Immunol 2016;27(6):612–9.

180. Forno E, Young OM, Kumar R, et al. Maternal obesity in pregnancy, gestational weight gain, and risk of childhood asthma. Pediatrics 2014;134(2):e535–46.

181. Hollingsworth JW, Maruoka S, Boon K, et al. In Utero supplementation with methyl donors enhances allergic airway disease in mice. J Clin Invest 2016;126(5):2012.

182. Grabenhenrich LB, Reich A, Fischer F, et al. The Novel 10-item asthma prediction tool: external validation in the German MAS birth cohort. PLoS One 2014;9(12):e115852.

Asthma over the Adult Life Course
Gender and Hormonal Influences

Joe G. Zein, MD, MBA[a], Joshua L. Denson, MD[b],
Michael E. Wechsler, MD, MMSc[b],*

KEYWORDS

- Asthma • Phenotype • Gender differences • Hormones • Aging • Autophagy

KEY POINTS

- At younger ages, asthma is more common among boys. After puberty, however, asthma becomes more common and more severe in women.
- The pathophysiology of asthma is complex and not fully defined. Epidemiologic data on asthma incidence, prevalence, and severity suggest an important role for sex hormones and lung aging in asthma pathogenesis.
- Age is an important determinant of asthma severity and response to asthma therapies. Older adults are more likely to be hospitalized and die from complications related to asthma.
- In the era of personalized medicine, a thorough evaluation of these gender differences in asthma severity and pathobiology across the life course will help optimize care for patients with this common disease.

INTRODUCTION

A major goal of current asthma treatment strategies is to provide a personalized approach to care. Instead of a 1-size-fits-all approach, efforts are being made to identify specific phenotypes and endotypes that may increase the likelihood of attaining asthma control in specific individuals. In that regard, it has long been recognized that there are gender and age differences in asthma incidence, prevalence, and severity worldwide.[1] Clinical observations suggest that a variety of factors related to gender, sex hormones, and aging mediate asthma severity. For example, older adults have been shown to have more frequent asthma exacerbations and tend to respond less well to inhaled corticosteroids.[2] Similarly, asthma is more prevalent and severe in young boys,[3–5] but after puberty, asthma is more severe and prevalent in women.[3,6] Girls with early menarche and multiparous women, who are exposed to higher estrogen levels and have greater cumulative exposure to sex hormones, have much higher risk for both asthma and severe asthma.[7,8] This article reviews factors related to gender, sex hormones, aging, and the interaction between such factors as they relate to the heterogeneity of asthma (**Fig. 1**).

GENDER AND ASTHMA
Epidemiology and Physiology

Gender can greatly influence lung health and plays a significant role in the development of lung diseases, including asthma, cancer, chronic bronchitis, and cystic fibrosis.[9] Asthma prevalence, health care utilization, and asthma severity are greater in boys ages 2 years to 13 years compared with girls but greater in girls and women ages 14 years to 22 years and even greater in women ages 23 years to 64 years.[6] Despite that asthma

Funding Support: Joe G. Zein: NIH-NHLBI K08HL133381.
[a] Respiratory Institute, Cleveland Clinic, 9500 Euclid Avenue, Cleveland, OH 44106, USA; [b] National Jewish Health, 1400 Jackson Street, Denver, CO 80206, USA
* Corresponding author.
E-mail address: WechslerM@NJHealth.org

Clin Chest Med 40 (2019) 149–161
https://doi.org/10.1016/j.ccm.2018.10.009

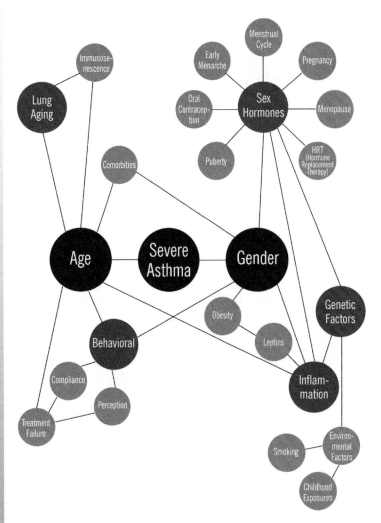

Fig. 1. The effect of age and gender on asthma severity is influenced by many internal and external factors. Epidemiologic data support a significant role for sex hormones. Gender differences in asthma across the life span are informing of unique features for women's health. Factors, such as puberty, pregnancy, menopause, hormonal contraception or replacement therapy, and hormonal variation during the menstrual cycle, are associated with changes in asthma severity and prevalence. Sex hormones interact with genetic and environmental factors to modulate inflammation and, consequently, asthma severity. Similarly, the interaction between fat distribution, airway and systemic inflammation, and gender underlies the gender dimorphism of the obese asthma phenotype. In the elderly, lung aging, immunosenescence, medication compliance, and treatment failure have an impact on asthma severity and control. Consequently, they lead to higher mortality and morbidity in this frail population. Understanding this network of complex interactions among these factors helps understanding of the pathobiology of asthma and generating a personalized approach to manage each individual patient.

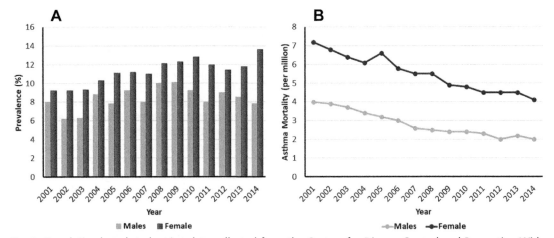

Fig. 2. Population-based study using data collected from the Centers for Disease Control and Prevention Wide-ranging Online data for Epidemiologic Research based on death certificates for US residents from 1999 to 2015 shows that although increasing asthma prevalence was slightly higher in girls and women as opposed to boys and men (*A*), decreasing asthma mortality continued to be twice as high in girls and women compared with boys and men (*B*).

prevalence has been increasing over time (**Fig. 2**A) and advances in asthma management have resulted in reduced mortality overall, mortality in women continues to exceed the mortality in men by a factor of 2^{10} (**Fig. 2**B). Although the exact mechanisms remain unknown, gender differences in asthma have been associated with immunologic, hormonal, or gender-specific environmental and/or occupational factors.[11–14] Differences in early life exposure, eating habits, and levels of physical activity also influence asthma incidence.[15] In that regard, the lower incidence of asthma seen in children living on farms[16] depends on environmental factors. Amish and Hutterite children, with similar genetic backgrounds but living in different farming communities, have variable asthma susceptibility that is inversely correlated to innate immune stimulation.[17] The cumulative asthma incidence, however, lower in girls compared with boys raised on a farm, suggests that gender influences the impact of farming exposures.[18]

The association between childhood obesity and asthma is also gender specific. Two large cross-sectional series from China and the Netherlands and 2 additional longitudinal cohorts from the United Kingdom and Taiwan reported that childhood asthma is only associated with obesity in young and adolescent girls but not in young boys.[19–22] One possible explanation for this may relate to leptins, key players in body weight regulation that increase helper T cell type 1 (T_H1) inflammation.[23] In a cross-sectional study of 114 children ages 5 years to 18 years, higher serum leptin levels were associated with obesity, female gender, and asthma.[23] Similarly, worse lung function was related to the interaction between fat distribution, airway and systemic inflammation, and gender (see **Fig. 1**), resulting in a gender dimorphism of the obese-asthma phenotype that is highest among women 12 years to 44 years of age.[24,25] The Severe Asthma Research Program (SARP) and the European Network for Understanding Mechanisms of Severe Asthma reported a higher female-to-male ratio (4.4:1) in severe asthma. A higher body mass index (BMI), however, was reported among women with severe asthma compared with nonsevere asthma but not in men.[5,26] Although the gender dimorphism of the obese-asthma phenotype is supported by most but not all reports,[27] it is unclear whether this is caused by sex hormones or other gender-specific factors.

Loss of lung function has also been associated with gender differences. Exposure to particulate matter and to second-hand smoking have both been associated with lower forced expiratory volume in the first second of expiration (FEV_1) in women but not in men ages 55 years and younger.[28] Additionally, although no gender difference has been observed in the incidence of atopic asthma, an association between BMI and nonatopic asthma in women of childbearing age compared with men has been reported.[29,30] Altogether, this suggests an interaction between gender, age, BMI, and asthma type (atopic vs nonatopic) on the response to risk factors and environmental exposures[31] (see **Fig. 1**).

Gender-specific asthma risks are frequently confounded by other comorbidities. Thus, appropriate statistical adjustments are frequently needed before confirming or dismissing any associations. For example, a higher prevalence of asthma was reported among same-sex partnered men and women. Such an association, however, may be hard to conclude in the setting of higher rate of obesity among same-sex partnered women and smoking among same-sex partnered men.[32] Similarly the higher asthma prevalence reported among women with attention-deficit/hyperactivity disorder (ADHD) compared with men with ADHD may be related to higher prevalence of smoking and obesity[33] in that patient population. The authors recently studied asthma prevalence among 7210 individuals with gender identity disorder and 490 who underwent gender-affirming surgery using a large clinical data set (Explorys, IBM Watson Health, Armonk, New York). Asthma risk was highest in male-to-female transgender individuals, including those with male-to-female gender-affirming surgery (odds ratio [OR] 3.49 and 3.73, respectively; $P<.001$). Asthma risk was also high in female-to-male transgender individuals and in those with female-to-male gender-affirming surgery (OR 2.62 and 2.65, respectively; $P<.001$). Contrary to the authors' hypothesis that androgens are protective and estrogens are detrimental, asthma prevalence was also high in female-to-male transgender individuals. Those findings are consistent with a previous report that cross-sex hormone therapy was associated with higher all-cause mortality, in both male-to-female and female-to-male groups.[34] Counterintuitively, in that report, estrogen therapy lacked cardiovascular protection. Those cumulative findings raise questions about the potential respiratory health consequences of cross-sex hormone therapy and suggest that the effect of exogenous and endogenous sex hormones may not be similar.

Differences in Perception, Behavior, and Response to Therapy in Men Versus Women

Asthma is more prevalent and severe in middle-aged women and is associated with higher mortality[5,35] (see **Fig. 1**). Direct hospitalization and medication costs are higher in women compared with men, even after adjusting for comorbidities and asthma severity.[35] This could be secondary to gender differences in symptom perception or health-seeking behaviors. Compared with men, women with comparable asthma severity and lung function report more dyspnea, score worse on asthma-related quality-of-life questionnaires, and require higher asthma-related health services.[36–41] Likewise, although the prevalence of asthma is similar in female and male swimmers (19%), gender differences in asthma-related symptoms have been described. Female swimmers report, in general, more coughing whereas males frequently complain of allergies.[42] In general, women with asthma report worse sleep quality and more anxiety.[43] Thus, a better knowledge of these female-specific aspects of asthma-related symptoms might result in improved quality of life and health of women with asthma.[44]

In the United States, many gender differences in occupational and environmental exposures exist among working adults. For example, smoking is less common among women compared with men (18.3% vs 22.8%), yet women who smoke have a 2.2 higher OR of carrying a diagnosis of asthma and report more asthma symptoms, such as wheezing.[45,46] This higher prevalence of adverse health outcomes among women who smoke is compounded by a higher risk of physical tobacco dependence among women with asthma compared with those without asthma.[46,47] The care of women with asthma cannot be planned independent of workplace exposures. Among adults with work-related asthma, women are more likely to work in health care, retail, and education.[48] These differences also extend into the house environment. Compared with nonasthmatics, patients with asthma, women in particular, are more likely to own furry pets (49.9% vs 44.8%; $P<.001$) and allow them into the bedroom (68.7%).[49] Understanding these gender differences in perception, behavior, and exposures helps educate asthmatics, in particular those with difficult-to-treat asthma, about triggers avoidance and asthma control.

Medication adherence, peak flow measurement, and behavior toward health care use also differ between men and women. For example, although women are more likely to have unscheduled office visits and carry a rescue inhaler than men (61% vs 30%), men were more likely to visit the emergency department because they ran out of their inhaled medication (OR 2.5; $P = .02$).[50–52] Recent data suggest that girls and women may benefit from antileukotriene therapy more than boys and men. In both humans and mice, lipoxygenase–activating protein and novel type 5-lipoxygenase inhibitors were found more potent in girls

and women, a response that was reversed by 5α-dihydrotestosterone.[53] Combined, these data suggest that gender differences in asthma also may be related to differences in health behaviors, adherence to treatment guidelines, and response of controller therapy.

Hormones Differences in Asthma

Although the etiology of many of these differences in asthma with regard to gender are multifactorial, issues related to hormonal factors, such as seen with puberty, during the menstrual cycle, and during pregnancy and menopause, explain some of the differences. During the luteal phase of the menstrual cycle, estradiol and progesterone levels are 2-fold to 7-fold higher and FEV_1 and forced vital capacity are lower in women with and without asthma.[54,55] Women with asthma, however, had lower FEV_1 and more respiratory symptoms in the premenstrual and menstrual period. This translates clinically into increased airway hyperresponsiveness and higher rate of urgent health care utilization.[55,56] To date, evidence-based therapy for premenstrual asthma is still lacking. A beneficial role of oral contraceptive pills (OCPs) was suggested in a small series of 18 women.[57] In women receiving OCPs, the suppression of the rise in luteal-phase sex hormones resulted in an attenuated cyclical change in airway hyperresponsiveness manifested by smaller variation in provocative concentration causing a 20% drop in FEV_1 and in peak expiratory flow rate.[57] Neither therapy with meclofenamic acid nor estradiol supplementation, however, was found beneficial in 2 separate randomized controlled trials.[58,59]

In addition to their beneficial effect in premenstrual asthma, hormonal contraceptives were associated with lower risk of current asthma (OR 0.68; 95% CI, 0.47–0.98) and fewer symptoms in women with asthma (OR, 0.18; 95% CI, 0.06–0.56).[8,60] Other studies, however, showed conflicting results. A cross-sectional Nordic-Baltic population survey that included 5791 women 25 years to 44 years of age demonstrated a higher risk for asthma (OR 1.42; 95% CI, 1.09–1.86) and wheeze with shortness of breath (OR 1.27; 95% CI, 1.02–1.60) among women using oral contraceptives.[61] The authors conducted a cross-sectional analysis on women ages 20 years to 50 years using a large clinical registry (Explorys). Of 6,524,990 women who met the inclusion criteria, 2,116,000 (32.4%) were using OCPs and 692,470 (10.6%) carried the diagnosis of lifetime asthma. Prevalence of asthma was higher in those taking OCPs (14.3% vs 8.8%; $P<.001$). OCP use was associated with increased risk of asthma (adjusted OR 1.77 [1.76–1.78]; $P<.001$) adjusting for age category, race, BMI category, and smoking.[62] This analysis did not take into consideration the dose, composition, or the route of administration of exogenous sex hormone. Those characteristics are extremely important in determining the optimal contraceptive modality in women with asthma.

Asthma During Pregnancy

Although asthma is commonly a serious condition, it frequently improves during pregnancy. Approximately one-third of pregnant women experience more asthma symptoms and increased bronchial hyper-responsiveness.[63] Consequently, severe maternal asthma is complicated by significant newborn comorbidities, such as respiratory complications, hyperbilirubinemia, and higher rates of prematurity and intrauterine growth retardation.[64] Remarkably, reduced birthweights were seen mainly in female newborns of asthmatic mothers but not in male newborns, suggesting gender-specific effect on maternal inflammation and placental function.[65] Although the exact mechanism remains unknown, both mechanical effects of the fetus on the airways and hormonal effects have been implicated. In addition, maternal asthma was linked to higher alteration in placental global gene expression in the female placenta compared with males, affecting pathways involved in immune regulation and cellular growth.[66]

Asthma and Menopause

The effect of menopause on asthma was best studied in a cohort of premenopausal and postmenopausal women 34 years to 68 years of age. Among the 121,700 girls and women participating in the Nurses' Health Study, postmenopausal women who never received hormonal replacement therapy had a lower incidence of asthma (age-adjusted relative risk of asthma incidence, 0.65; 95% CI, 0.46–0.92).[67] This protective effect of menopause was reversed by the use of estrogen-based hormone replacement therapy (age-adjusted relative risk of asthma, 1.49; 95% CI, 1.10–2.00).[67] Likewise, severe asthma may improve with menopausal transition when sex hormones wane.[67,68] The authors' recent work shows, for the first time, that there is a reversal of the gender switch at menopause: asthma once again becomes more severe in boys and men.[69] Further studies are needed to confirm these findings.

ASTHMA AND THE ELDERLY

In addition to gender-related and hormone-related asthma differences, age is an important determinant of asthma severity and response to asthma therapies. Older adults, in general, are more likely to be hospitalized and die from complications related to asthma,[70] yet the prevalence for adults over the age of 65 remains low—reported between 4% and 13%.[71–75] Reasons for this low prevalence are likely related to underdiagnosis or misdiagnosis (often as chronic obstructive pulmonary disease [COPD]) in this age group.[76–78] Although severe asthma has not increased in women over the age of 45,[69] mortality rates for asthmatics over the age of 65 have not decreased as they have in some other age groups.[79–81] In addition, some aging asthmatics seem to have a greater decline in lung function, less hyper-reactivity, and less atopy.[82–84] Unfortunately, elderly asthmatics are often excluded from clinical trials in asthma rendering the information available on asthma in the elderly inadequate.

The authors analyzed data on 1644 adult participants (age >18 years) from the SARP I and SARP II enrolled between 2002 and 2011.[85] The impact of age on asthma severity as defined by the proceedings of the American Thoracic Society[86] after adjustment for asthma duration and age-related comorbidities were assessed using a logistic regression. The probability of severe asthma increased directly with age until 45 years of age. Beyond 45 years, it increased in men but not in women, again suggesting an interaction between age and gender.[69]

Asthma Treatment in the Elderly

The increased disease burden and morbidity seen in elderly patients may have important treatment implications. Despite used less often in the elderly,[87,88] inhaled corticosteroids remain the cornerstone for therapy in this population with reduced mortality and hospitalizations.[89] In a 2015 study by Dunn and colleagues,[90] however, 1200 subjects previously enrolled in Asthma Clinical Research Network clinical trials were evaluated for the effect of age and gender on treatment failure to inhaled corticosteroids. A higher proportion of subjects greater than or equal to 30 years old experienced treatment failures (17.3% vs 10.3%; OR, 1.82; 95% CI, 1.30–2.54; P<.001), with rates increasing proportionally with increasing age (OR per year, 1.02 [95% CI, 1.01–1.04]; OR per 5 years, 1.13 [95% CI, 1.04–1.22]; P<.001). After stratification for specific therapy, inhaled corticosteroid treatment failures consistently increased with increasing age (OR per year, 1.03; 95% CI, 1.01–1.07). Although girls and women had an absolute increase in treatment failures compared with boys and men (15.2% vs 11.7%; P = .088), this was not statistically significant in this cohort.[90]

Pathophysiologic Mechanisms of Asthma in the Elderly

The pathophysiology for the differences noted with aging asthmatics remains unclear, but this population seems to have clear inflammatory and cellular alterations that could be contributing. Elderly asthmatics are noted to have alterations in their innate and adaptive immune systems, which may be contributing to their greater burden of disease. These changes, often termed, *immunosenescence*, seem driven by chronic, systemic, low-grade inflammation, with increased levels of interleukin (IL)-6, IL-1β, and tumor necrosis factor α.[91,92] The changes noted during aging, also termed, *inflamm-aging*,[93] are an area of active investigation.

One other possible explanation for some of the changes associated with aging in asthma relates to autophagy. Autophagy refers to the biological process of intracellular degradation that delivers cytoplasmic components to lysosomes within eukaryotic cells. Abnormal autophagy has been implicated in multiple diseases, including cancer, neurodegeneration, infection, COPD, pulmonary hypertension, cystic fibrosis and normal aging. Plasma marker of autophagy (LC3B) is increased in asthmatics and more severe airway inflammation (more autophagy in airways). Increased levels of LC3B are associated with lower FEV_1 and with increased age among asthmatics. Levels of LC3B vary depending on the type of airway inflammation present (eosinophilic vs noneosinophilic).

Another possible explanation for asthma in the elderly relates to shorter leukocyte telomere length, which has been associated independently with aging. Telomeres are protective caps at the end of the chromosomes and are shortened with each cell division, allowing them to be used as markers of cellular aging. This process is further accelerated by inflammation commonly seen in chronic diseases such as asthma. Accelerated aging has also been associated with blood eosinophilic inflammation and with life course–persistent asthma.[94] Whether studying asthma across the life span can inform studies of aging or if leukocyte telomere length can be used as a reliable biomarker to predict disease duration need further evaluation.[95]

Elderly adults have higher rates of airway neutrophils, with emerging data showing increased markers of neutrophilic inflammation in elderly asthmatics.[96–100] Immunosenescence is known to increase susceptibility to infections in the elderly, which may contribute to the increasing morbidity seen in asthma of the elderly or those with late-onset asthma.[101] In addition to changes noted in the immune system of the elderly, numerous structural alterations occur with increasing age in asthmatics that may contribute to this decline in function, including greater chest wall rigidity, less elastic recoil, and reduced respiratory muscle strength.[102–104] Furthermore, compared with younger asthmatics, elderly asthmatics have increased air trapping, more large airway wall thickening, and increased small airway resistance. These changes seen in both immune and structural lung function are complex and remain to be fully elucidated, but research is ongoing.

THE ROLE OF SEX HORMONES IN ASTHMA PATHOPHYSIOLOGY

Although several population-based epidemiologic studies suggest a gender discordance in severe asthma, little is known regarding the underlying mechanisms. Sex hormones have a wide variety of effects, for example, the progesterone receptor is expressed in airway epithelium and inhibits ciliary beat frequency, which may affect mucociliary clearance.[105] Men and women produce estrogens, progesterones, and testosterone, whose levels change at puberty (adrenarche and menarche), fluctuate over the reproductive life (menstrual cycle), and decline with aging in men and menopause in women.[106,107] In addition, women have cyclic changes in hormones, linked to asthma exacerbations.[108] Chronic airway inflammation, resulting from multiple immune cell activation, leads to airway remodeling and excess decline of FEV_1 of 33 mL/y in patients with asthma compared with nonasthmatics.[109] Estrogen receptors (ERs), expressed on the majority of immune cells, can regulate myriad immune functions, including adhesion, migration, and antibody and cytokine production in response to the hormone. For example, mast cells undergo degranulation in the presence of physiologic concentrations of 17β-estradiol and allergen cross-linking of surface IgE, suggesting that estradiol enhances IgE-dependent mast cell activation.[110] Similarly, higher IL-17A production and IL-23R expression were reported in helper T cell type 17–differentiated cells from women compared with men with severe asthma. Those results were replicated in ovariectomized mice receiving 17β-estradiol.[111] Collectively, these data suggest that estrogen signaling in airway inflammation may contribute to gender differences in asthma and allergy.[112] On the other hand, testosterone attenuates type 2 innate lymphoid cells (ILC2) function and proliferation, which explains why women with asthma have a higher number of circulating

ILC2 compared with men.[113] A small observational study involving 130 adult asthmatics found that testosterone is a negative predictor of percent sputum neutrophils, adjusting for gender and BMI, suggesting additional anti-inflammatory roles for testosterone.[114]

Genetics of Gender and Aging in Asthma

As with most complex diseases, a combination of genetic, environmental, and lifestyle factors cause asthma. So far, different genetic determinants for lung function T_H1 innate immunity have been associated with asthma progression and loss in lung function in both men and women.[115,116] Likewise, although helper T cell type 2 (T_H2) pathway genes, in general, are associated with asthma susceptibility, some T_H2-regulated genes, such as Arg 2, are associated with severe asthma.[117–120] The effect of asthma severity genes on asthma severity and lung function decline (ie, percent predicted FEV_1), however, between men and women remains unknown.

In cardiovascular diseases, the effect of gender on plasma lipid levels and coronary heart disease (CHD) is mediated through gender-specific effects of genes, such as the apolipoprotein E gene polymorphism; for example, gender strongly influences plasma lipid levels and the risk of CHD.[121] Likewise, hormone replacement therapy increases high-density lipoprotein and lowers E-selectin in women with CHD who have the ER-α IVS1–401 C/C genotype compared with other genotypes.[122,123] In asthma, gender may also influence genetic polymorphisms. Candidate gene analysis shows that single-nucleotide polymorphisms in the thymic stromal lymphopoietin gene are associated with a lower risk of asthma in men but a higher risk of asthma in women, although the underlying mechanisms are unclear.[124] Likewise, male-specific and female-specific genome-wide association studies identified 6 gender-specific asthma risk loci, of which 2 were male specific and 4 were female specific; all were ancestry specific.[125] The most significant gender-specific association in European Americans was at the interferon (IFN) regulatory factor 1 locus on 5q31.1. IFN regulatory factor 1 encodes a transcription factor that activates the transcription of the genes encoding IFN-α, IFN-β, and IFN-γ cytokines, all of which have been implicated in asthma pathogenesis.[126]

Genetic Effects on Hormones and Aging in Asthma

The binding of 17β-estradiol in the cytoplasm to ERα or ERβ results in receptor dimerization. Ligand-activated ER dimers translocate into the nucleus and recognize specific estrogen response elements located in or near promoter DNA regions of target genes to promote gene expression.[127] ER activation and/or repression, however, is much more complex and is tissue specific.[128] Ligand-bound ER can also regulate gene transcription indirectly by interacting with transcription factors, such as activator protein 1 or specificity protein 1.[129,130] In a study evaluating 200 asthma probands and their families (n = 1249), 5 variants in the ERα gene (*ESR1*) were found associated with bronchial hyper-responsiveness and rapid annual loss in lung function especially in female subjects.[131] Similarly altered estrogen action, which affects lung development and/or airway remodeling, was related to different ERα and ERβ isoforms generated through RNA alternative splicing processes. In asthma, airway inflammation causes a differential expression of these ERα and ERβ variants and results in modification in the estrogen-signaling pathway in tissues that express the ER, such as airway smooth muscle. Subsequently, this leads to alteration in intracellular calcium and airway smooth muscle contractility.[132]

ERs, expressed on a majority of immune cells, including alveolar macrophages, play an important role in allergic lung inflammation. In patients with asthma, a higher proportion of M2-polarized macrophages was isolated from bronchoalveolar lavage fluid and airway walls and was correlated with severe asthma and lower FEV_1.[133] Likewise, in an ovariectomized female mice model, estrogen supplementation enhanced M2 polarization after allergen challenge. This M2 polarization was impaired in macrophage-specific deletion of ERα.[112,134]

Similar to estrogens, the biological effect of androgens is mediated via the androgen receptor; a nuclear receptor expressed in many immune cells, such as neutrophils, macrophages, and B cells and T cells. Androgens can regulate gene transcription either by directly binding to DNA or indirectly in a non-DNA binding–dependent manner. In contrast to estrogen, androgens, such as testosterone, are believed to protect against type 2 airway inflammation by downregulating and inhibiting ILC2 proliferation in response to IL-33.[113,135] Dehydroepiandrosterone, an adrenal androgen, was also found to inhibit the phosphoinositide 3-kinase–dependent signal pathway and to prevent bronchial epithelial to mesenchymal transition, which is involved in airway remodeling.[136,137]

Both CD25(hi) Foxp3(+) and IL-10–producing regulatory T cells (Tregs) play an important role in preventing T_H2 responses to allergens, mostly due to the expression of high levels of the transcription factor Foxp3 by CD25(hi) Tregs.[138] In asthma, however, both Foxp3 expression and, consequently, CD25(hi) Treg number and suppressive function were decreased.[139] Low androgen levels secondary to medical castration significantly lowered the percentage of $CD4^+$ CD25(hi) T cells ($P<.05$).[140] In contrast to findings from rat models, however, androgen-dependent increases of Foxp3 expression in human CD25(hi) Tregs were seen only in women in the ovulatory phase of the menstrual cycle but not in men. This was correlated with the presence of an androgen response element (ARE) within the Foxp3 locus. During the menstrual cycle, free testosterone levels doubles during ovulation[141]; this may counteract the proinflammatory effects of the elevated estrogen levels. In a recent study, asthma complicated by ambient air pollutant exposure was associated with higher differentially methylated regions of Foxp3 promoter site in girls and women compared with boys and men. Differentially methylated regions were reported to decline with age.[142] Collectively these findings suggest that androgens modulate the differentiation of Tregs and may be a useful therapy for asthma.[143]

SUMMARY

Gender differences and aging both have a significant impact on asthma prevalence and severity. There is strong evidence to suggest that gender and sex hormones and their underlying genetics have an impact on asthma incidence and severity throughout the life course. These associations are confounded, however, by many internal and external factors, such as atopy, smoking, lung aging, obesity, and gender/age differences in behavior and environmental exposures. On the other hand, older adults have the highest mortality from asthma, even after adjusting for age-related comorbidities, and are more likely to experience treatment failure. Additional work is needed to establish the biological mechanisms through which gender and hormones influence asthma across the life span. These studies will lead to new knowledge on the genesis of asthma and help implement gender-based and age-based precision care in asthma.

REFERENCES

1. Masoli M, Fabian D, Holt S, et al. The global burden of asthma: executive summary of the GINA Dissemination Committee report. Allergy 2004; 59(5):469–78.
2. Banerji A, Clark S, Afilalo M, et al. Prospective multicenter study of acute asthma in younger versus older adults presenting to the emergency department. J Am Geriatr Soc 2006;54(1):48–55.
3. Zein JG, Udeh BL, Teague WG, et al. Impact of age and sex on outcomes and hospital cost of acute asthma in the United States, 2011-2012. PLoS One 2016;11(6):e0157301.
4. Dawson B, Illsley R, Horobin G, et al. A survey of childhood asthma in Aberdeen. Lancet 1969; 1(7599):827–30.
5. The ENFUMOSA cross-sectional European multi-centre study of the clinical phenotype of chronic severe asthma. European Network for Understanding Mechanisms of Severe Asthma. Eur Respir J 2003;22(3):470–7.
6. Schatz M, Camargo CA Jr. The relationship of sex to asthma prevalence, health care utilization, and medications in a large managed care organization. Ann Allergy Asthma Immunol 2003;91(6):553–8.
7. Jenkins MA, Dharmage SC, Flander LB, et al. Parity and decreased use of oral contraceptives as predictors of asthma in young women. Clin Exp Allergy 2006;36(5):609–13.
8. Salam MT, Wenten M, Gilliland FD. Endogenous and exogenous sex steroid hormones and asthma and wheeze in young women. J Allergy Clin Immunol 2006;117(5):1001–7.
9. Townsend EA, Miller VM, Prakash YS. Sex differences and sex steroids in lung health and disease. Endocr Rev 2012;33(1):1–47.
10. Yaqoob Z, Al-Kindi S. Trends in asthma mortality in the United States: a population-based study. Chest 2017;152(4):A27.
11. Becklake MR, Kauffmann F. Gender differences in airway behaviour over the human life span. Thorax 1999;54(12):1119–38.
12. Almqvist C, Worm M, Leynaert B, working group of GA2LEN WP 2.5 Gender. Impact of gender on asthma in childhood and adolescence: a GA2LEN review. Allergy 2008;63(1):47–57.
13. Vink NM, Postma DS, Schouten JP, et al. Gender differences in asthma development and remission during transition through puberty: the TRacking Adolescents' Individual Lives Survey (TRAILS) study. J Allergy Clin Immunol 2010;126(3):498–504.e1-6.
14. Melgert BN, Ray A, Hylkema MN, et al. Are there reasons why adult asthma is more common in females? Curr Allergy Asthma Rep 2007;7(2):143–50.
15. Kosti RI, Priftis KN, Anthracopoulos MB, et al. The association between leisure-time physical activities and asthma symptoms among 10- to 12-year-old children: the effect of living environment in the PANACEA study. J Asthma 2012;49(4):342–8.
16. Fuchs O, Genuneit J, Latzin P, et al. Farming environments and childhood atopy, wheeze, lung function, and exhaled nitric oxide. J Allergy Clin Immunol 2012;130(2):382–8.e6.

17. Stein MM, Hrusch CL, Gozdz J, et al. Innate immunity and asthma risk in amish and hutterite farm children. N Engl J Med 2016;375(5):411–21.

18. Genuneit J. Sex-specific development of asthma differs between farm and nonfarm children: a cohort study. Am J Respir Crit Care Med 2014; 190(5):588–90.

19. Wang D, Qian Z, Wang J, et al. Gender-specific differences in associations of overweight and obesity with asthma and asthma-related symptoms in 30 056 children: result from 25 districts of Northeastern China. J Asthma 2014;51(5):508–14.

20. Willeboordse M, van den Bersselaar DL, van de Kant KD, et al. Sex differences in the relationship between asthma and overweight in Dutch children: a survey study. PLoS One 2013;8(10):e77574.

21. Murray CS, Canoy D, Buchan I, et al. Body mass index in young children and allergic disease: gender differences in a longitudinal study. Clin Exp Allergy 2011;41(1):78–85.

22. Ho WC, Lin YS, Caffrey JL, et al. Higher body mass index may induce asthma among adolescents with pre-asthmatic symptoms: a prospective cohort study. BMC Public Health 2011;11:542.

23. Quek YW, Sun HL, Ng YY, et al. Associations of serum leptin with atopic asthma and allergic rhinitis in children. Am J Rhinol Allergy 2010;24(5):354–8.

24. Lang JE, Hossain J, Dixon AE, et al. Does age impact the obese asthma phenotype? Longitudinal asthma control, airway function, and airflow perception among mild persistent asthmatics. Chest 2011;140(6):1524–33.

25. Scott HA, Gibson PG, Garg ML, et al. Relationship between body composition, inflammation and lung function in overweight and obese asthma. Respir Res 2012;13:10.

26. Moore WC, Meyers DA, Wenzel SE, et al. Identification of asthma phenotypes using cluster analysis in the Severe Asthma Research Program. Am J Respir Crit Care Med 2010;181(4):315–23.

27. Tantisira KG, Colvin R, Tonascia J, et al. Airway responsiveness in mild to moderate childhood asthma: sex influences on the natural history. Am J Respir Crit Care Med 2008;178(4):325–31.

28. Comhair SA, Gaston BM, Ricci KS, et al. Detrimental effects of environmental tobacco smoke in relation to asthma severity. PLoS One 2011;6(5): e18574.

29. Beuther DA, Sutherland ER. Overweight, obesity, and incident asthma: a meta-analysis of prospective epidemiologic studies. Am J Respir Crit Care Med 2007;175(7):661–6.

30. Ma J, Xiao L. Association of general and central obesity and atopic and nonatopic asthma in US adults. J Asthma 2013;50(4):395–402.

31. Balmes JR, Cisternas M, Quinlan PJ, et al. Annual average ambient particulate matter exposure estimates, measured home particulate matter, and hair nicotine are associated with respiratory outcomes in adults with asthma. Environ Res 2014;129:1–10.

32. Blosnich JR, Lee JG, Bossarte R, et al. Asthma disparities and within-group differences in a national, probability sample of same-sex partnered adults. Am J Public Health 2013;103(9):e83–7.

33. Fasmer OB, Halmoy A, Eagan TM, et al. Adult attention deficit hyperactivity disorder is associated with asthma. BMC Psychiatry 2011;11:128.

34. Dhejne C, Lichtenstein P, Boman M, et al. Longterm follow-up of transsexual persons undergoing sex reassignment surgery: cohort study in Sweden. PLoS One 2011;6(2):e16885.

35. Serra-Batlles J, Plaza V, Morejon E, et al. Costs of asthma according to the degree of severity. Eur Respir J 1998;12(6):1322–6.

36. Sinclair AH, Tolsma DD. Gender differences in asthma experience and disease care in a managed care organization. J Asthma 2006; 43(5):363–7.

37. McCallister JW, Holbrook JT, Wei CY, et al. Sex differences in asthma symptom profiles and control in the American Lung Association Asthma Clinical Research Centers. Respir Med 2013;107(10): 1491–500.

38. Chhabra SK, Chhabra P. Gender differences in perception of dyspnea, assessment of control, and quality of life in asthma. J Asthma 2011; 48(6):609–15.

39. de Miguel Diez J, Hernandez Barrera V, Puente Maestu L, et al. Psychiatric comorbidity in asthma patients. Associated factors. J Asthma 2011; 48(3):253–8.

40. Lisspers K, Stallberg B, Janson C, et al. Sex-differences in quality of life and asthma control in Swedish asthma patients. J Asthma 2013;50(10):1090–5.

41. Woods SE, Brown K, Engel A. The influence of gender on adults admitted for asthma. Gend Med 2010;7(2):109–14.

42. Paivinen MK, Keskinen KL, Tikkanen HO. Swimming and asthma: differences between women and men. J Allergy 2013;2013:520913.

43. Sundberg R, Toren K, Franklin KA, et al. Asthma in men and women: treatment adherence, anxiety, and quality of sleep. Respir Med 2010;104(3): 337–44.

44. Clark NM, Gong ZM, Wang SJ, et al. From the female perspective: long-term effects on quality of life of a program for women with asthma. Gend Med 2010;7(2):125–36.

45. Syamlal G, Mazurek JM, Dube SR. Gender differences in smoking among U.S. working adults. Am J Prev Med 2014;47(4):467–75.

46. Bjerg A, Ekerljung L, Eriksson J, et al. Higher risk of wheeze in female than male smokers. Results from

the Swedish GA 2 LEN study. PLoS One 2013;8(1): e54137.

47. Guo SE, Ratner PA, Okoli CT, et al. The gender-specific association between asthma and the need to smoke tobacco. Heart Lung 2014;43(1):77–83.

48. White GE, Seaman C, Filios MS, et al. Gender differences in work-related asthma: surveillance data from California, Massachusetts, Michigan, and New Jersey, 1993-2008. J Asthma 2014; 51(7):691–702.

49. Downes MJ, Roy A, McGinn TG, et al. Factors associated with furry pet ownership among patients with asthma. J Asthma 2010;47(7):742–9.

50. Lindner PS, Lindner AJ. Gender differences in asthma inhaler compliance. Conn Med 2014; 78(4):207–10.

51. Heaney LG, Brightling CE, Menzies-Gow A, et al, British Thoracic Society Difficult Asthma Network. Refractory asthma in the UK: cross-sectional findings from a UK multicentre registry. Thorax 2010; 65(9):787–94.

52. Pai S, Mancuso CA, Loganathan R, et al. Characteristics of asthmatic patients with and without repeat emergency department visits at an inner city hospital. J Asthma 2014;51(6):627–32.

53. Pace S, Pergola C, Dehm F, et al. Androgen-mediated sex bias impairs efficiency of leukotriene biosynthesis inhibitors in males. J Clin Invest 2017;127(8):3167–76.

54. Farha S, Asosingh K, Laskowski D, et al. Effects of the menstrual cycle on lung function variables in women with asthma. Am J Respir Crit Care Med 2009;180(4):304–10.

55. Tan KS, McFarlane LC, Lipworth BJ. Loss of normal cyclical beta 2 adrenoceptor regulation and increased premenstrual responsiveness to adenosine monophosphate in stable female asthmatic patients. Thorax 1997;52(7):608–11.

56. Rao CK, Moore CG, Bleecker E, et al. Characteristics of perimenstrual asthma and its relation to asthma severity and control: data from the Severe Asthma Research Program. Chest 2013;143(4): 984–92.

57. Tan KS, McFarlane LC, Lipworth BJ. Modulation of airway reactivity and peak flow variability in asthmatics receiving the oral contraceptive pill. Am J Respir Crit Care Med 1997;155(4):1273–7.

58. Ensom MH, Chong G, Zhou D, et al. Estradiol in premenstrual asthma: a double-blind, randomized, placebo-controlled, crossover study. Pharmacotherapy 2003;23(5):561–71.

59. Eliasson O, Densmore MJ, Scherzer HH, et al. The effect of sodium meclofenamate in premenstrual asthma: a controlled clinical trial. J Allergy Clin Immunol 1987;79(6):909–18.

60. Nwaru BI, Sheikh A. Hormonal contraceptives and asthma in women of reproductive age: analysis of

data from serial national Scottish Health Surveys. J R Soc Med 2015;108(9):358–71.

61. Macsali F, Real FG, Omenaas ER, et al. Oral contraception, body mass index, and asthma: a cross-sectional Nordic-Baltic population survey. J Allergy Clin Immunol 2009;123(2):391–7.

62. Morales-Estrella JL, Boyle MB. Transgender status is associated with higher risk of lifetime asthma. American Thoracic Society International Conference. May 20, 2018 - San Diego Convention Center, San Diego, California.

63. Juniper EF, Daniel EE, Roberts RS, et al. Improvement in airway responsiveness and asthma severity during pregnancy. A prospective study. Am Rev Respir Dis 1989;140(4):924–31.

64. Mendola P, Mannisto TI, Leishear K, et al. Neonatal health of infants born to mothers with asthma. J Allergy Clin Immunol 2014;133(1):85–90.e1-4.

65. Murphy VE, Gibson PG, Giles WB, et al. Maternal asthma is associated with reduced female fetal growth. Am J Respir Crit Care Med 2003;168(11): 1317–23.

66. Osei-Kumah A, Smith R, Jurisica I, et al. Sex-specific differences in placental global gene expression in pregnancies complicated by asthma. Placenta 2011;32(8):570–8.

67. Troisi RJ, Speizer FE, Willett WC, et al. Menopause, postmenopausal estrogen preparations, and the risk of adult-onset asthma. A prospective cohort study. Am J Respir Crit Care Med 1995;152(4 Pt 1):1183–8.

68. O'Connor KA, Ferrell RJ, Brindle E, et al. Total and unopposed estrogen exposure across stages of the transition to menopause. Cancer Epidemiol Biomarkers Prev 2009;18(3):828–36.

69. Zein JG, Dweik RA, Comhair SA, et al. Asthma is more severe in older adults. PLoS One 2015; 10(7):e0133490.

70. Moorman JE, Akinbami LJ, Bailey CM, et al. National surveillance of asthma: United States, 2001-2010. Vital Health Stat 3 2012;(35):1–67.

71. McHugh MK, Symanski E, Pompeii LA, et al. Prevalence of asthma among adult females and males in the United States: results from the National Health and Nutrition Examination Survey (NHANES), 2001-2004. J Asthma 2009;46(8):759–66.

72. Malik A, Saltoun CA, Yarnold PR, et al. Prevalence of obstructive airways disease in the disadvantaged elderly of Chicago. Allergy Asthma Proc 2004;25(3):169–73.

73. Kim YK, Kim SH, Tak YJ, et al. High prevalence of current asthma and active smoking effect among the elderly. Clin Exp Allergy 2002;32(12): 1706–12.

74. Enright PL, McClelland RL, Newman AB, et al. Underdiagnosis and undertreatment of asthma in the elderly. Cardiovascular Health Study Research Group. Chest 1999;116(3):603–13.

75. Burrows B, Barbee RA, Cline MG, et al. Characteristics of asthma among elderly adults in a sample of the general population. Chest 1991;100(4): 935–42.

76. Mathur SK. Allergy and asthma in the elderly. Semin Respir Crit Care Med 2010;31(5):587–95.

77. Gonzalez-Garcia M, Caballero A, Jaramillo C, et al. Prevalence, risk factors and underdiagnosis of asthma and wheezing in adults 40 years and older: a population-based study. J Asthma 2015;52(8): 823–30.

78. Bellia V, Battaglia S, Catalano F, et al. Aging and disability affect misdiagnosis of COPD in elderly asthmatics: the SARA study. Chest 2003;123(4): 1066–72.

79. Tsai CL, Lee WY, Hanania NA, et al. Age-related differences in clinical outcomes for acute asthma in the United States, 2006-2008. J Allergy Clin Immunol 2012;129(5):1252–8.e1.

80. Tsai YC, Hsieh LF, Yang S. Age-related changes in posture response under a continuous and unexpected perturbation. J Biomech 2014;47(2): 482–90.

81. Moorman JE, Mannino DM. Increasing U.S. asthma mortality rates: who is really dying? J Asthma 2001; 38(1):65–71.

82. Lange P, Parner J, Vestbo J, et al. A 15-year follow-up study of ventilatory function in adults with asthma. N Engl J Med 1998;339(17):1194–200.

83. Hopp RJ, Bewtra A, Nair NM, et al. The effect of age on methacholine response. J Allergy Clin Immunol 1985;76(4):609–13.

84. Slavin RG, Haselkorn T, Lee JH, et al. Asthma in older adults: observations from the epidemiology and natural history of asthma: outcomes and treatment regimens (TENOR) study. Ann Allergy Asthma Immunol 2006;96(3):406–14.

85. Jarjour NN, Erzurum SC, Bleecker ER, et al. Severe asthma: lessons learned from the National Heart, Lung, and Blood Institute Severe Asthma Research Program. Am J Respir Crit Care Med 2012;185(4): 356–62.

86. Proceedings of the ATS workshop on refractory asthma: current understanding, recommendations, and unanswered questionss. American Thoracic Society. Am J Respir Crit Care Med 2000;162(6): 2341–51.

87. Sin DD, Tu JV. Underuse of inhaled steroid therapy in elderly patients with asthma. Chest 2001;119(3): 720–5.

88. Hartert TV, Togias A, Mellen BG, et al. Underutilization of controller and rescue medications among older adults with asthma requiring hospital care. J Am Geriatr Soc 2000;48(6):651–7.

89. Sin DD, Tu JV. Inhaled corticosteroid therapy reduces the risk of rehospitalization and all-cause

90. Dunn RM, Lehman E, Chinchilli VM, et al. Impact of age and sex on response to asthma therapy. Am J Respir Crit Care Med 2015;192(5):551–8.

91. Skloot GS, Busse PJ, Braman SS, et al. An official american thoracic society workshop report: evaluation and management of asthma in the elderly. Ann Am Thorac Soc 2016;13(11):2064–77.

92. Dunn RM, Busse PJ, Wechsler MF. Asthma in the elderly and late-onset adult asthma. Allergy 2018; 73(2):284–94.

93. Franceschi C, Campisi J. Chronic inflammation (inflammaging) and its potential contribution to age-associated diseases. J Gerontol A Biol Sci Med Sci 2014;69(Suppl 1):S4–9.

94. Belsky DW, Shalev I, Sears MR, et al. Is chronic asthma associated with shorter leukocyte telomere length at midlife? Am J Respir Crit Care Med 2014; 190(4):384–91.

95. Guerra S. New asthma biomarkers: shorter telomeres, longer disease? Am J Respir Crit Care Med 2014;190(4):356–8.

96. Meyer KC, Rosenthal NS, Soergel P, et al. Neutrophils and low-grade inflammation in the seemingly normal aging human lung. Mech Ageing Dev 1998; 104(2):169–81.

97. Meyer KC, Soergel P. Variation of bronchoalveolar lymphocyte phenotypes with age in the physiologically normal human lung. Thorax 1999;54(8): 697–700.

98. Mathur SK, Schwantes EA, Jarjour NN, et al. Age-related changes in eosinophil function in human subjects. Chest 2008;133(2):412–9.

99. Ducharme ME, Prince P, Hassan N, et al. Expiratory flows and airway inflammation in elderly asthmatic patients. Respir Med 2011;105(9):1284–9.

100. Busse PJ, Birmingham JM, Calatroni A, et al. Effect of aging on sputum inflammation and asthma control. J Allergy Clin Immunol 2017;139(6):1808–18. e6.

101. Bauer BA, Reed CE, Yunginger JW, et al. Incidence and outcomes of asthma in the elderly. A population-based study in Rochester, Minnesota. Chest 1997;111(2):303–10.

102. Estenne M, Yernault JC, De Troyer A. Rib cage and diaphragm-abdomen compliance in humans: effects of age and posture. J Appl Physiol (1985) 1985;59(6):1842–8.

103. Janssens JP. Aging of the respiratory system: impact on pulmonary function tests and adaptation to exertion. Clin Chest Med 2005;26(3): 469–84. vi-vii.

104. Enright PL, Kronmal RA, Manolio TA, et al. Respiratory muscle strength in the elderly. Correlates and reference values. Cardiovascular Health Study

Research Group. Am J Respir Crit Care Med 1994; 149(2 Pt 1):430–8.

105. Jain R, Ray JM, Pan JH, et al. Sex hormone-dependent regulation of cilia beat frequency in airway epithelium. Am J Respir Cell Mol Biol 2012;46(4):446–53.

106. Santoro N, Brown JR, Adel T, et al. Characterization of reproductive hormonal dynamics in the perimenopause. J Clin Endocrinol Metab 1996;81(4):1495–501.

107. Haggerty CL, Ness RB, Kelsey S, et al. The impact of estrogen and progesterone on asthma. Ann Allergy Asthma Immunol 2003;90(3):284–91 [quiz: 291–3], 347.

108. Chandler MH, Schuldheisz S, Phillips BA, et al. Premenstrual asthma: the effect of estrogen on symptoms, pulmonary function, and beta 2-receptors. Pharmacotherapy 1997;17(2):224–34.

109. Ulrik CS, Lange P. Decline of lung function in adults with bronchial asthma. Am J Respir Crit Care Med 1994;150(3):629–34.

110. Zaitsu M, Narita S, Lambert KC, et al. Estradiol activates mast cells via a non-genomic estrogen receptor-alpha and calcium influx. Mol Immunol 2007;44(8):1977–85.

111. Newcomb DC, Cephus JY, Boswell MG, et al. Estrogen and progesterone decrease let-7f microRNA expression and increase IL-23/IL-23 receptor signaling and IL-17A production in patients with severe asthma. J Allergy Clin Immunol 2015;136(4):1025–34.e1.

112. Keselman A, Heller N. Estrogen signaling modulates allergic inflammation and contributes to sex differences in asthma. Front Immunol 2015;6:568.

113. Cephus JY, Stier MT, Fuseini H, et al. Testosterone attenuates group 2 innate lymphoid cell-mediated airway inflammation. Cell Rep 2017;21(9):2487–99.

114. Scott HA, Gibson PG, Garg ML, et al. Sex hormones and systemic inflammation are modulators of the obese-asthma phenotype. Allergy 2016; 71(7):1037–47.

115. Li X, Hawkins GA, Ampleford EJ, et al. Genome-wide association study identifies TH1 pathway genes associated with lung function in asthmatic patients. J Allergy Clin Immunol 2013;132(2):313–20.e5.

116. Li X, Howard TD, Moore WC, et al. Importance of hedgehog interacting protein and other lung function genes in asthma. J Allergy Clin Immunol 2011;127(6):1457–65.

117. Li H, Romieu I, Sienra-Monge JJ, et al. Genetic polymorphisms in arginase I and II and childhood asthma and atopy. J Allergy Clin Immunol 2006; 117(1):119–26.

118. Salam MT, Islam T, Gauderman WJ, et al. Roles of arginase variants, atopy, and ozone in childhood asthma. J Allergy Clin Immunol 2009;123(3):596–602, 602.e1-8.

119. Vercelli D. Arginase: marker, effector, or candidate gene for asthma? J Clin Invest 2003;111(12):1815–7.

120. Vonk JM, Postma DS, Maarsingh H, et al. Arginase 1 and arginase 2 variations associate with asthma, asthma severity and beta2 agonist and steroid response. Pharmacogenet Genomics 2010;20(3):179–86.

121. Kolovou G, Damaskos D, Anagnostopoulou K, et al. Apolipoprotein E gene polymorphism and gender. Ann Clin Lab Sci 2009;39(2):120–33.

122. Herrington DM, Howard TD, Brosnihan KB, et al. Common estrogen receptor polymorphism augments effects of hormone replacement therapy on E-selectin but not C-reactive protein. Circulation 2002;105(16):1879–82.

123. Herrington DM, Howard TD, Hawkins GA, et al. Estrogen-receptor polymorphisms and effects of estrogen replacement on high-density lipoprotein cholesterol in women with coronary disease. N Engl J Med 2002;346(13):967–74.

124. Hunninghake GM, Soto-Quiros ME, Avila L, et al. TSLP polymorphisms are associated with asthma in a sex-specific fashion. Allergy 2010;65(12):1566–75.

125. Myers RA, Scott NM, Gauderman WJ, et al. Genome-wide interaction studies reveal sex-specific asthma risk alleles. Hum Mol Genet 2014;23(19):5251–9.

126. Loisel DA, Tan Z, Tisler CJ, et al. IFNG genotype and sex interact to influence the risk of childhood asthma. J Allergy Clin Immunol 2011;128(3):524–31.

127. Lodish HBA, Kaiser CA, Krieger M, et al. Molecular cell biology. 8th edition. New York: WH Freeman and Company; 2016.

128. Hall JM, Couse JF, Korach KS. The multifaceted mechanisms of estradiol and estrogen receptor signaling. J Biol Chem 2001;276(40):36869–72.

129. Kushner PJ, Agard DA, Greene GL, et al. Estrogen receptor pathways to AP-1. J Steroid Biochem Mol Biol 2000;74(5):311–7.

130. Safe S. Transcriptional activation of genes by 17 beta-estradiol through estrogen receptor-Sp1 interactions. Vitam Horm 2001;62:231–52.

131. Dijkstra A, Howard TD, Vonk JM, et al. Estrogen receptor 1 polymorphisms are associated with airway hyperresponsiveness and lung function decline, particularly in female subjects with asthma. J Allergy Clin Immunol 2006;117(3):604–11.

132. Aravamudan B, Goorhouse KJ, Unnikrishnan G, et al. Differential expression of estrogen receptor variants in response to inflammation signals in human airway smooth Muscle. J Cell Physiol 2017; 232(7):1754–60.

133. Melgert BN, ten Hacken NH, Rutgers B, et al. More alternative activation of macrophages in lungs of asthmatic patients. J Allergy Clin Immunol 2011; 127(3):831–3.

134. Keselman A, Fang X, White PB, et al. Estrogen signaling contributes to sex differences in macrophage polarization during asthma. J Immunol 2017;199(5):1573–83.

135. Laffont S, Blanquart E, Savignac M, et al. Androgen signaling negatively controls group 2 innate lymphoid cells. J Exp Med 2017;214(6):1581–92.

136. Hackett TL. Epithelial-mesenchymal transition in the pathophysiology of airway remodelling in asthma. Curr Opin Allergy Clin Immunol 2012; 12(1):53–9.

137. Xu L, Xiang X, Ji X, et al. Effects and mechanism of dehydroepiandrosterone on epithelial-mesenchymal transition in bronchial epithelial cells. Exp Lung Res 2014;40(5):211–21.

138. Wan YY, Flavell RA. Regulatory T-cell functions are subverted and converted owing to attenuated Foxp3 expression. Nature 2007;445(7129):766–70.

139. Hartl D, Koller B, Mehlhorn AT, et al. Quantitative and functional impairment of pulmonary CD4+CD25hi regulatory T cells in pediatric asthma. J Allergy Clin Immunol 2007;119(5): 1258–66.

140. Page ST, Plymate SR, Bremner WJ, et al. Effect of medical castration on CD4+ CD25+ T cells, CD8+ T cell IFN-gamma expression, and NK cells: a physiological role for testosterone and/or its metabolites. Am J Physiol Endocrinol Metab 2006; 290(5):E856–63.

141. Rothman MS, Carlson NE, Xu M, et al. Reexamination of testosterone, dihydrotestosterone, estradiol and estrone levels across the menstrual cycle and in postmenopausal women measured by liquid chromatography-tandem mass spectrometry. Steroids 2011;76(1–2):177–82.

142. Prunicki M, Stell L, Dinakarpandian D, et al. Exposure to NO2, CO, and PM2.5 is linked to regional DNA methylation differences in asthma. Clin Epigenetics 2018;10:2.

143. Walecki M, Eisel F, Klug J, et al. Androgen receptor modulates Foxp3 expression in CD4+CD25+ Foxp3+ regulatory T-cells. Mol Biol Cell 2015; 26(15):2845–57.

Asthma and Corticosteroid Responses in Childhood and Adult Asthma

Amira Ali Ramadan, MD, MSc[a,b],
Jonathan M. Gaffin, MD, MMsc[c], Elliot Israel, MD[d,e],
Wanda Phipatanakul, MD, MS[a,d],*

KEYWORDS

- Childhood asthma • Inhaled corticosteroids • Corticosteroid response • Corticosteroid resistance
- Adult asthma

KEY POINTS

- Corticosteroids are the most effective treatment for asthma; inhaled corticosteroids (ICSs) are the first-line treatment for children and adults with persistent asthma.
- The anti-inflammatory effects of corticosteroids are mediated by both genomic and nongenomic factors.
- Variation in the response to corticosteroids has been observed. Patient characteristics, biomarkers, and genetic features may be used to predict response to ICSs.
- Response to corticosteroids can be assessed through different measures.
- The existence of multiple mechanisms underlying glucocorticoid insensitivity raises the possibility that this might indeed reflect different diseases with a common phenotype.

INTRODUCTION

Asthma is a chronic respiratory disease affecting approximately 300 million people worldwide.[1] In the United States, an estimated 43.3 million people, including 9.3 million children, have asthma.[2] Asthma is characterized by chronic inflammation and airway obstruction. Corticosteroids, inhaled or systemic, are the most effective treatment for asthma in adults and children and they are recommended by many international asthma management guidelines.[1,3] Corticosteroids have anti-inflammatory properties, which account for their effectiveness in suppressing the underlying airway inflammatory process and controlling asthma symptoms.[4]

Inhaled corticosteroids (ICSs) are the mainstay treatment in patients with chronic persistent asthma,[4] whereas short courses of oral corticosteroids (OCSs) are effective to establish control of asthma exacerbations or during a period of gradual deterioration of asthma not responding to step-up controller therapy.[5] A large number of studies investigating ICSs in asthma have demonstrated improvement in symptoms, lung function, airway hyperresponsiveness, and exacerbation frequency[6,7]; however, the response to these

Disclosure Statement: Funding from NIH K24 AI 106822, UG1 HL139124 and the Allergy Asthma Awareness Initiative.
[a] Division of Allergy and Immunology, Boston Children's Hospital, 300 Longwood Avenue, Boston, MA 02115, USA; [b] Beth Israel Deaconess Center, Cardiovascular institute, 330 Brookline Avenue, Boston, MA 02215, USA; [c] Division of Respiratory Diseases, Boston Children's Hospital, Boston, MA, USA; [d] Harvard Medical School, 25 Shattuck Street, Boston, MA 02115, USA; [e] Brigham and Women's Hospital, 15 Francis Street, Boston, MA 02115, USA
* Corresponding author. Division of Allergy and Immunology, Boston Children's Hospital, 300 Longwood Avenue, Fegan Building, 6th Floor, Boston, MA 02115.
E-mail address: Wanda.Phipatanakul@childrens.harvard.edu

chestmed.theclinics.com

medications is highly variable, particularly when administered at moderate-to-high dosages.[8] The variability in response may be attributable to different mechanisms underlying the airway inflammation.[9]

INFLAMMATION IN ASTHMA

Most patients with asthma have underlying immune-mediated inflammation involving Type 2 helper T (TH2) cells and innate lymphoid cells of group 2 (ILC2) responses that result in production of cytokines, inflammatory peptides, chemokines, and growth factors.[10] This leads to production of immunoglobulin (Ig)E and subsequent activation of mast cells and activation and recruitment of eosinophils resulting in airway hyperresponsiveness, smooth-muscle hypertrophy, structural airway remodeling, and mucus secretion.[11] This chronic inflammation underlies the typical symptoms of asthma, which include intermittent wheezing, coughing, shortness of breath, and chest tightness. However, studies of the cellular components of airway inflammation have found increasing evidence that a significant proportion of human asthma may be driven by non-TH2 inflammation.[6,12] Asthma is classically divided into 3 main immunopathological phenotypes: eosinophilic, neutrophilic, and paucigranulocytic.

MECHANISM OF ACTION OF CORTICOSTEROIDS
Molecular Mechanism of Action

The anti-inflammatory effects of corticosteroids are mediated by both genomic and nongenomic effects.[13,14] ICSs target gene transcription through their interactions with the glucocorticoid receptor (GR) at the glucocorticoid response element.[15]

The airway inflammation in asthma is characterized by the increased expression of multiple inflammatory genes, including those encoding for cytokines, chemokines, adhesion molecules, and inflammatory enzymes and receptors. The major action of corticosteroids is to switch off these genes[16] by reversing histone acetylation of activated inflammatory genes (transrepression).[17] The anti-inflammatory effect of ICSs is mediated through their binding to the corticosteroid receptor, which can subsequently reduce inflammatory gene expression. This is often attributed to a direct inhibitory effect of the GR on inflammatory gene transcription.[18] This mechanism results in the suppression of proinflammatory molecules called transrepression and upregulation of many anti-inflammatory molecules called transactivation. Transrepression accounts for many of the desired GC effects.[19]

Cellular Effect of Corticosteroids

At a cellular level, corticosteroids reduce the number of inflammatory cells in the airways, including eosinophils, T lymphocytes, mast cells, and dendritic cells.[4] These effects of corticosteroids are produced through inhibiting the recruitment of inflammatory cells into the airway by suppressing the production of chemotactic mediators and adhesion molecules and by inhibiting the survival in the airways of inflammatory cells, such as eosinophils, T lymphocytes, and mast cells.[20] ICSs attenuate airway eosinophil numbers, reduce asthma exacerbations and mortality, and lead to improvements in lung function and health-related quality of life[21,22] (**Box 1**).

Criterion for Corticosteroid Responsiveness

Current asthma guidelines characterize treatment response as improved lung function, symptoms, or exacerbations.[1] Corticosteroid response can be assessed through normalization or improvement across multiple domains: airflow limitation measured by lung function testing, symptom scores, and airway inflammation.[23]

Assessment of Steroid Responsiveness

Asthma control should aim to achieve day-to-day (or current) asthma control, minimize activity limitation, prevent asthma exacerbations, and reduce decline in lung function over time, while minimizing the risk of side effects from medications required to achieve this control.[24] The British Thoracic Society guidelines describe the goal of total (or optimal) asthma control as comprising no daytime or nighttime symptoms, normal lung function, and no exacerbations.[25]

Response to ICSs should be examined across the domains of symptoms, lung function, exacerbation rate.[26] Direct and indirect measures of airway inflammation may also be considered. **Box 2** details subjective and objective measures of asthma control.

In children, the definition of corticosteroid responsiveness has been debated. Currently, there is no accepted definition of steroid response. A recent study in pediatric patients with severe asthma proposed the definition of steroid response in children[27,28] as $\geq$15% increase of forced expiratory volume in 1 second (FEV1)% predicted, bronchodilator reversibility (BDR) of 12% or greater (**Table 1**). However, it is acknowledged that this might not be an appropriate definition for children because many children with a confirmed diagnosis of severe asthma have normal spirometric results, but their symptoms remain poorly controlled.[29,30]

Box 1
Effects of corticosteroids

- Suppress multiple inflammatory genes that are activated in asthmatic airways by reversing histone acetylation.
- Increase messenger RNA degradation, thereby blocking production of proinflammatory cytokines.
- Increase the synthesis of anti-inflammatory proteins.
- Suppress the increased microvascular permeability and plasma leakage into the airway lumen that occur in asthma, which adds to the airway obstruction.
- Suppressing the production of chemotactic mediators and adhesion molecules and inhibiting its survival in the airways.
- Inhibit the remodeling process.
- Reduce the inflammatory cells in the airways, including eosinophils, T lymphocytes, mast cells, and dendritic cells.

Symptoms

Although symptoms may be of most importance to patients, symptom perception is often poor in asthmatic children,[31] making this less than ideal as a measure of response.

Box 2
Measures of assessment of steroid responsiveness in adults

Subjective measurement:

- Self-monitoring of symptoms, and activity limitations.
- Standardized asthma-specific questionnaire tools (Asthma Control Test, ACQ ATAC).
- Quality of life assessments: asthma quality of life questionnaire (AQLQ), pediatric AQLQ.

Objective measurement:

- Exacerbation rate
- Lung function spirometry (forced expiratory volume in 1 second)
- Peak expiratory flow
- Bronchodilator reversibility
- Inflammatory markers
- Sputum cytology
- Fraction of exhaled nitric oxide

Abbreviations: ACQ, asthma control questionnaire; ATAC, asthma therapy assessment questionnaire.

Lung function

Although studies in adults have relied on changes in lung function as an indicator of corticosteroid responsiveness,[32] children with severe asthma often have less airflow limitation than do adults[33–36] and do not always have concordance between lung function measures and symptoms.[35] Furthermore, spirometry is often normal in children even with quite severe asthma.[37] Lung function is only one component of asthma control and is best assessed in combination with current symptoms.[1]

However, studies have assessed complete corticosteroid responsiveness by selected cutpoints of symptoms, FEV1, bronchodilator reversibility, and exhaled nitric oxide.[36] In other studies, steroid sensitivity was defined by greater than 15% improvement in prebronchodilator FEV1, after a short course of OCSs.[38,39]

Factors Affecting Corticosteroid Response in Asthma in Both Children and Adults

Even though ICSs have been established as first-line treatment in adults and children with persistent asthma, there is substantial heterogeneity of responses to ICS therapy.[40] The change in lung function associated with asthma treatment administration follows a near-normal distribution, demonstrating substantial interindividual variability,[41] with a significant proportion of both nonresponders and high responders to therapy. This wide variability in interindividual response, combined with high intraindividual repeatability, suggests a genetic basis to the heterogeneity in asthma treatment response.[42] This heterogeneity is also influenced by other factors, including age, sex, socioeconomic status, race and/or ethnicity, and gene by environment interactions.[43] The multiple factors that appear to impact the effectiveness of ICS treatment can be characterized as either modifiable or nonmodifiable (**Tables 2 and 3**)

The modifiable factors must be assessed before consideration of response to treatment, for example, patients should be checked for adherence to treatment, coexisting conditions should be treated,[11] and the diagnosis of severe asthma must be kept in mind in some cases that do not respond to corticosteroids.

Potential modifiable/reversible factors are

Poor treatment adherence Suboptimal adherence leads to poorer clinical outcomes.[44] There are 2 forms of nonadherence: intentional and unintentional. Unintentional nonadherence can result

Table 1
Steroid responsiveness criteria in children with asthma

Steroid Response in Children	
ACT score[a]	>19/25 or 50% increase
FeNO	Normal (<24 ppb)
Morning FEV1[a]	FEV1 ≥80% of predicted value or ≥15% increase
Sputum eosinophil counts	<2.5%

Abbreviations: ACT, asthma control test; FeNO, fraction of exhaled nitric oxide; FEV1, forced expiratory volume in 1 second.
[a] ACT score.
Adapted from Bossley CJ, Fleming L, Ullmann N, et al. Assessment of corticosteroid response in pediatric patients with severe asthma by using a multidomain approach. J Allergy Clin Immunol 2016;138(2):418–9; with permission.

from the complexity of the treatment regimen or understanding of the medication.[45] Intentional barriers to adherence are driven by illness perceptions and medication beliefs, patients and parents deliberately choose not to follow the doctor's recommendations. Common nonintentional barriers are related to family routines, child-raising issues, and to social issues such as poverty.[46] A retrospective case-control survey identified poor adherence of 22% in 57 children with difficult-to-control asthma.[38]

Pitfalls in drug delivery One potential explanation of poor response to corticosteroid treatment could be the suboptimal prescribed dosing of ICS, particularly in young children who may receive less of the actuated medication delivered to the distal airways than older children and adults. Furthermore, even with appropriately chosen medication and delivery device, many people with asthma do not use their inhaler correctly.[47]

Comorbidities Comorbidities that have not been managed well and alternative diagnoses, such as inhaled foreign body and structural abnormalities, need to be addressed to optimize asthma management.

Environmental influences and allergen exposure Studies have shown that partial corticosteroid response may be due to ongoing exposure to environmental triggers[29] and that persistent allergen exposure in sensitized individuals can lead to an interleukin (IL)-2 and IL-4–mediated corticosteroid resistance.[48]

Cigarette smoking is also known to cause corticosteroid resistance.[28,29] In fact, tobacco smoke, even by passive exposure, leads to increased asthma symptoms and decreased response to ICSs. Studies found that asthmatic patients exposed to tobacco are refractory to standard controller therapies, namely ICSs.[49] Kobayashi and colleagues[50] demonstrated that passive smoke exposure impaired histone deacetylase-2 function, which could contribute to steroid resistance in children with asthma.

Stress Recently, stress-related glucocorticoid resistance of TH2 cytokine production by T cells was described in children with asthma who reported inadequate social support.[51] Although asthma exacerbation has long been thought to be affected by emotional states, evidence has only recently emerged to identify cellular and molecular mechanisms responsible for stress-induced glucocorticoid insensitivity.[52]

Nonmodifiable factors
Genetics Genetic variation may partly explain asthma treatment response heterogeneity.[53] Endogenous corticosteroid level and exogenous therapeutic response to corticosteroids are also strongly influenced by genetics.[54] Previous studies have suggested that 60% to 80% of patients with asthma have different responses to corticosteroid treatment due to genetic factors,[55] highlighting the importance of gene polymorphisms for the interindividual variability in a patient's response to medication.[56] Among children participating in the CAMP study, a variation in TBX21 coding (replacement of histidine 33 with glutamine) affected the effect of ICSs on airway hyperresponsiveness,[57] whereas a functional variant in glucocorticoid-induced transcript 1 gene (GLCCI1) was associated with a decreased response to corticosteroids.[58] TBX21 encodes for the transcription factor T-bet (T-box expressed in T cells), which influences naive T lymphocyte development and has been implicated in asthma pathogenesis.[57]

A review done by Duong-Thi-Ly and colleagues,[56] found that various potential genetic factors associated with the response to ICSs, and that they could be used to predict the individual therapeutic response of children with asthma to ICS. Among the genes identified, variants in T-box 21 (TBX21) and Fc fragment of IgE receptor II (FCER2) contribute indirectly to the variability in the response to ICSs by altering the inflammatory mechanisms in asthma, whereas other genes, such as

Table 2
Modifiable factors that, in patients with severe asthma, may contribute to poor symptom control and/or exacerbations, with diagnostic investigations, and effective intervention strategies

	Modifiable Risk Factors	Diagnosis	Intervention Strategies
Medication and Delivery	Incorrect inhaler technique Poor adherence with controller therapy	Check technique against a device-specific checklist	Physical demonstration and regular rechecking Identify adherence barriers, including cost; simplify treatment regimen; electronic inhaler reminders for missed doses; refill reminders
Exposure	Smoking or environmental tobacco smoke; biomass fuel exposure Allergen exposure in sensitized patients (house dust mite, cat, mold, cockroach)	History, urinary cotinine Skin prick testing, history	Smoking cessation advice; alternative cooking or heating methods Selected avoidance strategies if shown to be effective
	Indoor or outdoor air pollution, extreme weather	Specific questioning, seasonal or event related	Ventilate dwelling; alternative cooking/heating methods; avoid running during outdoor air pollution or extreme weather
	Occupational exposure to allergens or irritants	Occupational history, peak expiratory flow on work/non–work days	Early withdrawal from exposure
	Respiratory viruses including rhinovirus, respiratory syncytial virus, influenza	History, serology	Consider avoiding close contact with children when they have respiratory infections; influenza vaccination
Comorbidities	Obesity Gastroesophageal reflux disease Rhinosinusitis ± nasal polyposis COPD (ie, asthma-COPD overlap) Anxiety, depression Vocal cord dysfunction Bronchiectasis ABPA Pregnancy	Body mass index Usually only relevant when symptomatic; 24-hour pH monitoring including acid and non-acid reflux ENT evaluation, nasal endoscopy and/or CT sinuses Smoking history, diffusing capacity, lung volumes, ± HRCT chest Inspiratory/expiratory flow-volume loops, functional laryngoscopy (±with exercise), HRCT larynx HRCT chest, sputum culture, investigate for immunodeficiency and ABPA Serum IgE, skin test/specific IgE for aspergillus, IgG Aspergillus precipitins Pregnancy test	Diet and exercise; bariatric surgery Lifestyle changes, proton pump inhibitor, reduce medications that predispose to reflux; treatment of asymptomatic reflux may not improve asthma control Nasal corticosteroids (spray or wash), surgery if needed; consider leukotriene modifier if aspirin exacerbated respiratory disease Smoking cessation, pulmonary rehabilitation, long-acting muscarinic antagonist, check for cardiac

(continued on next page)

Table 2
(continued)

	Modifiable Risk Factors	Diagnosis	Intervention Strategies
Social	Socioeconomic problems Illicit drug use At-risk populations (adolescents, elderly)	Empathic questioning about cost barriers to adherence; social work consultation Blood/urine testing Assess adherence, inhaler technique, comorbidities (especially in elderly), medication interactions	Community/government support; medication samples; choose lowest cost medication regimen Refer for withdrawal strategies and support

Abbreviations: ABPA, allergic bronchopulmonary aspergillosis; COPD, chronic obstructive pulmonary disease; CT, computed tomography; ENT, ear nose throat; HRCT, high-resolution computed tomography; Ig, immunoglobulin.
   Data from Israel E, Reddel HK. Severe and difficult-to-treat asthma in adults. N Engl J Med 2017;377(10):965–76.

corticotropin-releasing hormone receptor 1 (CRHR1), nuclear receptor subfamily 3 group C member 1 (NR3C1), stress-induced phosphoprotein 1 (STIP1), dual-specificity phosphatase 1 (DUSP1), glucocorticoid-induced 1 (GLCCI1), histone deacetylase 1 (HDAC), ORMDL sphingolipid biosynthesis regulator 3 (ORMDL3), and vascular endothelial growth factors directly affect this variability through the anti-inflammatory mechanisms of ICSs.[56] The effect of genetic variants on treatment outcome might occur through differences in disease subtypes or through influences on drug level or drug target.[26]

Studies have investigated the genetic influences on the ICS response in chronic treatment of asthma.[23,36] ICS response studies, such as those implicating genetic variants, are STIP1,[59] TBX21,[57,60] and WDR21A,[61] GLCCI1,[58] FBXL7,[62] 9T,10 CRHR1, and MAPT.[63]

On the contrary, a recent study reported no evidence to confirm previously reported associations between candidate genetic variants and ICS response (ie, change of FEV1 from baseline) in patients with asthma.[64]

Epigenetics In asthmatic children, treatment response to systemic corticosteroid is heterogeneous and may be mediated by an epigenetic mechanism.[3]

Recently, DNA methylation has been increasingly explored due to its important role in the regulation of gene expression.[65] DNA methylation (DNAm) is the modification of cytosine by adding a methyl group to the 5′ position of C. DNAm mostly occurs in the context of CpG dinucleotides and represents an important epigenetic mechanism that regulates gene expression.[66] Several studies have successfully identified DNAm of certain nucleotides as a biomarker for asthma.[67,68] These epigenetic biomarkers may be used to distinguish children who do not respond to steroid treatment well.[65]

Table 3
Monitoring corticosteroids using different measures: clinical, pulmonary function, and evidence of airway inflammation

Clinical Measures	Pulmonary Function Measures	Challenge Techniques	Airway Inflammation	Distal Lung or Small Airways
Symptoms Exacerbations Asthma control and quality of life questionnaires	Change in FEV1 Change in % predicted FEV1, especially in children Post-bronchodilator FEV1	Airway hyperresponsiveness: methacholine, histamine, or cold air Exercise challenge	Induced sputum cytology Exhaled nitric oxide	Closing volume Imaging (air trapping) – high-resolution CT scan Hyperpolarized helium FEF_{25-75}

Abbreviation: FEF_{25-75}, the forced expiratory flow at 25–75% of forced vital capacity (FVC) (FEF25–75%).
   Adapted from Szefler SJ, Martin RJ. Lessons learned from variation in response to therapy in clinical trials. J Allergy Clin Immunol 2010;125(2):285–92; [quiz: 93–4]; with permission.

Patient characteristics/phenotypes and biomarkers Asthma encompasses a broad collection of heterogeneous disease subtypes with different underlying pathophysiological mechanisms.[69] Simpson and colleagues,[70] described 4 inflammatory subtypes of asthma based on the immune cell profile of sputum taken from patients. These subtypes include eosinophilic (eosinophils >3%), neutrophilic (neutrophils >61%), mixed granulocytic (increased eosinophils and neutrophils), and paucigranulocytic asthma (normal levels of both of these specific immune cell types). The neutrophilic and eosinophilic phenotype usually do not respond well to corticosteroids.[71]

In clinical practice, variable responses to corticosteroid treatment have been observed. Phenotypic presentations in young children with asthma are varied and might contribute to differential responses to asthma controller medications. Treatment response to inhaled corticoids is clearly dependent on certain asthma phenotypes.[72,73] Szefler and Martin[74] found that treatment response was highly variable even in adults with mild to moderate persistent asthma and that there was some potential to relate treatment response to patient characteristics and biomarkers. Specifically, allergies and high levels of exhaled nitric oxide (eNO) indicated a favorable response to corticosteroids.[73]

Race Race and ethnicity may influence the response to treatment in patients with asthma[75]; black patients may have a diminished response to glucocorticoids.[70] Koo and colleagues[76] reported that black children with severe asthma had less improvement in FeNO than white children and were more likely to experience exacerbations. Although these data suggest a differential response to therapy between patients with asthma by race and ethnicity, the evidence regarding ethnic variations in response to steroid treatment is still limited. Evidence suggests that black individuals have a racial predisposition to diminished glucocorticoid responsiveness, which may contribute to their heightened asthma morbidity.[77] Although disparities in access to care and quality of care have been implicated in the racial differential outcomes,[78] it is also possible that there are inherent pathophysiologic or even pharmacogenomic differences between white and African American individuals that result in these discrepancies.[79]

Microbiome Early evidence suggests that there may be a relationship between the airway microbiome and physiologic response to corticosteroids. Evidence showed that strains of streptococci can influence the response of bronchial epithelial cells to corticosteroids[80] and *Haemophilus* and parainfluenzae species have been shown to inhibit corticosteroid response of asthmatic alveolar macrophages and peripheral blood monocytes.[80,81]

Predictors of Asthma Response to Corticosteroid

As the response to ICS is not uniform and shows variability among individuals, it would be highly desirable to identify a subgroup of patients who show a favorable (or worse) response to ICSs.

In the current guidelines for asthma treatment, therapeutic strategy is adjusted on the basis of symptoms, lung function, and acute exacerbations; however, the relationship between these key components of the disease may vary among different asthmatic patients.[82] Thus, predictors such as baseline pulmonary function and levels of markers of allergic inflammation could be used to predict response to ICSs. Lower prebronchodilator lung function and higher BDR of FEV1, as well as degree of airway hyperresponsiveness to methacholine is associated with more favorable response to ICSs.[83,84] Further, positive ICS response has also been associated with biomarkers of TH2 inflammation, such as FeNO levels, total eosinophil count, IgE levels, and Eosinophilic cationic protein (ECP) levels.[73]

Biomarkers

Biomarkers known to be useful for the diagnosis of asthma, as well as being relevant to the response to treatment, may be useful in personalizing care of the asthmatic patient.[85] The utility of biomarkers in asthma for predicting future exacerbations, response to treatment, or lung function decline is a topic of growing interest.[86] Cowan and colleagues[87] suggested that baseline inflammatory biomarkers enable prediction of ICS responsiveness in asthma.

Specific inflammatory biomarkers could potentially serve as corticosteroid response predictors (eg, fraction of nitric oxide in exhaled breath) and eosinophilic markers (exhaled NO or sputum eosinophils).[87] Approximately 50% of asthma cases are attributable to eosinophilic airway inflammation. ICSs are particularly effective in combating Th2-driven inflammation featuring mast cell and eosinophilic airway infiltration.[88] Eosinophilic phenotype usually responds well to corticosteroids, except for a small subgroup with severe asthma in whom even in the presence of eosinophils the ICS seem to have a less responsive role.[84]

Predictors of response in adults

- FeNO
- FEV1
- Smoking
- *Gender*

Fraction of exhaled nitric oxide Over the past decade, fraction of exhaled nitric oxide (FeNO) values and sputum eosinophil counts have been used as biomarkers of airway inflammation and predictors of steroid responsiveness.[28,87] FeNO values are correlated with airway eosinophilia[89] and associated with airway hyperresponsiveness.[90] FeNO values are high in asthmatic patients.[91,92] Furthermore, studies indicate that high FeNO values in asthmatic patients indicate an at-risk phenotype for exacerbation and predict clinical response to ICSs or OCSs.[92] Multiple studies have found that a favorable response to fluticasone was associated with higher levels of FeNO, as well as total eosinophil counts and levels of serum IgE.[83,84,93] Evidence indicates that FeNO, which is a marker of T-helper cell type 2 (Th2)-mediated airway inflammation, has a high positive and negative predictive value for identifying corticosteroid-responsive airway.[94] FeNO production is very sensitive to ICS therapy because ICS therapy can directly inhibit FeNO production by modulation of inducible nitric oxide synthase.[95] In fact, studies have found that sputum eosinophils and FeNO are the best predictors of favorable response to oral prednisolone in patients with severe asthma.[96] High FeNO (>50 parts per billion) strongly suggests airway eosinophilia and hence steroid responsiveness.[97]

The combination of high FeNO and high urinary bromotyrosine (BrTyr), which is a biochemical fingerprint of eosinophil activation, were reported in a study to predict a favorable clinical response to ICSs with improvement in ACQ, FEV1, or airway reactivity.[87]

Forced expiratory volume in 1 second Evidence concluded that short-term response to ICSs with regard to FEV1 improvement predicts long-term control from the Predicting Response to Inhaled Corticosteroid Efficacy (PRICE) trial.[74] It is reported that favorable corticosteroid response was associated with lower levels of methacholine provocation concentration causing a 20% fall in FEV1.[73,98] Similarly, bronchodilator reversibility was highly predictive to significant response to triamcinolone actinide injection in the Severe Asthma Research Program (SARP III) study.[99]

Smoking Another predictor of long-term controller response in adults was identified in the Smoking Modulates Outcomes of Glucocorticoid Therapy (SMOG) study,[49] in which the response to ICS was attenuated in subjects with mild asthma who smoke, suggesting that adjustments to standard therapy may be required to attain asthma control[49,74] in this population. Smoking is a strong predictor of poor response to ICS.

Gender The influence of sex on ICS response has been inconsistent.[82] Galant and colleagues[100] found that female sex was associated with a higher likelihood of responding to ICS therapy, defined as greater than 7.5% increase in FEV1 from baseline.

Predictors of response in children

- Baseline low pulmonary function
- Inflammatory markers
- Gene expression
- Aeroallergen sensitization
- Others

Baseline pulmonary function In children, baseline parameters, favoring a greater differential response for ICS, includes decreased pulmonary function, increased FEV1 response to a bronchodilator, airway hyperresponsiveness, and markers of allergic inflammation (eNO and ECP).[73] A recent study of a SARP III cohort of adults and children with severe asthma found that baseline bronchodilator response and fractional exhaled nitric oxide had good sensitivity and specificity for predicting response in all groups except children with nonsevere asthma.[99] The Childhood Asthma Research and Education Network's Best Add-On Giving Effective Response (BADGER) study suggested that children who responded best to low-dose ICSs had worse asthma control, lower pulmonary function, and lower PC20 levels, which indicate greater bronchial reactivity.[101]

Inflammatory markers Biomarkers associated with differential responses to asthma treatments have been studied in children.[65] Szefler and colleagues[73] found that higher exhaled nitric oxide (eNO), blood eosinophil counts, and serum IgE were associated with a better FEV1 response to ICS.

As in adults, children with predominately allergic airway inflammation or eosinophilic phenotypes are likely to have a beneficial response to ICS.[73,74,101,102]

Gene expression Transcriptional profiling of individual responses is a necessary and fundamental step to better understand the individual variation and identify biomarkers of systemic corticosteroid treatment response.[103] A recent study used genome-wide expression profiling of nasal epithelial cells to identify genes with temporal expression patterns among children with asthma before and after treatment with systemic corticosteroids, concluded that vanin-1 (VNN1) contributes to corticosteroid responsiveness, and that changes in VNN1 nasal epithelial mRNA expression and VNN1 promoter methylation might be clinically useful biomarkers of treatment response in asthmatic children.

Aeroallergen sensitization Among other markers of allergic inflammation, children who have specific IgE or skin prick allergen sensitivity have been found to be ICS responders.[73,101] Studies suggest that children with markers of allergic asthma may experience greater benefits from ICS treatment than children without such markers.[74] Bacharier and colleagues conducted secondary analysis in the CARE Network revealed that preschool children at high risk for asthma experience favorable responses to ICS therapy, particularly when indicators of greater disease severity and aeroallergen sensitization are present.[104] Fitzpatrick and colleagues[105] reported best response to daily ICS in children with both aeroallergen sensitization and blood eosinophil counts of $\geq$300/μL; they demonstrated more asthma control days and fewer exacerbations.

Others Severe other clinical features have been reported to be associated with ICS sensitivity. Knuffman and colleagues[98] identified that parental history of asthma strongly suggested ICS response in the asthmatic child. Female sex[100] and normal body weight[106] have also been shown to be associated with a favorable response to ICSs. In addition, obesity is another factor that might influence the response to ICS.[107] In the TREXA trial, male sex was reported to be associated with greater duration of asthma control as a result of daily treatment with ICS.[108]

Monitoring Response

Response to corticosteroids is monitored by the assessment of clinical symptoms, which only partially correlates with underlying airway inflammation.[109] Several biomarkers have been assessed following treatment with corticosteroids, including measures of lung function, peripheral blood and sputum indices of inflammation, exhaled gases, and breath condensates.[110] Some of these inflammatory biomarkers are

already finding their way into clinical practice (eg, fraction of nitric oxide in exhaled breath).[109]

Petsky and colleagues[93] found that the use of FeNO to guide asthma therapy in children might be beneficial in a subset of children. However, interpretation of low FeNO in children receiving ICS therapy may not correlate with improved inflammation or good control.[101]

A recent study recommended monitoring eosinophils in the sputum of patients with severe, prednisone-dependent, asthma as a means to maintain symptom control, reduce exacerbations, and preserve FEV1 in these patients[111]; however, this remains technically difficult in clinical practice.

Failure to Respond/Nonresponders

Although ICS is currently recommended as the first-line therapy, the significant heterogeneity in response to asthma treatment is evident with as much as 22% to 60% of nonresponder rate in both asthmatic children and adults treated with ICS.[73,112–114] Approximately, 5% to 15% of asthmatic children fail to respond to ICSs and they are often treated with high doses of ICSs, which then has the potential to cause significant side effects.[115,116]

Several inflammatory phenotypes have been identified by the use of biomarkers. Most of them are based on the predominant type of cells in different biological fluids with sputum to be remained the most representative one.[84] Lack of response to corticosteroids in asthma might be seen in patients who do not have a responsive endotype (Th2-low asthma), or a subset of patients who have Th2-high asthma.[117] Patients with a neutrophilic phenotype, assessed by sputum cytology, frequently shows inadequate response to corticosteroid treatment,[118,119] even in mild asthma.[84]

The existence of multiple mechanisms underlying glucocorticoid insensitivity raises the possibility that this might indeed reflect different diseases with a common phenotype.[120]

Several mechanisms have been proposed to account for a failure to respond to corticosteroids, including a reduced number of GR, altered affinity of the ligand for GR, reduced ability of the GR to bind to DNA, or increased activation of transcription factors, such as activator protein-1 (AP-1), that compete for DNA binding.[121]

A study found that oxidation of the amino acid cysteine is associated with decreased responsiveness to systemic glucocorticoids in children with difficult-to-treat asthma.[122]

Corticosteroid Resistance

Corticosteroid-resistant (CR) asthma was first described by Schwartz and colleagues[123] in

1967. A common definition of GC resistance is the failure of an asthmatic patient to improve FEV1 by 15% from a baseline of less than 75% predicted after an adequate dose (eg, >40 mg prednisolone) for an adequate duration of time (eg, 1–2 weeks).[42]

Although the prevalence of corticosteroid resistance among children is very low, these children account for a disproportionate health care spending.[124] Identification of corticosteroid resistance is important, allowing delivering alternative therapies; conversely, in the corticosteroid-sensitive patient, the dose of therapy should be minimized to avoid unwanted side effects.[29]

Tobacco smoke–induced steroid resistance

Adult patients with asthma who currently smoke have relative steroid resistance,[125] and require increased doses of corticosteroids for asthma control.[126] The mechanisms of tobacco smoke–induced steroid resistance has been associated with a neutrophilic inflammatory phenotype.[124] Neutrophilia in the airways is associated with a poor response to ICSs in asthma,[118] and the increase in sputum neutrophils in smokers with asthma compared with nonsmokers with asthma[127] may account for the impaired response to corticosteroids.

Raised tumor necrosis factor-α levels in smokers[128] may also cause an increase in the number of glucocorticoid β receptors,[129] which have been associated with corticosteroid resistance.

Even passive smoking may contribute to corticosteroid-insensitive inflammation in children with severe asthma by impairing histone deacetylase protein expression and activity.[50] This stresses the need for a smoke-free environment for asthmatic children.[50]

Mechanisms for resistance Several molecular mechanisms have been identified to account for corticosteroid resistance in asthma,[124] including overexpression of proinflammatory transcription factors, phosphorylation of GRs, and increases in the decoy GR-β.7 histone deacetylase.[50]

Persistent immune activation and airway inflammation, which to varying degrees is resistant to glucocorticoid therapy, appears to define the immunologic abnormality underlying steroid-resistant asthma.[130]

1. Certain cytokines (particularly interleukins 2, 4, and 13, which show increased expression in bronchial biopsy samples from patients with steroid-resistant asthma) may induce a reduction in affinity of GRs in inflammatory cells, such as T lymphocytes, resulting in local resistance to the anti-inflammatory actions of corticosteroids.[131,132]

2. Impaired nuclear localization of GRs in response to a high concentration of corticosteroids and defective acetylation of histone-4, interfering with the anti-inflammatory actions of corticosteroids.[133]

3. Immunomodulation: TH2 cytokines have also been proposed to play a role in severe CR asthma. A study has shown that CD41 T cells from patients with CR asthma are less able to produce the anti-inflammatory cytokine IL-10 in response to dexamethasone than cells from patients with CS asthma.[134]

4. A subset of subjects with CR asthma demonstrates airway expansion of specific gram-negative bacteria, which triggers TAK1/mitogen-activated protein kinase activation and induce corticosteroid resistance.[81]

EFFECTS OF AGE AND DISEASE SEVERITY ON SYSTEMIC CORTICOSTEROID RESPONSES IN ASTHMA

Phipatanakul and colleagues,[99] in the SARP III cohort of adult and children with severe asthma, describe a distinction between adults and children with severe asthma in terms of their response to parenteral corticosteroids. The study reported that adults, but not children, with severe asthma remain phenotypically distinct from those with nonsevere asthma. The baseline FEV1 response to bronchodilator and baseline fractional exhaled nitric oxide were good predictors of an FEV1 corticosteroid response. These findings suggest differences between children and adults in the pathobiologic underpinnings of severe asthma that require further investigation. The difference in persistence of the phenotype after corticosteroids and bronchodilator in adults and children is interesting and suggests that as patients move to adulthood their asthma may be a less reversible disease.[99]

A recent meta-analysis also showed that in mild persistent asthma, response to steroids was different in adults than in children. In adult patients with mild intermittent asthma, ICS improves lung function and alleviates airway hyperresponsiveness and airway inflammation, but did influence symptom scores. However, in children, the benefit of ICSs in symptom control was more significant.[7]

SUMMARY

Corticosteroids are the most effective therapy for asthma. Corticosteroids suppress inflammation via several molecular mechanisms. Baseline features may identify ICS responsiveness and thus determine patients who would most likely to benefit from ICS treatment. Heterogeneity of the response to corticosteroids exists in adult and pediatric asthma with few biomarkers consistently indicating favorable response before treatment. Monitoring responses by using biomarkers as sputum eosinophils, exhaled breath condensates, and have been used as tools primarily in research studies. Using symptom assessment tools, exacerbation rate, lung function, and clinically available markers of airway inflammation can help identify individual patient response in clinical practice. Patients with asthma have different responses to corticosteroids due to multiple factors. CR asthma is uncommon and presents a clinical challenge because alternative treatment choices are limited. Asthma response to steroids was found to be different in adults than in children.

REFERENCES

1. Global strategy for asthma management and prevention. 2017. Available at: http://ginasthma.org/gina-reports/. Accessed September 1, 2018.
2. CDC. NHIS Data. Table 3-1. 2016. Lifetime asthma population estimates by age. United States: National Health Interview Survey, 2016.
3. Lougheed MD, Lemiere C, Ducharme FM, et al. Canadian Thoracic Society 2012 guideline update: diagnosis and management of asthma in preschoolers, children and adults: executive summary. Can Respir J 2012;19(6):e81–8.
4. Barnes PJ. Inhaled corticosteroids. Pharmaceuticals (Basel) 2010;3(3):514–40.
5. Fergeson JE, Patel SS, Lockey RF. Acute asthma, prognosis, and treatment. J Allergy Clin Immunol 2017;139(2):438–47.
6. Haldar P, Pavord ID. Noneosinophilic asthma: a distinct clinical and pathologic phenotype. J Allergy Clin Immunol 2007;119(5):1043–52 [quiz: 53–4].
7. Du W, Zhou L, Ni Y, et al. Inhaled corticosteroids improve lung function, airway hyperresponsiveness and airway inflammation but not symptom control in patients with mild intermittent asthma: a meta-analysis. Exp Ther Med 2017;14(2):1594–608.
8. Kelly HW. Inhaled corticosteroid dosing: double for nothing? J Allergy Clin Immunol 2011;128(2):278–81.e2.
9. Deykin A, Lazarus SC, Fahy JV, et al. Sputum eosinophil counts predict asthma control after discontinuation of inhaled corticosteroids. J Allergy Clin Immunol 2005;115(4):720–7.
10. Vijverberg SJ, Hilvering B, Raaijmakers JA, et al. Clinical utility of asthma biomarkers: from bench to bedside. Biologics 2013;7:199–210.
11. Israel E, Reddel HK. Severe and difficult-to-treat asthma in adults. N Engl J Med 2017;377(10):965–76.
12. Woodruff PG, Modrek B, Choy DF, et al. T-helper type 2-driven inflammation defines major subphenotypes of asthma. Am J Respir Crit Care Med 2009;180(5):388–95.
13. Rhen T, Cidlowski JA. Antiinflammatory action of glucocorticoids–new mechanisms for old drugs. N Engl J Med 2005;353(16):1711–23.
14. de Benedictis FM, Bush A. Corticosteroids in respiratory diseases in children. Am J Respir Crit Care Med 2012;185(1):12–23.
15. Trevor JL, Deshane JS. Refractory asthma: mechanisms, targets, and therapy. Allergy 2014;69(7):817–27.
16. Barnes PJ. How corticosteroids control inflammation: Quintiles Prize Lecture 2005. Br J Pharmacol 2006;148(3):245–54.
17. Barnes PJ. Glucocorticosteroids. Handb Exp Pharmacol 2017;237:93–115.
18. Kelly MM, King EM, Rider CF, et al. Corticosteroid-induced gene expression in allergen-challenged asthmatic subjects taking inhaled budesonide. Br J Pharmacol 2012;165(6):1737–47.
19. Gensler LS. Glucocorticoids: complications to anticipate and prevent. Neurohospitalist 2013;3(2):92–7.
20. Barnes PJ, Adcock IM. How do corticosteroids work in asthma? Ann Intern Med 2003;139(5 Pt 1):359–70.
21. Suissa S, Ernst P, Benayoun S, et al. Low-dose inhaled corticosteroids and the prevention of death from asthma. N Engl J Med 2000;343(5):332–6.
22. Pauwels RA, Pedersen S, Busse WW, et al. Early intervention with budesonide in mild persistent asthma: a randomised, double-blind trial. Lancet 2003;361(9363):1071–6.
23. Bossley CJ, Fleming L, Ullmann N, et al. Assessment of corticosteroid response in pediatric patients with severe asthma by using a multidomain approach. J Allergy Clin Immunol 2016;138(2):413–20.e6.
24. O'Byrne PM. Global guidelines for asthma management: summary of the current status and future challenges. Pol Arch Med Wewn 2010;120(12):511–7.
25. British guideline on the management of asthma. Thorax 2014;69(Suppl 1):1–192.
26. Vijverberg SJH, Farzan N, Slob EMA, et al. Treatment response heterogeneity in asthma: the role of genetic variation. Expert Rev Respir Med 2018;12(1):55–65.
27. Adcock IM, Ito K. Steroid resistance in asthma: a major problem requiring novel solutions or a non-issue? Curr Opin Pharmacol 2004;4(3):257–62.
28. Little SA, Chalmers GW, MacLeod KJ, et al. Noninvasive markers of airway inflammation as

predictors of oral steroid responsiveness in asthma. Thorax 2000;55(3):232–4.

29. Bossley CJ, Saglani S, Kavanagh C, et al. Corticosteroid responsiveness and clinical characteristics in childhood difficult asthma. Eur Respir J 2009; 34(5):1052–9.

30. Fitzpatrick AM, Teague WG. Severe asthma in children: insights from the National Heart, Lung, and Blood Institute's Severe Asthma Research Program. Pediatr Allergy Immunol Pulmonol 2010; 23(2):131–8.

31. Rietveld S, Everaerd W. Perceptions of asthma by adolescents at home. Chest 2000;117(2):434–9.

32. Martin RJ, Szefler SJ, King TS, et al. The predicting response to inhaled corticosteroid efficacy (PRICE) trial. J Allergy Clin Immunol 2007;119(1):73–80.

33. Gupta A, Gupta LK, Rehan HS, et al. Response to inhaled corticosteroids on serum CD28, quality of life, and peak expiratory flow rate in bronchial asthma. Allergy Asthma Proc 2017;38(2):13–8.

34. Wang G, Baines KJ, Fu JJ, et al. Sputum mast cell subtypes relate to eosinophilia and corticosteroid response in asthma. Eur Respir J 2016;47(4): 1123–33.

35. Keskin O, Uluca U, Birben E, et al. Genetic associations of the response to inhaled corticosteroids in children during an asthma exacerbation. Pediatr Allergy Immunol 2016;27(5):507–13.

36. Fitzpatrick AM, Stephenson ST, Brown MR, et al. Systemic corticosteroid responses in children with severe asthma: phenotypic and endotypic features. J Allergy Clin Immunol Pract 2017;5(2):410–9.e4.

37. Bacharier LB, Strunk RC, Mauger D, et al. Classifying asthma severity in children: mismatch between symptoms, medication use, and lung function. Am J Respir Crit Care Med 2004;170(4): 426–32.

38. Ranganathan SC, Payne DN, Jaffe A, et al. Difficult asthma: defining the problems. Pediatr Pulmonol 2001;31(2):114–20.

39. Chan MT, Leung DY, Szefler SJ, et al. Difficult-to-control asthma: clinical characteristics of steroid-insensitive asthma. J Allergy Clin Immunol 1998; 101(5):594–601.

40. Anderson WJ, Short PM, Williamson PA, et al. Inhaled corticosteroid dose response using domiciliary exhaled nitric oxide in persistent asthma: the FENOtype trial. Chest 2012;142(6):1553–61.

41. Kainu A, Lindqvist A, Sarna S, et al. FEV1 response to bronchodilation in an adult urban population. Chest 2008;134(2):387–93.

42. Drazen JM, Silverman EK, Lee TH. Heterogeneity of therapeutic responses in asthma. Br Med Bull 2000;56(4):1054–70.

43. Lemanske RF Jr, Busse WW. Asthma: clinical expression and molecular mechanisms. J Allergy Clin Immunol 2010;125(2 Suppl 2):S95–102.

44. Normansell R, Kew KM, Stovold E. Interventions to improve adherence to inhaled steroids for asthma. Cochrane Database Syst Rev 2017;(4):CD012226.

45. Lee JX, Wojtczak HA, Wachter AM, et al. Understanding asthma medical nonadherence in an adult and pediatric population. J Allergy Clin Immunol Pract 2015;3(3):436–7.

46. Klok T, Kaptein AA, Brand PLP. Nonadherence in children with asthma reviewed: the need for improvement of asthma care and medical education. Pediatr Allergy Immunol 2015;26(3):197–205.

47. Normansell R, Kew KM, Mathioudakis AG. Interventions to improve inhaler technique for people with asthma. Cochrane Database Syst Rev 2017;(3):CD012286.

48. Kam JC, Szefler SJ, Surs W, et al. Combination IL-2 and IL-4 reduces glucocorticoid receptor-binding affinity and T cell response to glucocorticoids. J Immunol 1993;151(7):3460–6.

49. Lazarus SC, Chinchilli VM, Rollings NJ, et al. Smoking affects response to inhaled corticosteroids or leukotriene receptor antagonists in asthma. Am J Respir Crit Care Med 2007;175(8):783–90.

50. Kobayashi Y, Bossley C, Gupta A, et al. Passive smoking impairs histone deacetylase-2 in children with severe asthma. Chest 2014;145(2):305–12.

51. Miller GE, Gaudin A, Zysk E, et al. Parental support and cytokine activity in childhood asthma: the role of glucocorticoid sensitivity. J Allergy Clin Immunol 2009;123(4):824–30.

52. Haczku A, Panettieri RA. Social stress and asthma: the role of corticosteroid insensitivity. J Allergy Clin Immunol 2010;125(3):550–8.

53. Leusink M, Vijverberg SJ, Koenderman L, et al. Genetic variation in uncontrolled childhood asthma despite ICS treatment. Pharmacogenomics J 2016;16(2):158–63.

54. Inglis GC, Ingram MC, Holloway CD, et al. Familial pattern of corticosteroids and their metabolism in adult human subjects–the Scottish Adult Twin Study. J Clin Endocrinol Metab 1999;84(11): 4132–7.

55. Baye TM, Abebe T, Wilke RA. Genotype-environment interactions and their translational implications. Per Med 2011;8(1):59–70.

56. Duong-Thi-Ly H, Nguyen-Thi-Thu H, Nguyen-Hoang L, et al. Effects of genetic factors to inhaled corticosteroid response in children with asthma: a literature review. J Int Med Res 2017;45(6):1818–30.

57. Tantisira KG, Hwang ES, Raby BA, et al. TBX21: a functional variant predicts improvement in asthma with the use of inhaled corticosteroids. Proc Natl Acad Sci U S A 2004;101(52):18099–104.

58. Tantisira KG, Lasky-Su J, Harada M, et al. Genome-wide association between GLCCI1 and response to glucocorticoid therapy in asthma. N Engl J Med 2011;365(13):1173–83.

59. Hawkins GA, Lazarus R, Smith RS, et al. The glucocorticoid receptor heterocomplex gene STIP1 is associated with improved lung function in asthmatic subjects treated with inhaled corticosteroids. J Allergy Clin Immunol 2009;123(6):1376–83.e7.

60. Lopert A, Rijavec M, Žavbi M, et al. Asthma treatment outcome in adults is associated with rs9910408 in TRX21 gene. Sci Rep 2013;3:2915.

61. Cho SH, Park BL, Shin SW, et al. Association between WDR21A polymorphisms and airway responsiveness to inhaled corticosteroids in asthmatic patients. Pharmacogenet Genomics 2012;22(5):327–35.

62. Park HW, Dahlin A, Tse S, et al. Genetic predictors associated with improvement of asthma symptoms in response to inhaled corticosteroids. J Allergy Clin Immunol 2014;133(3):664–9.e5.

63. Tantisira KG, Lazarus R, Litonjua AA, et al. Chromosome 17: association of a large inversion polymorphism with corticosteroid response in asthma. Pharmacogenet Genomics 2008;18(8):733–7.

64. Mosteller M, Hosking L, Murphy K, et al. No evidence of large genetic effects on steroid response in asthma patients. J Allergy Clin Immunol 2017;139(3):797–803.e7.

65. Zhang X, Biagini Myers JM, Yadagiri VK, et al. Nasal DNA methylation differentiates corticosteroid treatment response in pediatric asthma: a pilot study. PLoS One 2017;12(10):e0186150.

66. Feinberg AP. Genome-scale approaches to the epigenetics of common human disease. Virchows Arch 2010;456(1):13–21.

67. Begin P, Nadeau KC. Epigenetic regulation of asthma and allergic disease. Allergy Asthma Clin Immunol 2014;10(1):27.

68. Yang IV, Richards A, Davidson EJ, et al. The nasal methylome: a key to understanding allergic asthma. Am J Respir Crit Care Med 2017;195(6):829–31.

69. Haldar P, Pavord ID, Shaw DE, et al. Cluster analysis and clinical asthma phenotypes. Am J Respir Crit Care Med 2008;178(3):218–24.

70. Simpson JL, Scott R, Boyle MJ, et al. Inflammatory subtypes in asthma: assessment and identification using induced sputum. Respirology 2006;11(1):54–61.

71. Alangari AA. Corticosteroids in the treatment of acute asthma. Ann Thorac Med 2014;9(4):187–92.

72. Zeiger RS, Szefler SJ, Phillips BR, et al. Response profiles to fluticasone and montelukast in mild-to-moderate persistent childhood asthma. J Allergy Clin Immunol 2006;117(1):45–52.

73. Szefler SJ, Phillips BR, Martinez FD, et al. Characterization of within-subject responses to fluticasone and montelukast in childhood asthma. J Allergy Clin Immunol 2005;115(2):233–42.

74. Szefler SJ, Martin RJ. Lessons learned from variation in response to therapy in clinical trials. J Allergy Clin Immunol 2010;125(2):285–92 [quiz: 93–4].

75. Koo S, Gupta A, Fainardi V, et al. Ethnic variation in response to im triamcinolone in children with severe therapy-resistant asthma. Chest 2016;149(1):98–105.

76. Leong AB, Ramsey CD, Celedon JC. The challenge of asthma in minority populations. Clin Rev Allergy Immunol 2012;43(1–2):156–83.

77. Federico MJ, Covar RA, Brown EE, et al. Racial differences in T-lymphocyte response to glucocorticoids. Chest 2005;127(2):571–8.

78. Ford JG, McCaffrey L. Understanding disparities in asthma outcomes among African Americans. Clin Chest Med 2006;27(3):423–30, vi.

79. Wechsler ME, Castro M, Lehman E, et al. Impact of race on asthma treatment failures in the asthma clinical research network. Am J Respir Crit Care Med 2011;184(11):1247–53.

80. Goleva E, Harris JK, Robertson CE, et al. Airway microbiome and responses to corticosteroids in corticosteroid-resistant asthma patients treated with acid suppression medications. J Allergy Clin Immunol 2017;140(3):860–2.e1.

81. Goleva E, Jackson LP, Harris JK, et al. The effects of airway microbiome on corticosteroid responsiveness in asthma. Am J Respir Crit Care Med 2013;188(10):1193–201.

82. Wu YF, Su MW, Chiang BL, et al. A simple prediction tool for inhaled corticosteroid response in asthmatic children. BMC Pulm Med 2017;17(1):176.

83. Carmichael J, Paterson IC, Diaz P, et al. Corticosteroid resistance in chronic asthma. Br Med J (Clin Res Ed) 1981;282(6274):1419–22.

84. Perlikos F, Hillas G, Loukides S. Phenotyping and endotyping asthma based on biomarkers. Curr Top Med Chem 2016;16(14):1582–6.

85. Szefler SJ, Wenzel S, Brown R, et al. Asthma outcomes: biomarkers. J Allergy Clin Immunol 2012;129(3):S9–23.

86. Buhl R, Korn S, Menzies-Gow A, et al. Assessing biomarkers in a real-world severe asthma study (ARIETTA). Respir Med 2016;115:7–12.

87. Cowan DC, Taylor DR, Peterson LE, et al. Biomarker-based asthma phenotypes of corticosteroid response. J Allergy Clin Immunol 2015;135(4):877–83.e1.

88. Schleich F, Sophie D, Renaud L. Biomarkers in the management of difficult asthma. Curr Top Med Chem 2016;16(14):1561–73.

89. Berry MA, Shaw DE, Green RH, et al. The use of exhaled nitric oxide concentration to identify eosinophilic airway inflammation: an observational study in adults with asthma. Clin Exp Allergy 2005;35(9):1175–9.

90. Jatakanon A, Lim S, Kharitonov SA, et al. Correlation between exhaled nitric oxide, sputum eosinophils, and methacholine responsiveness in patients with mild asthma. Thorax 1998;53(2): 91–5.

91. Dweik RA, Comhair SA, Gaston B, et al. NO chemical events in the human airway during the immediate and late antigen-induced asthmatic response. Proc Natl Acad Sci U S A 2001;98(5):2622–7.

92. Dweik RA, Sorkness RL, Wenzel S, et al. Use of exhaled nitric oxide measurement to identify a reactive, at-risk phenotype among patients with asthma. Am J Respir Crit Care Med 2010; 181(10):1033–41.

93. Petsky HL, Kynaston JA, Turner C, et al. Tailored interventions based on sputum eosinophils versus clinical symptoms for asthma in children and adults. Cochrane Database Syst Rev 2007;(2): CD005603.

94. Donohue JF, Jain N. Exhaled nitric oxide to predict corticosteroid responsiveness and reduce asthma exacerbation rates. Respir Med 2013;107(7): 943–52.

95. Radomski MW, Palmer RM, Moncada S. Glucocorticoids inhibit the expression of an inducible, but not the constitutive, nitric oxide synthase in vascular endothelial cells. Proc Natl Acad Sci U S A 1990;87(24):10043–7.

96. Kupczyk M, Haque S, Middelveld RJ, et al. Phenotypic predictors of response to oral glucocorticosteroids in severe asthma. Respir Med 2013; 107(10):1521–30.

97. Wadsworth S, Sin D, Dorscheid D. Clinical update on the use of biomarkers of airway inflammation in the management of asthma. J Asthma Allergy 2011;4:77–86.

98. Knuffman JE, Sorkness CA, Lemanske RF Jr, et al. Phenotypic predictors of long-term response to inhaled corticosteroid and leukotriene modifier therapies in pediatric asthma. J Allergy Clin Immunol 2009;123(2):411–6.

99. Phipatanakul W, Mauger DT, Sorkness RL, et al. Effects of age and disease severity on systemic corticosteroid responses in asthma. Am J Respir Crit Care Med 2017;195(11):1439–48.

100. Galant SP, Morphew T, Guijon O, et al. The bronchodilator response as a predictor of inhaled corticosteroid responsiveness in asthmatic children with normal baseline spirometry. Pediatr Pulmonol 2014;49(12):1162–9.

101. Rabinovitch N, Mauger DT, Reisdorph N, et al. Predictors of asthma control and lung function responsiveness to step 3 therapy in children with uncontrolled asthma. J Allergy Clin Immunol 2014;133(2):350–6.

102. Zacharasiewicz A, Wilson N, Lex C, et al. Clinical use of noninvasive measurements of airway inflammation in steroid reduction in children. Am J Respir Crit Care Med 2005;171(10):1077–82.

103. Xiao C, Biagini Myers JM, Ji H, et al. Vanin-1 expression and methylation discriminate pediatric asthma corticosteroid treatment response. J Allergy Clin Immunol 2015;136(4):923–31.e3.

104. Bacharier LB, Guilbert TW, Zeiger RS, et al. Patient characteristics associated with improved outcomes with use of an inhaled corticosteroid in preschool children at risk for asthma. J Allergy Clin Immunol 2009;123(5):1077–82, 82.e1-5.

105. Fitzpatrick AM, Jackson DJ, Mauger DT, et al. Individualized therapy for persistent asthma in young children. J Allergy Clin Immunol 2016;138(6): 1608–18.e12.

106. Forno E, Lescher R, Strunk R, et al. Decreased response to inhaled steroids in overweight and obese asthmatic children. J Allergy Clin Immunol 2011;127(3):741–9.

107. Peters-Golden M, Swern A, Bird SS, et al. Influence of body mass index on the response to asthma controller agents. Eur Respir J 2006;27(3): 495–503.

108. Gerald JK, Gerald LB, Vasquez MM, et al. Markers of differential response to inhaled corticosteroid treatment among children with mild persistent asthma. J Allergy Clin Immunol Pract 2015;3(4): 540–6.e3.

109. Vijverberg SJ, Koenderman L, Koster ES, et al. Biomarkers of therapy responsiveness in asthma: pitfalls and promises. Clin Exp Allergy 2011;41(5): 615–29.

110. Brightling CE, Green RH, Pavord ID. Biomarkers predicting response to corticosteroid therapy in asthma. Treat Respir Med 2005;4(5):309–16.

111. Aziz-Ur-Rehman A, Dasgupta A, Kjarsgaard M, et al. Sputum cell counts to manage prednisone-dependent asthma: effects on FEV1 and eosinophilic exacerbations. Allergy Asthma Clin Immunol 2017;13(1):17.

112. Malmstrom K, Rodriguez-Gomez G, Guerra J, et al. Oral montelukast, inhaled beclomethasone, and placebo for chronic asthma. A randomized, controlled trial. Montelukast/Beclomethasone Study Group. Ann Intern Med 1999;130(6): 487–95.

113. Szefler SJ, Martin RJ, King TS, et al. Significant variability in response to inhaled corticosteroids for persistent asthma. J Allergy Clin Immunol 2002;109(3):410–8.

114. Bateman ED, Boushey HA, Bousquet J, et al. Can guideline-defined asthma control be achieved? The Gaining Optimal Asthma ControL study. Am J Respir Crit Care Med 2004;170(8):836–44.

115. Adcock IM, Lane SJ. Corticosteroid-insensitive asthma: molecular mechanisms. J Endocrinol 2003;178(3):347–55.

116. Weiss ST, Litonjua AA, Lange C, et al. Overview of the pharmacogenetics of asthma treatment. Pharmacogenomics J 2006;6(5):311–26.

117. Dunican EM, Fahy JV. Asthma and corticosteroids: time for a more precise approach to treatment. Eur Respir J 2017;49(6).

118. Green RH, Brightling CE, Woltmann G, et al. Analysis of induced sputum in adults with asthma: identification of subgroup with isolated sputum neutrophilia and poor response to inhaled corticosteroids. Thorax 2002;57(10):875–9.

119. Moore WC, Hastie AT, Li X, et al. Sputum neutrophils are associated with more severe asthma phenotypes using cluster analysis. J Allergy Clin Immunol 2014;133(6):1557–63.e5.

120. Ito K, Chung KF, Adcock IM. Update on glucocorticoid action and resistance. J Allergy Clin Immunol 2006;117(3):522–43.

121. Ramamoorthy S, Cidlowski JA. Exploring the molecular mechanisms of glucocorticoid receptor action from sensitivity to resistance. Endocr Dev 2013;24:41–56.

122. Stephenson ST, Brown LA, Helms MN, et al. Cysteine oxidation impairs systemic glucocorticoid responsiveness in children with difficult-to-treat asthma. J Allergy Clin Immunol 2015;136(2):454–61.e9.

123. Schwartz HJ, Lowell FC, Melby JC. Steroid resistance in bronchial asthma. Ann Intern Med 1968;69(3):493–9.

124. Adcock IM, Barnes PJ. Molecular mechanisms of corticosteroid resistance. CHEST 2008;134(2):394–401.

125. Clearie KL, McKinlay L, Williamson PA, et al. Fluticasone/Salmeterol combination confers benefits in people with asthma who smoke. Chest 2012;141(2):330–8.

126. Thomson NC, Spears M. The influence of smoking on the treatment response in patients with asthma. Curr Opin Allergy Clin Immunol 2005;5(1):57–63.

127. Chalmers GW, MacLeod KJ, Thomson L, et al. Smoking and airway inflammation in patients with mild asthma. Chest 2001;120(6):1917–22.

128. Churg A, Dai J, Tai H, et al. Tumor necrosis factor-alpha is central to acute cigarette smoke-induced inflammation and connective tissue breakdown. Am J Respir Crit Care Med 2002;166(6):849–54.

129. Webster JC, Oakley RH, Jewell CM, et al. Proinflammatory cytokines regulate human glucocorticoid receptor gene expression and lead to the accumulation of the dominant negative beta isoform: a mechanism for the generation of glucocorticoid resistance. Proc Natl Acad Sci U S A 2001;98(12):6865–70.

130. Leung DY, Bloom JW. Update on glucocorticoid action and resistance. J Allergy Clin Immunol 2003;111(1):3–22 [quiz: 3].

131. Szefler SJ, Leung DY. Glucocorticoid-resistant asthma: pathogenesis and clinical implications for management. Eur Respir J 1997;10(7):1640–7.

132. Spahn JD, Szefler SJ, Surs W, et al. A novel action of IL-13: induction of diminished monocyte glucocorticoid receptor-binding affinity. J Immunol 1996;157(6):2654–9.

133. Matthews JG, Ito K, Barnes PJ, et al. Defective glucocorticoid receptor nuclear translocation and altered histone acetylation patterns in glucocorticoid-resistant patients. J Allergy Clin Immunol 2004;113(6):1100–8.

134. Hawrylowicz C, Richards D, Loke TK, et al. A defect in corticosteroid-induced IL-10 production in T lymphocytes from corticosteroid-resistant asthmatic patients. J Allergy Clin Immunol 2002;109(2):369–70.

Immunomodulators and Biologics
Beyond Stepped-Care Therapy

Mauli Desai, MD[a], John Oppenheimer, MD[b],
David M. Lang, MD[c],*

KEYWORDS

- Asthma • Benralizumab • Omalizumab • Reslizumab • Mepolizumab • Dupilumab

KEY POINTS

- Biological agents offer promise for patients with severe persistent asthma that is poorly controlled despite appropriate "stepped care" management.
- Improved understanding of asthma endotypes, and use of biomarkers to predict treatment response, will facilitate our ability to prescribe biologics more effectively to treat patients with severe asthma that is poorly controlled.
- Antiimmunoglobulin E has been associated with statistically and clinically significant benefit in properly selected patients in randomized, double-blind, placebo-controlled trials.
- In asthmatic patients with poorly controlled asthma who have an eosinophilic phenotype, humanized monoclonal antibodies directed against interleukin 5 (IL-5), and a monoclonal antibody binding to IL-5 receptor alpha on eosinophils and basophils, have been associated with statistically and clinically significant benefit in randomized, double-blind, placebo-controlled trials.
- Blockade of IL-4 receptor alpha has been associated with statistically and clinically significant benefit in randomized, double-blind, placebo-controlled trials.
- In the future, additional biological therapies will be available for the treatment of asthma. Likely targets include thymic stromal lymphopoietin and IL-33.

INTRODUCTION

We have seen rapid advancements in recent years with the discovery of targeted therapeutics for severe asthma. Biologics offer promise for patients with refractory, severe asthma who otherwise depend on chronic or frequent use of oral corticosteroids.[1] As described in previous articles, significant progress has been achieved in our understanding of the complex underpinnings of Type 2 (T2) asthma. Until recently, the same level of effort was not directed to develop pharmacotherapeutic agents for non-T2 asthma; consequently, there are relatively greater unmet needs for treatment of patients with this phenotype.[2] Asthma can also be described phenotypically as

Conflicts of Interest: Medscape (reviewer); Med Learning Group (cme speaker) (M. Desai). Adjudication: Astra Zeneca, Teva, Novartis, Abbvie; DSMB: GSK; Consultant: Astra Zeneca, GSK, Sanofi, Teva, Kaleo; Annals of Allergy Asthma and Immunology and Allergy Watch: Associate Editor; Medscape: Editor (pulmonary); Current Allergy and Asthma Reports: section editor; Up to Date (reviewer) (J. Oppenheimer). D.M. Lang has received honoraria from, has served as a consultant for, and/or has carried out clinical research with: AstraZeneca, Genentech/Novartis, Hycor; Journal of Asthma (Associate Editor), Allergy and Asthma Proceedings (Editorial Board), AllergyWatch (Assistant Editor), DynaMed (Topic Editor) (D.M. Lang).
[a] Division of Allergy and Clinical Immunology, Icahn School of Medicine at Mount Sinai, 1425 Madison Avenue Box 1089, New York, NY 10029, USA; [b] Department of Medicine UMDNJ - Rutgers, Pulmonary and Allergy Assoc, 1 Springfield Avenue, Summit, NJ 07901, USA; [c] Department of Allergy and Clinical Immunology, Cleveland Clinic, Respiratory Institute, 9500 Euclid Avenue – A90, Cleveland, OH 44195, USA
* Corresponding author.
E-mail address: langd@ccf.org

Clin Chest Med 40 (2019) 179–192
https://doi.org/10.1016/j.ccm.2018.10.011
0272-5231/19/© 2018 Elsevier Inc. All rights reserved.

eosinophilic or noneosinophilic.[3] In patients with an eosinophilic phenotype, remarkable levels of eosinophils are seen in sputum, airway, and peripheral blood; in asthmatics who exhibit a noneosinophilic phenotype, eosinophils may be present, but another inflammatory cell (eg, neutrophil) is the predominant inflammatory cell observed.

The discovery of biologics has narrowed the gap between conventional management and an era of precision medicine, which will involve choosing the right drug for the right patient at the right time. Understanding asthma endotypes and their pathophysiologic processes, as well as phenotypes and biomarkers to predict treatment response, will facilitate our ability to prescribe biologics more effectively to treat patients with severe asthma that is poorly controlled.

In this article, the authors describe available and experimental biological therapies for T2 asthma and briefly discuss the potential agents for non-T2 asthma. They also address gaps in our understanding of biologics as well as future directions.

BIOLOGICS FOR T2 ASTHMA

T-helper cell type-2 (Th2) cells, B cells, eosinophils, epithelial cells, type-2 innate lymphoid (ILC2) cells and others, as well as the interleukin signaling molecules IL-4, IL-5, IL-13, and immunoglobulin E (IgE) are important in the inflammatory cascade of T2 asthma. Many patients with T2 asthma are responsive to inhaled corticosteroids (ICS). For those, however, whose asthma remains poorly controlled despite using conventional controller therapies, monoclonal antibodies blocking one or more of these pathways may restore asthma control. Proposed biomarkers of T2 asthma include IgE, blood and lung eosinophils, exhaled nitric oxide, serum IgE, serum periostin, urine leukotriene E4, and others.[4]

Biological drugs are therapeutic agents synthesized from biological sources and directed against a specific target. Clinical trials of targeted monoclonal antibodies to IgE, IL-5, IL-5 receptor, IL-4 receptor alpha (IL-4rα), and thymic stromal lymphopoietin (TSLP) have shown promising results in the reduction of asthma exacerbations when given as add-on therapy versus placebo, with overall favorable safety profiles.[3] Clinical trials of selected biological agents are summarized in **Table 1**. One biologic drug is currently approved by the Food and Drug Administration (FDA) for allergic (IgE-mediated) asthma, and 3 anti-IL 5 drugs are available at this time for eosinophilic asthma; several other biological drugs are in the development pipeline.

Omalizumab

Omalizumab is a chimeric human-mouse recombinant antibody that binds to the domain at which IgE binds to FCeRI on mast cells and basophils.[5,6] Its primary mechanism of action is binding of free IgE in the circulation, forming biologically inert, small complexes that do not activate complement and are cleared by the reticuloendothelial system.[6] Omalizumab was approved by the FDA in 2003 for management of patients aged 12 years and older with moderate-severe persistent asthma not achieving asthma control despite use of ICS, who exhibit wheal/flare reaction to a perennial allergen, and whose IgE is in the range of 30 to 700 IU/mL. In 2016, omalizumab was approved for children aged 6 to 11 years.[5] Weight and serum IgE level determine dose and interval (ie, every 2 weeks vs 4 weeks).[5]

Omalizumab has demonstrated statistically and clinically significant benefit in randomized, double-blind, placebo-controlled trials. Randomized controlled trials of omalizumab in which patients were enrolled who were not well controlled on combination controller therapy with ICS and long-acting beta agonists (LABA) are described in **Table 1**. Omalizumab was associated with a statistically significant reduction in the rate of asthma exacerbations and severe asthma exacerbations, as well as statistically significant improvements in asthma-related quality of life, reliance on reliever medication, and asthma symptom scores.[7,8] It should be noted that one of the randomized controlled trials enrolled subjects who did not receive high-dose ICS,[7] and one was a relatively small study focused on evaluating FcεRI expression on basophils and plasmacytoid dendritic cells as a prognostic factor for clinical improvement.[9] The study by Hanania and colleagues[8] demonstrated a statistically significant reduction in asthma exacerbations (0.66 vs 0.88 per patient, $P = .006$), reflecting a 25% relative risk reduction.

The salutary response to omalizumab observed in patients with refractory asthma exhibits a gradual pattern of onset: 38% responding in 4 weeks, 62% after 16 weeks.[10,11] In pivotal trials, the potential for benefit could not reliably be predicted based on demographic characteristics (eg, age, gender) or total serum IgE level.[6] However, evidence suggests that higher levels of T2 biomarkers, including not only peripheral eosinophil counts but also exhaled nitric oxide and serum periostin, increase the likelihood of clinical benefit.[12,13] Omalizumab may be efficacious for patients fulfilling label criteria who have high or low levels of eosinophils.[14] A post hoc analysis of

Table 1
Sentinel phase 2 & 3 clinical trials of drugs approved and under investigation for T2 asthma

Drug	First author/Year	Journal	Inclusion Criteria (Phenotype)	Number of Randomized Subjects	Age Eligibility (years)	Dosing	Duration of Treatment Period	Primary Endpoint	Key Secondary Endpoints	Significant Findings
Omalizumab	Humbert et al,[7] 2005	Allergy	Not adequately controlled on high dose ICS and LABA, history of exacerbation	482	12–75	According To Label	28 wk	Rate of exacerbations	AQLQ, Total asthma Symptom scores	25% relative reduction in exacerbations, improved AQLQ and asthma symptom scores
	Hanania et al,[8] 2011	Ann Intern Med	Not adequately controlled on high dose ICS and LABA, history of exacerbation	850	12–75	According to label	48 wk	Rate of exacerbations	AQLQ, Total asthma Symptom scores	25% relative reduction in exacerbations, improved AQLQ and asthma symptom scores
	Chanez et al,[9] 2010	Respir Med	Not adequately controlled on high dose ICS and LABA, history of exacerbation	31	≥18	According to label	16 wk	FcεRI expression on basophils and plasmacytoid dendritic cells as determined by flow cytometry	Nocturnal awakenings, impairment in daily activities	FcεRI expression did not correlate with clinical response
Mepolizumab	Nair et al,[25] 2009	N Engl J Med	Not adequately controlled despite oral corticosteroids, sputum eosinophilia	20	≥18	Mepolizumab 750 mg Q4W IV vs placebo	5 mo	Rate of exacerbations and mean reduction in the steroid dose as a percentage of the maximum possible reduction	Effect on sputum and blood eosinophils, symptoms, and airflow limitation	Significant reduction in eosinophils, decreased exacerbations, reduction in OCS requirements
	Haldar et al,[26] 2009	N Engl J Med	Refractory eosinophilic asthma and a history of recurrent severe exacerbations	61	≥18	Mepolizumab 750 mg Q4W IV vs placebo	52 wk	Number of severe exacerbations per subject during the treatment phase	Change in asthma symptoms, AQLQ scores, lung function, airway hyperresponsiveness, and blood and sputum eosinophil counts	A significant reduction in severe exacerbations in the active treatment arm vs placebo, and improved AQLQ scores
	Pavord et al,[27] 2012	Lancet	>2 severe asthma exacerbations in the previous year and eosinophilic inflammation	621	≥12	Mepolizumab 75 mg IV vs 250 mg IV vs 750 mg IV vs placebo	52 wk	Rate of clinically significant asthma exacerbations	Rate of hospital admissions, visits to the emergency department, blood and sputum eosinophil counts, prebronchodilator FEV1, and scores on AQLQ and ACQ	Significant reductions in exacerbations (39%–52%) in all active treatment arms compared to placebo

(continued on next page)

Table 1
(continued)

Drug	First author/Year	Journal	Inclusion Criteria (Phenotype)	Number of Randomized Subjects	Age Eligibility (years)	Dosing	Duration of Treatment Period	Primary Endpoint	Key Secondary Endpoints	Significant Findings
	Ortega et al,[28] 2014	N Engl J Med	Recurrent asthma exacerbations and evidence of eosinophilic inflammation despite high doses of inhaled glucocorticoids	576	12–82	Mepolizumab 75 mg IV vs 100 mg SC vs placebo	32 wk	Rate of clinically significant asthma exacerbations	Change in FEV1 and symptom scores	Comparable reductions in exacerbations in both active treatment arms of 75 mg IV and 100 mg subcutaneous (47% and 53%) compared to placebo
	Bel et al,[29] 2014	N Engl J Med	Severe eosinophilic asthma and maintenance treatment with systemic glucocorticoids before entering the study	135	≥12	Mepolizumab 100 mg subq vs placebo	20 wk	Degree of reduction in the glucocorticoid dose, a lack of asthma control during weeks 20–24, or withdrawal from treatment	Rate of asthma exacerbations, asthma control, and safety	Significant reduction from baseline in glucocorticoid dose in the mepolizumab group, and a decrease in exacerbation rate compared to placebo
Reslizumab	Corren et al,[33] 2016	Chest	Not adequately controlled despite at least a medium-dose inhaled corticosteroid, unselected for eosinophil counts	492	18–65	Reslizumab (3 mg/kg) IV vs placebo	16 wk	Change in baseline FEV1 from baseline to week 16	ACQ-7 scores, use of short-acting β-agonists, and FVC	In the subgroup with eosinophilic count >400 cells/µL, there were clinically meaningful effects on lung function and symptom scores
	Castro et al,[34] 2015	Lancet	Asthma was inadequately controlled by medium-to-high doses of ICS, blood eosinophils of 400 cells per µL or higher, and one or more exacerbations in the previous year	953 total	12–75	Reslizumab (3 mg/kg) IV vs placebo	52 wk	Annual frequency of clinical asthma exacerbations	Change from baseline in FEV1,symptom scores, rescue use of short-acting β-agonist, and blood eosinophil count	Significant reduction in the frequency of asthma exacerbations in both studies (rate ratio 0.5, 0.41) compared with placebo

Drug	Study	Journal	Population	N	Age	Intervention	Duration	Primary outcome	Secondary measures	Results
Benralizumab	Bleeker et al,[39] 2016	Lancet	Asthma for at least 1 year and at least two exacerbations while on high-dosage ICS plus LABA in the previous year	1205	12–75	Benralizumab 30 mg subq q4w vs q8w (first 3 doses q4w) vs placebo	48 wk	Annual exacerbation rate ratio vs placebo	Prebronchodilator FEV1 and total asthma symptom score at week 48, for patients with blood eosinophil counts of at least 300 cells per µL	Benralizumab reduced the annual asthma exacerbation rate over 48 wk when given Q4W (RR 0·55) or Q8W (RR 0·49)
	FitzGerald et al,[40] 2016	Lancet	Severe asthma uncontrolled by medium-dosage to high-dosage ICS plus LABA, and a history of two or more exacerbations in the previous year	1306	12–75	Benralizumab 30 mg subq q4w vs q8w (first 3 doses q4w) vs placebo	56 wk	Annual exacerbation rate ratio vs placebo for patients receiving high-dosage ICS plus LABA with baseline blood eosinophils 300 cells per µL or greater	Pre-bronchodilator FEV1 and total asthma symptom score	Benralizumab resulted in significantly lower annual exacerbation rates with the Q4W regimen (RR 0·64 and Q8W regimen [RR 0·72) compared with placebo
	Nair et al,[41] 2017	N Engl J Med	Severe eosinophilic asthma, 6 mo oral steroids before enrollment	220	>18	Benralizumab 30 mg subq q4w vs q8w (first 3 doses q4w) vs placebo	28 wk	Percentage change in the oral glucocorticoid dose from baseline to week 28	Annual asthma exacerbation rates, lung function, symptoms, and safety	Benralizumab showed significant, clinically relevant benefits, as compared with placebo, on oral glucocorticoid use and exacerbation rates
Dupilumab	Wenzel et al,[43] 2013	N Engl J Med	Moderate-to-severe uncontrolled eosinophilic asthma on ICS/LABA, at least 1 exacerbation within 2 y of randomization	52	18–65	Dupilumab 300 mg weekly vs placebo	12 wk	Occurrence of asthma exacerbation	Time to exacerbation, change in lung function symptom scores, rescue inhaler use	The treatment arm had a reduction in exacerbations
	Wenzel et al,[44] 2016	Lancet	Moderate-to-severe uncontrolled asthma despite ICS/LABA with at least 1 exacerbation in previous year	769	≥18	Dupilumab 200 mg Q2W vs 300 mg Q2W vs 200 mg Q4W vs 300 mg Q4W vs placebo	24 wk	ΔFEV1 in week 12 in the subpopulation with eos >300	Annualized asthma exacerbation rate, time to severe exacerbation symptoms scores, rescue inhaler use	Statistically significant increase in FEV1 for all dosing regimens except 200 mg Q4wk

(continued on next page)

Table 1
(continued)

Drug	First author/Year	Journal	Inclusion Criteria (Phenotype)	Number of Randomized Subjects	Age Eligibility (years)	Dosing	Duration of Treatment Period	Primary Endpoint	Key Secondary Endpoints	Significant Findings
	Rabe et al,[47] 2018	N Engl J Med	Severe, glucocorticoid-treated asthma	210	≥12	Dupilumab 300 mg Q2W vs placebo	24 wk	Percent reduction of glucocorticoid dose at 24 wk	Proportion of patients at week 24 with a glucocorticoid steroid dose reduction of at least 50% and the proportion of patients with a reduction of glucocorticoid steroid dose of less than 5 mg per day	The percentage change in the glucocorticoid dose was −70.1% in the dupilumab group as compared with −41.9% in the placebo group
	Castro et al,[46] 2018	N Engl J Med	Uncontrolled asthma despite ICS/LABA plus additional controllers	1902	≥12	Dupilumab 200 mg Q2W vs 300 mg Q2W vs placebo	52 wk	Annualized rate of severe exacerbations and the absolute change from baseline to week 12 in the FEV1 before bronchodilator use	Exacerbation rate and FEV1 in patients with an eosinophil count of 300 or more per cubic millimeter	The annualized rate of severe exacerbation was 47.7% lower in the dupilumab group compared with placebo. At week 12, the FEV1 had increased by 0.32 L in the dupilumab group.
Tezepelumab	Corren et al,[48] 2017	N Engl J Med	History of exacerbations and uncontrolled asthma despite ICS/LABA	584	18–75	Tezepelumab 70 mg every 4 wk, 210 mg every 4 wk, or 280 mg every 2 wk, or placebo	52 wk	Annualized rate of asthma exacerbations	Changes from baseline in FEV1, symptom scores, time to exacerbation, percentage with severe exacerbations	Exacerbation rates in the respective tezepelumab groups were lower by 61%, 71%, and 66% than the rate in the placebo group

Abbreviations: AQLQ, asthma quality of life questionnaire; FEV1, forced expiratory volume in one second.

pooled data from 2 pivotal randomized controlled trials of omalizumab found a greater reduction in exacerbation rates in subjects with higher baseline levels of blood eosinophils.[15] These findings are consistent with data from other studies, which demonstrate that high baseline eosinophil counts can serve to identify an exacerbation-prone subgroup[12,13]; such patients would be more likely to experience clinically meaningful improvement with administration of biological agents.

In pivotal trials,[5] omalizumab was associated with a substantial rate of local reactions. A rate of anaphylaxis of approximately 1 in 1000 was observed; this has been confirmed by surveillance data recorded since approval of the drug in June 2003. Based on the observed risk of anaphylaxis, in July 2007, the FDA added a black box warning to the omalizumab label and stipulated that a Medication Guide should be provided for patients.[5] The warning indicates that health care providers administering omalizumab should be prepared to manage anaphylaxis and that patients should be closely observed for an appropriate period after omalizumab administration.

The package insert for omalizumab describes a numerical, but not statistically significant, increased rate of malignancy in patients receiving omalizumab.[5] Of 4127 subjects who received omalizumab, 20 (0.5%) developed malignancy; of 2236 who received placebo injections, 5 (0.2%) developed malignancy. Because these malignancies were diagnosed over a shorter period than the time oncogenesis requires to develop (ie, 6 months in 60% of cases), and because heterogeneity of tumors was observed, the causal relationship of these tumors with omalizumab was uncertain. A longitudinal study[16] with a median follow-up time of approximately 5 years compared the safety of omalizumab in 5007 asthmatics receiving omalizumab with 2829 asthmatics not receiving omalizumab. Rates of malignancy were similar: 12.3 per 1000 patient years for omalizumab, compared with 13.0 per 1000 patient years in asthmatics who did not receive omalizumab. This implies omalizumab is not associated with an increased risk for malignancy. This study found a higher rate of cardiovascular events in asthmatics receiving omalizumab (13.4 per 1000 patient years)—including myocardial infarction and cerebrovascular events—compared with non–omalizumab-treated asthmatics (8.1 per 1000 patient years). Although these results suggest omalizumab is associated with an increased risk of cardiovascular events, there were aspects of the study design that would imply this is not the case, including baseline differences in cardiovascular risk factors. An analysis of 25 randomized controlled trials found no remarkable difference in rates of cardiovascular events in 3342 omalizumab-treated asthmatics compared with 2895 asthmatics who did not receive omalizumab.[5] Efforts to further understand possible risks for malignancy and for cardiovascular disease are continuing during postmarketing surveillance.

Benefit has also been reported with use of omalizumab for patients with allergic bronchopulmonary aspergillosis,[17] asthma with concomitant nasal polyposis,[18] and blocking aspirin-provoked respiratory reaction during desensitization in aspirin-exacerbated respiratory disease.[19] Preseasonal treatment with omalizumab has also been shown to reduce asthma exacerbation typically observed in schoolchildren during the fall; this may be related to a potentially important effect of omalizumab on restoration of interferon production in the setting of viral upper respiratory infection.[20]

Mepolizumab

Mepolizumab, a humanized monoclonal antibody (IgG$_1$ kappa) against the IL-5 molecule, was the first antieosinophil-targeted biologic to enter the US market. IL-5 is a key driver of eosinophil maturation, proliferation, and effector functions; it binds to the IL-5 receptor complex on the eosinophil cell surface. The FDA-approved mepolizumab, dosed 100 mg subcutaneous every 4 weeks, in November 2015, is an add-on treatment for patients aged 12 years and older with severe asthma and an eosinophilic phenotype.[21] Mepolizumab also has demonstrated efficacy in the treatment of eosinophilic granulomatosis with polyangiitis and was FDA approved for this condition in December 2017, at a dose of 300 mg (3 separate 100 mg injections subcutaneously) every 4 weeks.[22]

Initial studies of mepolizumab failed to show significant improvement in clinical measures of asthma, despite successfully reducing blood and sputum eosinophil counts. In one randomized, double-blind, parallel group study, 24 patients with mild asthma received intravenous (IV) mepolizumab, 750 mg, for 3 doses or placebo for more than 20 weeks.[23] Mepolizumab reduced blood and sputum eosinophil counts, but had no significant impact on airway hyperresponsiveness, forced expiratory volume in one second (FEV1), or peak flow. In another multicenter, randomized, double-blind, placebo-controlled study, 362 patients with poorly controlled asthma despite daily ICS were randomized to receive IV mepolizumab, 250 mg, mepolizumab, 750 mg, or placebo at monthly intervals.[24] Despite reducing blood and sputum eosinophil counts, mepolizumab therapy did not improve lung function tests, symptom scores, beta agonist use, exacerbation rates, or quality of life measures.

Subsequently, using an alternative approach, with subjects preselected with an eosinophilic phenotype despite oral corticosteroid (OCS) use, the results were encouraging. Two small randomized, double-blind, parallel-group trials published in 2009 showed statistically significant reductions in annual rate of exacerbations.[25,26] As shown in **Table 1**, Nair and colleagues[25] identified a subgroup of patients with sputum eosinophilia and airway symptoms despite continued treatment with prednisone and assigned them to receive 750 mg IV mepolizumab (N = 8) or placebo (N = 11) for 5 monthly infusions. Subjects randomized to mepolizumab exhibited a significant reduction in eosinophils, decreased exacerbations, and were able to reduce their OCS requirements (84% of the maximum possible reduction per protocol compared with 48%) (P = .04). A larger study of patients with refractory eosinophilic asthma and a history of recurrent exacerbations (N = 61) with the same mepolizumab dosing, given for more than 50 weeks, had a significant reduction in severe exacerbations in the active treatment arm versus placebo (2.0 vs 3.4 mean exacerbations per subject; relative risk 0.57; confidence interval [CI] 0.32–0.92; P = .02) and a significant improvement in the Asthma Quality of Life Questionnaire.[26] Significant improvement was not seen in the secondary outcomes of lung function and symptom scores.

The Dose Ranging Efficacy and Safety with Mepolizumab in Severe Asthma (DREAM) study, a dose-ranging efficacy study of mepolizumab with more than 600 subjects, demonstrated that 75 mg, 250 mg, and 750 mg of IV mepolizumab produced similar clinical benefits, with significant reductions in clinically significant exacerbations ranging from 39% to 52% compared with placebo over the course of 50 weeks.[27] The Mepolizumab as Adjunctive Therapy in Patients with Severe Asthma (MENSA) study by Ortega and colleagues[28] was a 32-week multicenter randomized, double-blind trial of mepolizumab, 75 mg, IV versus, 100 mg, subcutaneous versus placebo in 576 patients with severe eosinophilic asthma. Comparable (47% and 53%) reductions in the treatment arms were observed compared with placebo (P<.001).

Treatment with mepolizumab has also been shown to be steroid-sparing. The Steroid Reduction with Mepolizumab Study (SIRIUS) enrolled 135 patients with severe eosinophilic asthma. Mepolizumab treatment at a dose of 100 mg subcutaneously every 4 weeks for 20 weeks resulted in a 50% reduction from baseline in glucocorticoid dosing, compared with no reduction in the placebo arm.[29] Despite this, the treatment arm had a relative reduction of 32% in the annualized rate of exacerbations (1.44 vs 2.12, P = .04), with a similar safety profile.

In pivotal trials of mepolizumab, the drug had an acceptable adverse-event and side-effect profile. In a 2009 study, the only serious adverse events reported were hospitalizations for acute asthma exacerbation.[26] One subject withdrew from the study due to a transient maculopapular rash, and in another study, one subject withdrew due to progressive shortness of breath, likely cardiac in cause.[25] Three patients died in the DREAM study but these deaths were categorized as unrelated to treatment (one fatal severe acute pancreatitis, one fatal asthma exacerbation, and a suicide). The overall frequency of serious adverse events was similar across treatment groups, with the most frequently reported adverse events being headache (17% placebo arm, 21% in mepolizumab arms) and nasopharyngitis (15% placebo arm, 19%–22% mepolizumab arms).[27] There were no reported life-threatening anaphylactic reactions. In both the MENSA and SIRIUS studies, the safety profile of mepolizumab was similar to placebo; most frequently reported adverse events were headache and nasopharyngitis.[28,29]

A recent study suggests mepolizumab may be efficacious in chronic rhinosinusitis with nasal polyposis (CRSwNP), a frequently co-occurring, comorbid condition in patients with severe asthma. In a randomized, double-blind, placebo-controlled trial, 105 adult patients with severe bilateral nasal polyposis requiring surgery[30] were randomized to receive mepolizumab, 750 mg, IV every 4 weeks or placebo, in addition to daily topical corticosteroid treatment. At week 25, more subjects randomized to mepolizumab (N = 54) had symptomatic improvement and fewer required sinus surgery compared with placebo.

Reslizumab

Reslizumab is also a humanized monoclonal antibody directed against IL-5, blocking binding of IL-5 to IL-5R on eosinophils. Unlike mepolizumab, reslizumab is given by an intravenous route (over 20–50 minutes); dosing is based on body weight. Reslizumab received FDA approval in March 2016 for patients aged 18 years and older with an eosinophilic asthma phenotype, as add-on therapy.[31] The recommended dosage is 3.0 mg/kg every 4 weeks.

In an initial 2011 study of reslizumab, as described in **Table 1**, patients were randomized to receive monthly infusions of reslizumab at 3.0 mg/kg dosing or placebo for 12 weeks (n = 106).[32] The primary endpoint was change in Asthma Control Questionnaire (ACQ) scores from baseline to week 15. The study found a trend toward greater asthma control with reslizumab; mean changes from baseline to end of therapy ACQ score were −0.7 in the treatment arm and −0.3 in the placebo group and improvements in airway function. Improvement was greater in subjects with nasal polyps.

In a Phase 3 study, 492 subjects with varying eosinophil counts were randomly assigned to receive IV reslizumab (3 mg/kg) or placebo monthly for 16 weeks.[33] The primary endpoint was change in FEV1 from baseline to week 16. No statistically significant difference in lung function was found; however, in the subgroup with eosinophil counts greater than 400 cells/μL, there were clinically meaningful improvements in lung function and symptom scores, implying this group is most likely to respond.

Two duplicate, multicenter, parallel, double-blind, parallel-group, randomized, placebo-controlled phase 3 trials of IV reslizumab (3.0 mg/kg) administered every 4 weeks for 1 year enrolled patients with eosinophilic asthma (eosinophils >400 cells/μL) inadequately controlled with medium-to-high dose ICS and with history of one or more exacerbations in the previous year. Both trials found subjects randomized to reslizumab had significant reductions in the primary endpoint of asthma exacerbations (study 1 [n = 477]: rate ratio (RR) of 0.5 (CI 0.37–0.67); study 2 [n = 476]: 0.41 [0.28–0.59]; $P<.0001$) compared with placebo.[34]

Reslizumab has been well tolerated. In one trial, the reslizumab group had fewer adverse events than placebo (55% vs 73%).[33] The most frequently reported adverse events were worsening asthma, upper respiratory infection, and sinusitis. Because of a black box warning of anaphylaxis, reslizumab is administered in a health care setting in which personnel, equipment, and supplies are present to manage anaphylaxis.[35] Two subjects had anaphylaxis (one deemed related to allergen immunotherapy, another related to reslizumab). The reslizumab-related reaction included symptoms of shortness of breath; wheezing and flushing shortly after infusion; and required treatment with epinephrine, salbutamol, antihistamine, and prednisone. In another trial, common adverse events were also similar with placebo.[34] The most common adverse events were worsening asthma, upper respiratory tract infections, and nasopharyngitis. Two patients had anaphylactic reactions.

There are no head-to-head comparison studies of anti-IL5 drugs. However, one small study evaluated the use of weight-based IV reslizumab in 10 prednisone-dependent patients with severe asthma, with elevated eosinophils (>3%) and persistent blood eosinophilia (>300 cells/uL) despite treatment with subcutaneous mepolizumab (100 mg SC q 4 weeks) for at least 1 year.[36] Subjects received 2 infusions of placebo monthly, followed by 4 infusions of reslizumab (3.0 mg/kg) monthly. Reslizumab was associated with reduction of sputum eosinophils by 91.2% ($P = .002$) and blood eosinophils by 87.4% ($P = .004$). This was also associated with significant improvements in lung function and symptom scores. These data suggest a fixed-dose strategy with mepolizumab may not lead to improvement of airway eosinophilia in some patients.

Benralizumab

Benralizumab is a monoclonal antibody that binds to the IL-5rα on eosinophils and basophils (rather than the IL-5 antibody itself). Receptor blockade on the eosinophil is thought to lead to cell apoptosis and to near complete depletion of eosinophils.

Benralizumab received FDA approval in late 2017 for add-on maintenance therapy for patients with severe asthma 12 years and older, with an eosinophilic phenotype. The recommended dose is 30 mg every 4 weeks for the first 3 doses, followed by once every 8 weeks.[37]

In a phase 2b randomized, controlled, double-blind study, subjects aged 18 to 75 years with uncontrolled asthma despite ICS and LABA use, and 2 to 6 exacerbations in the past year, were enrolled, as described in **Table 1**.[38] Subjects were randomly assigned to receive placebo or benralizumab at varying doses. In eosinophilic subjects (>300 cells/uL), annual exacerbation rates were lower in the benralizumab, 20 mg and 100 mg, groups than in the placebo group.

The efficacy and safety of benralizumab for patients with severe asthma uncontrolled with high-dosage ICS and long-acting β2-agonists (SIROCCO) trial was a 48-week randomized, double-blind, parallel-group, placebo-controlled multicenter study comparing benralizumab, 30 mg, subcutaneously every 4 weeks for the first 3 doses, then every 8 weeks thereafter versus benralizumab, 30 mg, or placebo subcutaneously every 4 weeks in 1204 patients aged 12 to 75 years.[39] Compared with placebo, benralizumab was associated with reductions in annual exacerbation rates when given every 4 weeks (RR 0.55, 95% CI 0.42–0.71; $P<.0001$) or every 8 weeks

(RR 0.49, 0.37–0.64; $P<.0001$) for more than 48 weeks. The active treatment arms also showed significant improvement in prebronchodilator FEV1 versus placebo.

Another randomized, double-blind, parallel-group, placebo-controlled phase 3 study (CALIMA) was undertaken in patients aged 12 to 75 years with severe asthma uncontrolled with ICS and LABA, plus a history of 2 or more exacerbations in the previous year (n = 1306). Subjects were randomized with a 1:1:1 assignment to receive benralizumab, 30 mg, subcutaneously every 4 weeks or every 8 weeks (after an initial 3 doses given every 4 weeks) or to placebo. The primary endpoint was annual exacerbation RR versus placebo for patients with baseline blood eosinophils 300 cells per μL or greater. Subjects randomized to active treatment every 4 weeks (RR 0.64 [95% CI 0.49–0.85], P = .0018, n = 241) and every 8 weeks (RR 0.72 [95% CI 0.54–0.95], P = .0188, n = 239) had lower exacerbation rates compared with placebo (RR 0.93 [95% CI 0.77–1.12], n = 248).[40]

The Oral Glucocorticoid-Sparing Effect of Benralizumab in Severe Asthma trial was a 28-week randomized controlled trial of benralizumab administered every 4 weeks or every 8 weeks (after 3 initial doses given every 4 weeks) versus placebo. The 2 benralizumab dosing regimens were associated with significant reductions in median final oral steroid dose from baseline: by 75% compared with 25% in the placebo arm ($P<.001$).[41]

Benralizumab has demonstrated a favorable safety profile. In the SIROCCO study, the most common adverse events were worsening of asthma and nasopharyngitis; adverse events were similar to placebo.[39] Five patients died in the placebo and benralizumab groups and one posttreatment; these deaths were not considered to be treatment related. In the CALIMA study,[40] adverse events were similar to placebo; a positive antidrug antibody response was reported in 15% of patients receiving benralizumab. Four patients died during treatment, and 2 died posttreatment; these deaths were categorized as unrelated to treatment.

Dupilumab

Dupilumab is a humanized monoclonal antibody targeting IL-4rα, shared by both IL-4 and IL-13, currently approved for severe atopic dermatitis. The FDA has recently approved Dupilumab as add-on maintenance therapy in patients 12 years and older with moderate-to-severe asthma with an eosinophilic phenotype or with oral corticosteroid-dependent asthma.[42] The 2 currently published studies regarding this agent for use in asthma are described in **Table 1**.

In a phase 2a study, Wenzel and colleagues[43] recruited subjects with moderate-to-severe persistent asthma and a blood eosinophil count of greater than 300 cells/μL or a sputum eosinophil level of at least 3%, who used medium-dose or high-dose ICS with LABA. Subjects were randomized to receive dupilumab (300 mg) or placebo subcutaneously once weekly, then discontinued their LABA at week 4 and tapered to discontinuation of their ICS during weeks 6 through 9. All subjects received study drug for 12 weeks or until a protocol-defined asthma exacerbation occurred. The primary end point was occurrence of an asthma exacerbation (defined as 2 or more day predefined drop in peak expiratory flow measurement or rescue β-2 agonist, need for predefined escalation of ICS, need for oral corticosteroids or hospitalization due to asthma). A total of 52 patients were assigned to dupilumab and 52 to placebo. Although 6% of subjects stratified to active therapy had an asthma exacerbation, 44% receiving placebo had an exacerbation and 87% reduction with dupilumab (odds ratio, 0.08; 95% CI, 0.02–0.28; $P<.001$). Significant improvements were also observed in secondary endpoints of lung function, ACQ5, nocturnal awakenings, and FeNO levels in those receiving dupilumab compared with placebo.

A second randomized, double-blind, placebo-controlled, parallel-group (phase 2b) trial enrolled 769 subjects with uncontrolled asthma and at least one exacerbation in the previous year despite treatment with medium-to-high dose ICS plus an LABA.[44] Subjects were randomly assigned to receive subcutaneous dupilumab, 200 mg or 300 mg, every 2 weeks or every 4 weeks, versus placebo for 24 weeks; randomization was stratified based on baseline eosinophil count. The primary outcome was change in FEV1 at week 12 in subjects with baseline blood eosinophils greater than or equal to 300 per uL. They found that in the subgroup with elevated eosinophils, all dupilumab dose regimens, except for 200 mg every 4 weeks, demonstrated significant increases in FEV1 compared with placebo, with these increases maintained throughout the 24 weeks of this study. Even in the group with lower eosinophil counts, dupilumab every 2 weeks resulted in significant improvements in lung function.

The rates of overall treatment-emergent adverse events were similar across all treatment groups with dupilumab versus placebo. Reported adverse events of greater than 10% included upper respiratory tract infection, injection site erythema, and headache for dupilumab and placebo, respectively. A clear dose–response association in injection-site reaction was seen with observed rates with dupilumab being 13% for 200 mg and 300 mg every 4 weeks, 20% for 200 mg every 2 weeks, 26% for 300 mg every 2 weeks, and 13% for placebo. Dupilumab did not increase the incidence of bacterial or opportunistic herpes viral infections, with rates across all dose regimens similar to those observed in the placebo group. Serious treatment-emergent adverse events were similar between dupilumab (7%) and placebo (6%). Two subjects in the 300 mg every 4 weeks regimen died during the study due to causes considered by the investigator and sponsor to be unrelated to study medication (acute cardiac failure, metastatic gastric cancer, organizing pneumonia, with cor pulmonale).

As previously mentioned, chronic sinusitis is associated with asthma and may be a trigger of worsening asthma control. A proof of concept study by Bachert and colleagues[45] explored the utility of dupilumab in 60 subjects with chronic rhinosinusitis with nasal polyposis, via performance of a randomized, double-blind, placebo-controlled parallel group study comparing 300 mg of dupilumab (following a 600 mg loading dose) versus placebo, in tandem with the use of nasal steroids for 16 weeks. Thirty subjects randomized to active therapy demonstrated a significant improvement in the primary endpoint of bilateral nasal polyp score compared with the 30 subjects randomized to placebo [baseline compared with 16 week least squares mean difference (-1.6, CI -2.4 to -0.7), $P<.001$]. Secondary endpoints, including change in Lung-McKay CT total score, morning peak nasal inspiratory flow, and SNOT-22, also demonstrated significant improvement with use of dupilumab compared with placebo. In the group of subjects with concomitant asthma, both improvements in endoscopic nasal polyp score, as well as asthma control and lung functions were seen.

A recent phase 3 study published by Castro and colleagues, demonstrated that 300 mg of dupilumab dosed every 2 weeks for 52 weeks resulted in a 47.7% reduction in severe asthma attacks in the overall group, with a 65.8% reduction in subjects with baseline eosinophil counts of >300 cells/uL, a 44.3% reduction in subjects with baseline eosinophil counts of 150 cells to <300 per cubic millimeter, while similar exacerbation rates were seen between active and placebo groups in subjects with a baseline blood eosinophil count of less than 150 per cubic millimeter. Similarly, the magnitude of improvement in lung function followed baseline eosinophil counts [overall population/9% ($P<.001$)], with the greatest improvement in FEV1 seen among patients with a blood eosinophil counts of 300 or more per cubic millimeter.[46] Lastly, a study by Rabe and colleagues demonstrated in a 24 week study of oral corticosteroid dependent asthmatics that the addition of Dupilumab 300 mg every 2 weeks resulted in a reduction in oral glucocorticoid use ($P<0.001$) while decreasing the rate of severe exacerbations by 59% and increasing the FEV1 by 0.22 liters compared to placebo.[47]

Tezepelumab

A more recent addition to the T2 treatment paradigm is a monoclonal antibody that targets TSLP, an upstream molecule secreted by epithelial cells with effector functions on many cells, including eosinophils, mast cells, Th2 cells, basophils, and others. In a randomized, double-blind, placebo-controlled (phase 2) trial of tezepelumab, an investigational human IgG2 monoclonal antibody that binds to TSLP, subjects with uncontrolled asthma receiving LABA, and medium-to-high dose ICS were randomized (in a 1:1:1:1 ratio) to receive tezepelumab (low dose, 70 mg every 4 weeks; medium dose, 210 mg q 4 weeks; high dose, 280 mg q 4 weeks) or placebo, as detailed in **Table 1**. Tezepelumab treatment resulted in annualized rate of exacerbations at week 52 of 0.26, 0.19, and 0.22, respectively, compared with 0.67 in the placebo arm. This reduction was seen independent of baseline eosinophil counts.[48] The incidence of reported adverse events was similar across the trial arms. Based on its upstream site of action, tezepelumab may exert efficacy for a broader population of severe, uncontrolled asthmatics, including those with non-T2 asthma.

BIOLOGICS UNDER INVESTIGATION FOR T2 ASTHMA

Several drugs, which are not yet FDA approved for severe asthma as of this article being written, merit mention.

Additional Biologics

Biologic molecules targeted against the IL-13 pathway, such as lebrikizumab and tralokinumab did not meet primary endpoints and are no longer under investigation for asthma.[49,50] These agents may create redundancy with an agent such as dupilumab, which essentially blocks both the IL-4 and IL-13 pathways. The IL-33 pathway, thought to play a role in respiratory allergy and asthma, and other pathways such as IL-6, may be other potential targets investigated in the future.

BIOLOGICS FOR NON-T2 ASTHMA

At present, there are no biologic agents approved specifically for patients with non-T2 asthma. Patients without evidence of elevated T2 biomarkers generally fall into the category of non-T2 asthma, which may represent a neutrophilic or paucicellular disease process. This phenotype is seen in patients with severe, refractory asthma, which underscores the importance of investigating non-T2 inflammatory pathways and targeted therapeutics.

Previous trials of biologics, such as antitumor necrosis factor (TNF) agents that block Th1 pathways, did not show promising results. In one trial, golimumab, a fusion protein that can bind TNF-α and is used to treat rheumatoid arthritis, was studied in a randomized, double-blind, placebo-controlled study of patients with severe uncontrolled asthma despite high-dose ICS and LABA.[51] Subjects (N = 309) were randomized in a 1:1:1:1 fashion to receive monthly subcutaneous injections of placebo or golimumab (50, 100, or 200 mg) through week 52. No significant differences were found in the coprimary endpoints of change in lung function and severe asthma exacerbations through week 24. Patients treated with golimumab experienced serious adverse events more frequently than placebo; because of an unfavorable risk-benefit profile, the study was discontinued early.

It is not yet clear, but some early clinical trials of biological therapies targeting severe T2 asthma have shown some efficacy in patients without apparent elevations in T2 biomarkers, albeit smaller than that seen with T2 asthma. This was seen in the Phase 2 randomized placebo controlled trials of dupilumab in severe asthma and the phase 2 trial of tezepelumab.[44,48] Treatment options for non-T2 asthma, which can be refractory to currently available pharmacotherapeutic agents, warrant further investigation.

Other pathways beyond the Th1/Th2 paradigm, such as Th17 and others, may add additional layers of complexity to the inflammatory cascade, but perhaps may yield novel drug targets for patients with non-T2 asthma. A randomized, double-blind, placebo-controlled study of brodalumab, a human anti-IL17rα monoclonal antibody, examined the role of blocking the IL-17 pathway in subjects with inadequately controlled moderate to severe asthma despite taking regular ICS.[52] Subjects (N = 302) were randomized to receive brodalumab (at doses of 140, 210, or 280 mg) or placebo. No significant improvement was found in the primary endpoint of change in ACQ score from baseline to week 12.

SUMMARY

Much remains to be determined to foster more optimal use of biological agents for patients with severe asthma, including use of validated biomarkers and other criteria for patient selection and assessment of treatment response. At present, these biotherapeutics remain very costly; better predictors of response will be required to achieve more favorable cost-effectiveness.[53] Alternative administration methods (such as decreasing frequency of administration or intermittent use), tailoring therapy more precisely based on phenotypes/endotypes, and prompt identification of nonresponders offer the potential for improved cost-efficacy.[20] Identifying prognostic factors and accurate measures of treatment response will facilitate more personalized treatment for severe asthma in the future.

REFERENCES

1. Darveaux J, Busse WW. Biologics in asthma–the next step toward personalized treatment. J Allergy Clin Immunol Pract 2015;3(2):152–60.
2. Fahy JV. Asthma was talking, but we weren't listening. Missed or ignored signals that have slowed treatment progress. Ann Am Thorac Soc 2016;13(Suppl 1):S78–82.
3. Carr TF, Zeki AA, Kraft M. Eosinophilic and noneosinophilic asthma. Am J Respir Crit Care Med 2018; 197(1):22–37.
4. Szefler SJ, Wenzel S, Brown R, et al. Asthma outcomes: biomarkers. J Allergy Clin Immunol 2012; 129(3 Suppl):S9–23.
5. Omalizumab, Xolair, label. Available at: https://www. gene.com/download/pdf/xolair_prescribing.pdf. Accessed April 22, 2018.
6. Rambasek TE, Lang DM, Kavuru MS. Omalizumab: where does it fit into current asthma management? Cleve Clin J Med 2004;71(3):251–61.
7. Humbert M, Beasley R, Ayres J, et al. Benefits of omalizumab as add-on therapy in patients with severe persistent asthma who are inadequately controlled despite best available therapy (GINA 2002 step 4 treatment): innovate. Allergy 2005; 60(3):309–16.
8. Hanania NA, Alpan O, Hamilos DL, et al. Omalizumab in severe allergic asthma inadequately controlled with standard therapy: a randomized trial. Ann Intern Med 2011;154(9):573–82.
9. Chanez P, Contin-Bordes C, Garcia G, et al. Omalizumab-induced decrease of FcξRI expression in patients with severe allergic asthma. Respir Med 2010; 104(11):1608–17.
10. Bousquet J, Rabe K, Humbert M, et al. Predicting and evaluating response to omalizumab in patients

with severe allergic asthma. Respir Med 2007;
101(7):1483–92.

11. Holgate S, Buhl R, Bousquet J, et al. The use of
omalizumab in the treatment of severe allergic
asthma: a clinical experience update. Respir Med
2009;103(8):1098–113.

12. Zeiger RS, Schatz M, Li Q, et al. High blood eosinophil count is a risk factor for future asthma exacerbations in adult persistent asthma. J Allergy Clin
Immunol Pract 2014;2(6):741–50.

13. Price DB, Rigazio A, Campbell JD, et al. Blood
eosinophil count and prospective annual asthma
disease burden: a UK cohort study. Lancet Respir
Med 2015;3(11):849–58.

14. Humbert M, Taillé C, Mala L, et al. Omalizumab
effectiveness in patients with severe allergic
asthma according to blood eosinophil count: the
STELLAIR study. Eur Respir J 2018;51(5) [pii:
1702523].

15. Hanania NA, Wenzel S, Rosén K, et al. Exploring the
effects of omalizumab in allergic asthma: an analysis
of biomarkers in the EXTRA study. Am J Respir Crit
Care Med 2013;187(8):804–11.

16. Long A, Rahmaoui A, Rothman KJ, et al. Incidence
of malignancy in patients with moderate-to-severe
asthma treated with or without omalizumab.
J Allergy Clin Immunol 2014;134(3):560–7.e4.

17. Li JX, Fan LC, Li MH, et al. Beneficial effects of Omalizumab therapy in allergic bronchopulmonary
aspergillosis: a synthesis review of published literature. Respir Med 2017;122:33–42.

18. Bidder T, Sahota J, Rennie C, et al. Omalizumab
treats chronic rhinosinusitis with nasal polyps and
asthma together-a real life study. Rhinology 2018;
56(1):42–5.

19. Lang DM, Aronica MA, Maierson ES, et al. Omalizumab can inhibit respiratory reaction during aspirin
desensitization. Ann Allergy Asthma Immunol 2018;
121:98–104.

20. Teach SJ, Gill MA, Togias A, et al. Preseasonal treatment with either omalizumab or an inhaled corticosteroid boost to prevent fall asthma exacerbations.
J Allergy Clin Immunol 2015;136(6):1476–85.

21. Nucala (Mepolizumab) Prescribing Information. Available at: https://www.gsksource.com/pharma/content/
dam/GlaxoSmithKline/US/en/Prescribing_Information/
Nucala/pdf/NUCALA-PI-PIL.PDF. Accessed April 26,
2018.

22. FDA Press Announcement. 2017. Mepolizumab.
Available at: https://www.fda.gov/NewsEvents/
Newsroom/PressAnnouncements/ucm588594.htm.
Accessed April 26, 2018.

23. Flood-Page PT, Menzies-Gow AN, Kay AB, et al.
Eosinophil's role remains uncertain as anti-
interleukin-5 only partially depletes numbers in
asthmatic airway. Am J Respir Crit Care Med
2003;167(2):199–204.

24. Flood-Page P, Swenson C, Faiferman I, et al. A study
to evaluate safety and efficacy of mepolizumab in
patients with moderate persistent asthma. Am J Respir Crit Care Med 2007;176(11):1062–71.

25. Nair P, Pizzichini MM, Kjarsgaard M, et al. Mepolizumab for prednisone-dependent asthma with sputum
eosinophilia. N Engl J Med 2009;360(10):985–93.

26. Haldar P, Brightling CE, Hargadon B, et al. Mepolizumab and exacerbations of refractory eosinophilic
asthma. N Engl J Med 2009;360(10):973–84.

27. Pavord ID, Korn S, Howarth P, et al. Mepolizumab for
severe eosinophilic asthma (DREAM): a multicentre,
double-blind, placebo-controlled trial. Lancet 2012;
380(9842):651–9.

28. Ortega HG, Liu MC, Pavord ID, et al. Mepolizumab
treatment in patients with severe eosinophilic
asthma. N Engl J Med 2014;371(13):1198–207.

29. Bel EH, Wenzel SE, Thompson PJ, et al. Oral
glucocorticoid-sparing effect of mepolizumab in
eosinophilic asthma. N Engl J Med 2014;371(13):
1189–97.

30. Bachert C, Sousa AR, Lund VJ, et al. Reduced need
for surgery in severe nasal polyposis with mepolizumab: randomized trial. J Allergy Clin Immunol 2017;
140(4):1024–31.e4.

31. FDA Press Announcement, Reslizumab. Available
at: https://www.fda.gov/NewsEvents/Newsroom/
PressAnnouncements/ucm491980.htm. Accessed
March 26, 2018.

32. Castro M, Mathur S, Hargreave F, et al. Reslizumab
for poorly controlled, eosinophilic asthma: a randomized, placebo-controlled study. Am J Respir
Crit Care Med 2011;184(10):1125–32.

33. Corren J, Weinstein S, Janka L, et al. Phase 3 study
of reslizumab in patients with poorly controlled
asthma: effects across a broad range of eosinophil
counts. Chest 2016;150(4):799–810.

34. Castro M, Zangrilli J, Wechsler ME, et al. Reslizumab for inadequately controlled asthma with
elevated blood eosinophil counts: results from two
multicentre, parallel, double-blind, randomised,
placebo-controlled, phase 3 trials. Lancet Respir
Med 2015;3(5):355–66.

35. Cinqair (Reslizumab) Prescribing Information. Available at: http://cinqair.com/pdf/PrescribingInformation.
pdf. Accessed April 26, 2018.

36. Mukherjee M, Aleman Paramo F, Kjarsgaard M, et al.
Weight-adjusted intravenous reslizumab in severe
asthma with inadequate response to fixed-dose subcutaneous mepolizumab. Am J Respir Crit Care
Med 2018;197(1):38–46.

37. Fasenra (benralizumab) Prescribing Information.
Available at: https://www.azpicentral.com/fasenra/
fasenra_pi.pdf. Accessed April 26, 2018.

38. Castro M, Wenzel SE, Bleecker ER, et al. Benralizumab, an anti-interleukin 5 receptor α monoclonal
antibody, versus placebo for uncontrolled

eosinophilic asthma: a phase 2b randomised dose-ranging study. Lancet Respir Med 2014;2(11): 879–90.

39. Bleecker ER, FitzGerald JM, Chanez P, et al. Efficacy and safety of benralizumab for patients with severe asthma uncontrolled with high-dosage inhaled corticosteroids and long-acting β2-agonists (SIROCCO): a randomised, multicentre, placebo-controlled phase 3 trial. Lancet 2016;388(10056): 2115–27.

40. FitzGerald JM, Bleecker ER, Nair P, et al. Benralizumab, an anti-interleukin-5 receptor α monoclonal antibody, as add-on treatment for patients with severe, uncontrolled, eosinophilic asthma (CALIMA): a randomised, double-blind, placebo-controlled phase 3 trial. Lancet 2016;388(10056):2128–41.

41. Nair P, Wenzel S, Rabe KF, et al. Oral glucocorticoid-sparing effect of benralizumab in severe asthma. N Engl J Med 2017;376(25):2448–58.

42. Available at: https://www.regeneron.com/sites/default/files/Dupixent_FPI.pdf.

43. Wenzel S, Ford L, Pearlman D, et al. Dupilumab in persistent asthma with elevated eosinophil levels. N Engl J Med 2013;368(26):2455–66.

44. Wenzel S, Castro M, Corren J, et al. Dupilumab efficacy and safety in adults with uncontrolled persistent asthma despite use of medium-to-high-dose inhaled corticosteroids plus a long-acting β2 agonist: a randomised double-blind placebo-controlled pivotal phase 2b dose-ranging trial. Lancet 2016;388(10039):31–44.

45. Bachert C, Mannent L, Naclerio RM, et al. Effect of subcutaneous dupilumab on nasal polyp burden in patients with chronic sinusitis and nasal polyposis:

a randomized clinical trial. JAMA 2016;315(5): 469–79.

46. Castro M, Corren J, Pavord I, et al. Dupilumab efficacy and safety in moderate-to-severe uncontrolled asthma. N Engl J Med 2018;378:2486–96.

47. Rabe K, Nair P, Brusselle G, et al. Efficacy and safety of dupilumab in glucocorticoid-dependent severe asthma. N Engl J Med 2018;378:2475–85.

48. Corren J, Parnes JR, Wang L, et al. Tezepelumab in adults with uncontrolled asthma. N Engl J Med 2017; 377(10):936–46.

49. Hanania NA, Korenblat P, Chapman KR, et al. Efficacy and safety of lebrikizumab in patients with uncontrolled asthma (LAVOLTA I and LAVOLTA II): replicate, phase 3, randomised, double-blind, placebo-controlled trials. Lancet Respir Med 2016; 4(10):781–96.

50. Piper E, Brightling C, Niven R, et al. A phase II placebo-controlled study of tralokinumab in moderate-to-severe asthma. Eur Respir J 2013; 41(2):330–8.

51. Wenzel SE, Barnes PJ, Bleecker ER, et al. A randomized, double-blind, placebo-controlled study of tumor necrosis factor-alpha blockade in severe persistent asthma. Am J Respir Crit Care Med 2009;179(7):549–58.

52. Busse WW, Holgate S, Kerwin E, et al. Randomized, double-blind, placebo-controlled study of brodalumab, a human anti-IL-17 receptor monoclonal antibody, in moderate to severe asthma. Am J Respir Crit Care Med 2013;188(11):1294–302.

53. Whittington MD, McQueen RB, Ollendorf DA, et al. Assessing the value of mepolizumab for severe eosinophilic asthma: a cost-effectiveness analysis. Ann Allergy Asthma Immunol 2017;118(2):220–5.

Bronchial Thermoplasty

Anne S. Mainardi, MD[a], Mario Castro, MD[b], Geoffrey Chupp, MD[a],*

KEYWORDS

- Bronchial thermoplasty • Radiofrequency ablation • Severe asthma • Airway smooth muscle

KEY POINTS

- Bronchial thermoplasty is the only device-based therapy for severe asthma that remains uncontrolled despite optimal medical management.
- Bronchial thermoplasty is performed by introducing a catheter through the working channel of a standard bronchoscope and delivering radiofrequency energy directly to the airway wall.
- Bronchial thermoplasty results in the reduction of smooth muscle mass in the airway wall.
- Several large human trials have shown that bronchial thermoplasty reduces asthma exacerbation rates and improves quality of life.
- More studies are needed to understand the physiologic mechanisms of bronchial thermoplasty and the ideal patient population to target for this therapy.

INTRODUCTION

Airway smooth muscle (ASM) plays a critical structural and immunomodulatory role in the airway and contributes to exacerbations and chronic airway remodeling in asthma.[1] Bronchial thermoplasty (BT), a therapeutic procedure that targets the ASM by applying radiofrequency energy to the airway wall, reduces ASM mass and function, which improves asthma disease activity and exacerbations. BT is indicated for patients with severe asthma that remains symptomatic despite compliant, maximal use of high-dose inhaled corticosteroids (ICS) and long-acting bronchodilators (LABA) (equivalent of Step 5 GINA guidelines therapy[2]).

SEVERE ASTHMA
Target Population of Bronchial Thermoplasty

Asthma is a chronic inflammatory disease estimated to affect more than 250 million people worldwide.[3] In the United States, asthma prevalence increased in the second half of the twentieth century[4,5] and is currently estimated to have a prevalence that approaches 8%.[6] The economic burden associated with the disease encompasses medical costs, mortality, and missed work and school days, and cost the US economy $81.9 billion in 2013. Medical spending significantly rises with increasing disease severity mostly attributable to prescription medications.[6,7] BT targets severe uncontrolled asthma. The American Thoracic

Disclosure Statement: A.S. Mainardi has no financial relationships to disclose. Dr. Castro receives University Grant Funding from NIH, American Lung Association, PCORI. He receives Pharmaceutical Grant Funding from AstraZeneca, Boeringer Ingelheim, Chiesi, GSK, Novartis, Sanofi Aventis. He is a consultant for Aviragen, Boston Scientific, Genentech, Nuvaira, Neutronic, Therabron, Theravance, Vectura, 4D Pharma, VIDA, Mallincrodt, Teva, Sanofi-Aventis. He is a speaker for Astra-Zeneca, Boeringer Ingelheim, Boston Scientific, Genentech, Regeneron, Sanofi, Teva. He receives royalties from Elsevier. G. Chupp reports receiving honoraria for advisory board and speaker bureau activity from Astra Zeneca, Glaxo-Smith-Kline, Genentech, Teva, Boehringer-Ingelheim, and Circassia.

a Department of Internal Medicine, Division of Pulmonary, Critical Care, and Sleep Medicine, Yale University School of Medicine, 300 Cedar Street, New Haven, CT 06520, USA; b Department of Internal Medicine, Division of Pulmonary and Critical Care Medicine, Washington University School of Medicine, 4523 Clayton Avenue, St Louis, MO 63110, USA

* Corresponding author. Division of Pulmonary, Critical Care, and Sleep Medicine, PO Box 208057, 300 Cedar Street, New Haven, CT 06520-8057.
E-mail address: geoffrey.chupp@yale.edu

Society/European Respiratory Society guidelines consider asthma to be severe if the patient requires treatment with high-dose ICS and LABA or leukotriene modifier/theophylline and/or systemic steroids for most of the past year to prevent asthma from becoming uncontrolled, or if it remains uncontrolled despite this therapy. Uncontrolled asthma may manifest as poor symptom control, frequent or severe exacerbations, and airflow limitation on bronchodilator withdrawal.[8] Severe asthma is distinct from difficult-to-control asthma, in which poor control is caused by medication nonadherence, medical comorbidities, airborne exposures, or other environmental or social factors.[9–11] Asthma management regimens target excessive inflammation and bronchoconstriction with the goal of obtaining control; maintaining normal activity levels; and minimizing the risks of exacerbations, fixed airflow limitation, and side effects.[2] ICS have been shown to reduce symptom frequency[12] and exacerbation rates,[13] but may not be as effective in patients with severe asthma, who show corticosteroid insensitivity,[8] with poor control despite high ICS doses.[14] Both severe and difficult-to-control patients that remain uncontrolled are candidates for BT.

Targeting Airway Smooth Muscle

It is important to consider the structure of the airway wall in asthma to understand the mechanism of BT. The airway wall consists of the mucosa, composed of an epithelial layer on a basement membrane; the submucosa, which is predominantly ASM; and the adventitia, which is made of connective tissue.[15,16] Alterations in the components of these structures and therefore function are physiologic or pathologic[17] and occur across the span of life in response to developmental abnormalities, allergens, infectious agents, and environmental factors.[18] Irreversible alterations to multiple aspects of the airway wall have been observed in those with asthma for nearly a century and termed airway remodeling.[19,20] Features of airway remodeling include airway wall thickening,[21] subepithelial fibrosis,[22] fibroblast hyperplasia,[23,24] and increased ASM mass.[24,25]

However, the pathobiology of asthma is also complex, particularly given the clinical phenotypic heterogeneity associated with this disease.[26] Many patients with severe asthma demonstrate type 2 inflammation, which is characterized by the inappropriate release of a particular cytokine profile that includes interleukin-4, -5, and -13.[27–29] Phenotype-targeted management is emerging as an important strategy in severe asthma,[30–34] and guidelines now advocate for biomarker testing, such as IgE or blood/sputum eosinophil levels to help guide targeted biologic treatments for patients with severe type 2 inflammation disease.[2,8] BT trials have not selected or identified a particular subtype of disease to target because ASM seems to be important in all subtypes.

Increased ASM mass caused by hyperplasia and hypertrophy has been observed in asthmatic airways.[35] The migration of ASM cells from the surrounding interstitium or from the circulating hematopoietic stem cell compartment may be responsible in the case of hyperplasia.[36] The increased size of large airways ASM cells compared with control subjects has been seen in nonfatal and fatal asthma cases, whereas hyperplasia in the small and large airways has been seen only in fatal asthma cases.[37] ASM contraction reduces the airway diameter, leading to increased airflow resistance.[38] Airway hyperresponsiveness, a key component of asthma, is not fully understood, but is thought to result from increased ASM mass and abnormal ASM contraction dynamics,[39] such as increased shortening capacity and velocity.[40] The role of ASM in the pathophysiology of asthma, however, may not be purely contractile.[41] ASM cells produce and secrete a variety of immunomodulatory mediators including cytokines, chemokines, and cell adhesion molecules; these mediators recruit airway inflammatory cells[42] and contribute to a proremodeling milieu.[20] The interaction between ASM and mast cells generates high levels of activated matrix metalloproteinase-1, which is associated with bronchial hyperresponsiveness.[43] By targeting ASM, BT may attenuate these structural and inflammatory effects.[44]

THE BRONCHIAL THERMOPLASTY PROCEDURE

BT is a procedure in which radiofrequency energy is applied to the airway wall. As with the energy used in radio broadcasting, this electromagnetic wave frequency lies between audio and infrared frequencies. Because biologic tissues are poor conductors, the application of current through an active electrode to the airway wall results in the generation of heat and subsequent dissipation of energy toward the grounding pad.[45] The heat generated is the mechanism of action of BT and preferentially affects and reduces the mass of ASM in treated and nontreated areas.

Initial Observations in Animals

The initial application of radiofrequency energy to the airways of mammals resulted in decreased airway wall thickness. In 2004, Danek, and colleagues[46] used radiofrequency energy in canine airways. The group hypothesized that the reduction in ASM would attenuate the airway responsiveness to a pharmacologic bronchoconstrictor as measured by change in airway diameter. The experiment involved 11 dogs. Radiofrequency energy was applied bronchoscopically to the left upper, left lower, right upper, or right lower lung regions. The energy was delivered at 55°C, 65°C, or 75°C to different regions in different dogs. The results showed a significant and persistent reduction in airway hyperresponsiveness to methacholine in airways treated at 65°C and 75°C. This outcome correlated histologically with a reduction in smooth muscle and its replacement by mature collagen.[46]

Procedure Details

This early study of BT informed today's procedural standards. Airways that are distal to the lobar bronchi and larger than 3 mm are treated, consistent with Danek's canine study and informed by early fluid mechanics models demonstrating that the greatest airflow resistance is in airways larger than 3 mm.[47] The treatment consists of three bronchoscopic procedures at least 3 weeks apart: one each to treat the two lower lobes and one to treat both upper lobes. The right middle lobe is not treated out of concern that its long and narrow bronchus could render it susceptible to chronic damage or collapse,[48] a theoretic concern[49] that has not been seen with BT.

The Alair Bronchial Thermoplasty System (Boston Scientific, Marlborough, MA) was Food and Drug Administration (FDA) approved in 2010 and remains the only system available for carrying out the procedure. It is a single-use system manufactured by Asthmatx, Inc (Sunnydale, CA) that consists of the Alair Catheter and the Alair Controller System. The catheter is used through the working channel of a standard flexible bronchoscope. The catheter contains a four-electrode array that is deployed in the airway by squeezing a hand trigger. The controller system includes the radiofrequency controller, which applies low-power, temperature-controlled radiofrequency energy to the catheter. The correct intensity and duration of energy transmission is ensured by algorithms that control energy parameters during delivery. The controller system also includes a footswitch, with which the controller is activated, and the patient return electrode, to which the electrical current returns (Alair Catheter Model ATS 2–5 Instructions for Use).

In accordance with prior studies[50] and manufacturer guidelines, 50 mg/d of prednisone (or

equivalent) is given on each of the 3 days leading up to the procedure and the day of and the day after the procedure (or longer) to prevent excessive inflammation. The patient is prepared for bronchoscopy according to the institution's practices. Once the bronchoscope is positioned in the distal airway, the catheter is advanced into the working channel until it is visualized at the tip of the bronchoscope. The hand trigger is used to deploy the electrode array, which is then arranged such that all electrodes are in contact with the airway wall (**Fig. 1**). The initiation of energy delivery is activated by the footswitch. After the energy is delivered, the catheter electrode array is retracted by 5 mm and energy is delivered again. To adjust the bronchoscope, the catheter is retracted into it to allow for safe repositioning. This process continues until the contiguous length of the airway has been incrementally treated, after which the bronchoscope is withdrawn. Patients are monitored after the procedure to ensure clinical stability.

Exploratory Studies in Humans

Following the canine study described previously, a human feasibility study was conducted by Miller and colleagues[51] to confirm that the effects of BT were reproducible in humans. The subjects in this study were eight patients with malignancy who were scheduled to undergo wedge resection, lobectomy, or pneumonectomy. Radiofrequency energy was applied using the Alair system. The airways treated were in the regions to be subsequently removed, which allowed for histologic examination 5 to 20 days after the thermoplasty procedure. Consistent with the animal studies, airways treated at 55°C showed minimal histologic

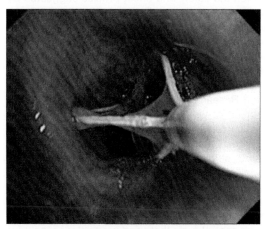

Fig. 1. Bronchial thermoplasty catheter with electrode array deployed in a segmental bronchus. The catheter is used in the working channel of a flexible bronchoscope. (*Courtesy of* Jonathan Puchalski, MD, Yale University School of Medicine, New Haven, CT.)

changes, whereas those treated at 65°C showed marked reduction in ASM compared with untreated nearby airways. The epithelium throughout was either normal or regenerative.[51] Therefore, this study demonstrated that the BT procedure delivered at 65°C was safe in humans and was effective at reducing ASM.

A subsequent human proof-of-concept single arm study was performed in 2006 by Cox and colleagues.[50] This study enrolled 16 patients with mild-to-moderate asthma to undergo a series of three BT procedures, one each to treat each lower lobe and one to treat both upper lobes. There was at least 3 weeks between procedures. The subjects were followed for 2 years. Daily symptom diaries for the first 12 weeks showed a significant improvement in symptom-free days compared with preprocedure baseline. Mean airway hyperresponsiveness, as measured by the concentration of methacholine that provokes a 20% reduction in FEV1 (PC20), was significantly improved at each of the prespecified time points of 12 weeks, 1 year, and 2 years post-procedure. There were 155 adverse events during the study period, most of which were mild and occurred a mean of 1 to 5 days after the procedure. The most frequent adverse events included cough (94% of subjects), dyspnea (69%), bronchospasm (63%), and chest discomfort (56%). The study was limited by its small sample size and lack of a control group, but demonstrated that BT improves airway hyperresponsiveness.[50]

PIVOTAL HUMAN TRIALS

Given the safety and effect profiles suggested by the early studies outlined previously, three randomized trials sought to demonstrate the clinical efficacy of BT (**Table 1**). These included the Asthma Intervention Research (AIR) Trial, published in 2007[52]; the Research in Severe Asthma (RISA) Trial in 2007[53]; and the Asthma Intervention Research 2 (AIR2) Trial in 2010.[54] Different outcomes were studied: AIR focused on exacerbation rates, RISA on safety, and AIR2 on self-reported asthma control. Of the three, only the AIR2 study included a control arm, in which subjects were blinded and underwent a sham procedure that included a BT catheter and actuations without radiofrequency applied to the airway wall. AIR and RISA studies included standard of care control arms that used medical management without a bronchoscopic procedure control. This lack of placebo/sham control has raised concerns about the validity of efficacy end points in these trails.

Asthma Intervention Research Trial

The AIR Trial was a multicenter study of 112 adults with moderate to severe persistent asthma managed with an ICS and LABA. Inclusion required a forced expiratory volume in 1 second (FEV₁) of 60% to 85% of predicted and a decline in asthma control after abstention of LABA during a 2-week baseline period. Participants were randomized to a treatment group or a control group. The treatment group underwent three BT procedures during a 6- to 9-week treatment period. The control group did not undergo procedures but received standard maintenance medication therapy. The study period consisted of the 12 months following the treatment period. At 3, 6, and 12 months, LABA therapy was withdrawn for 2 weeks in both groups during which time subjects self-monitored for signs and symptoms of exacerbation.

The primary outcome of the study was the difference between the control and treatment arms in the change in mild exacerbation rates between the baseline and the LABA withdrawal time periods. A mild exacerbation was defined as a period of at least 2 days during which morning peak flow was reduced, the need for rescue medication was increased, or the subject experienced nocturnal awakenings because of symptoms. Exacerbations were determined based on review of daily diary entries. The results showed that the average number of exacerbations during the LABA withdrawal periods at 3, 6, and 12 months compared with baseline was -0.16 ± 0.37 exacerbations per subject per week in the BT group versus 0.04 ± 0.29 in the control group ($P = .005$) demonstrating that BT reduces mild exacerbation rates.

In addition to reaching the primary end point, multiple secondary outcomes were positive, including change in morning peak expiratory flow (PEF) rescue medication puffs per week, and change in Asthma Quality of Life Questionnaire (AQLQ) and Asthma Control Questionnaire (ACQ) scores in the BT group compared with the control group at some, but not all time points. In contrast to the earlier canine study, BT did not result in a significant change in hyperresponsiveness, as measured by PC₂₀, or obstruction, as measured by FEV₁. There were significantly more adverse events during the treatment period in the BT group compared with the control group. Most of these were mild and occurred within 1 day of the procedure. There was no significant difference in adverse events between the control and BT treated groups in the post-treatment period. The primary limitation of the study was the lack of blinding in the study design, allowing for positive end points to be attributable to a procedure-related placebo effect.[52]

Table 1
Summary of pivotal human trials

Trial, Publication Year	Design	Control Group	Duration	Subject Number	Mean Prebronchodilator FEV$_1$, BT Versus Control	Primary Outcome	Result
AIR, 2007	Multicenter, randomized trial	Usual medical management	6- to 9-wk treatment period followed by 12-mo study period during which LABA withdrawn for 2-wk periods at 3, 6, and 9 mo	112	72.65 ± 10.41 vs 76.12 ± 9.28	Difference between study groups in change in mild exacerbation rate during scheduled LABA abstinence periods compared with baseline	Significant difference at 3 and 12 mo
RISA, 2007	Multicenter, randomized trial	Usual medical management	6-wk treatment period followed by 46-wk study period during which OCS or ICS weaned as able	32	62.9 ± 12.2 vs 66.4 ± 17.8	Difference between study groups in frequency of adverse events during treatment or study periods	Significant difference in frequency of multiple respiratory adverse effects during treatment period, no difference in post-treatment study period
AIR2, 2010	Multicenter, randomized trial	Sham procedure	12-wk treatment period followed by 46-wk study period with assessments at 3, 6, 9, and 12 mo	288	77.8 ± 15.65 vs 79.7 ± 15.14	Difference between study groups in achievement of AQLQ score change of at least 0.5 from baseline to the average of the 6-, 9-, and 12-mo scores	Achieved significance for both ITT and PP analyses

Abbreviations: AQLQ, asthma quality of life questionnaire; FEV$_1$, forced expiratory volume in 1 second; ITT, intention to treat; OCS, oral corticosteroids; PP, per protocol.

Research in Severe Asthma Trial

The RISA Trial was a multicenter study of 32 adults with symptomatic, severe asthma that was poorly controlled despite maintenance therapy. The study included patients with a baseline FEV_1 as low as 50%. About half of the subjects were taking oral corticosteroids (OCS) in addition to ICS and LABA. The treatment group underwent three BT procedures during a 6-week treatment period. The control group was treated with medications alone and did not undergo a bronchoscopic procedure. Following the 6-week treatment period, there was a 46-week post-treatment period that was divided into three phases: (1) a steroid stable phase, (2) a steroid wean phase, and (3) a reduced steroid phase. During the steroid wean phase, OCS or ICS were weaned if possible according to a specified protocol.

The objective of the study was to determine the safety of BT as measured by the frequency of adverse events in the treatment and post-treatment period. The primary analysis compared adverse events in the BT group versus control group for each period. During the treatment period, there were more total respiratory adverse events in the BT group. The subject frequencies of cough, wheezing, chest discomfort, and sputum discoloration were significantly higher in the BT group. There were seven serious events requiring short-term hospitalizations during this period, accounted for by four patients in the BT group and none in the control group. During the post-treatment study period, there was no significant difference in the frequency of adverse events between the BT and control groups.

Efficacy outcomes were reported although the study was not powered to measure them. During the steroid wean phase, four of eight BT subjects and one of seven control subjects were able to wean off OCS and remain off for the duration of the post-treatment period. Subjects were able to reduce their OCS dose by a mean of 63.5% in the BT group versus 26.2% in the control group and their ICS dose by 28.6% versus 20.0%, although the differences between groups were not significant. At the conclusion of the reduced steroid phase, the BT subjects showed a significantly greater improvement from baseline in short-acting bronchodilators use, AQLQ, and ACQ compared with the control subjects. There were no significant differences in change in PEF, symptom scores, symptom-free days, PC_{20}, or post-bronchodilator FEV_1. This study, like AIR1, was not blinded, so the treatment group may have experienced a placebo effect that influenced the outcomes.[53]

Asthma Intervention Research 2 Trial

The AIR2 Trial was a multicenter, randomized, sham-controlled study of 288 adults with asthma maintained on an ICS and LABA with evidence of obstruction (but FEV_1 not <60%) and airway hyperresponsiveness. The treatment group underwent three BT procedures 3 weeks apart during a 12-week treatment period. The control group underwent three sham procedures that mimicked the true procedures in every way except that no energy was delivered on activation of the electrode array within the airway. The post-treatment study period was the year following the treatment period, with assessments made at the beginning and then at 3, 6, 9, and 12 months. Results were analyzed for intention to treat (ITT)[30] groups, which included subjects who underwent at least one bronchoscopy, and prespecified per protocol (PP) groups, comprised of subjects who underwent all procedures and completed follow-up. Of the enrolled subjects, 190/196 in the BT group and 98/101 in the control group met ITT criteria; of these, 173 subjects in the BT group and 95 in the control group qualified for inclusion in the PP population.

The primary outcome was the difference between groups in the proportion of subjects whose integrated AQLQ score, measured at 6, 9, and 12 months, improved by at least 0.5. Statistics were analyzed with Bayesian analysis, which uses the posterior probability of superiority (PPS) to determine significance. In the ITT analysis, the primary end point was reached by 79% of subjects in the BT group compared with 64% in the sham group, which was significant with a PPS of 99.6%. In the PP population, 81% of subjects reached the primary end point, compared with 63% in the sham group (PPS, 99.9%). This result indicated that BT improved quality of life compared with a sham procedure. A subsequent analysis of subjects who have undergone BT suggested that those whose AQLQ score improved by at least 0.5 (responders) had significantly lower AQLQ scores at baseline (4.1 ± 1.1 for responders vs 5.1 ± 1.1 for nonresponders; $P<.001$). Analyses like this may help to guide proper patient selection for this procedure and suggest that there may be a quantifiable level of control that will enrich for a positive response to BT.

Statistically significant secondary end points, as measured by comparing the ITT groups, included rate of severe exacerbations and number of work/school days lost, with better outcomes in the BT group. Secondary outcomes including morning PEF, symptom-free days, symptom score, ACQ, and rescue medication use, were not significantly different between the BT and control groups.

The adverse events recorded in AIR2 included worsening asthma symptoms, emergency department (ED) presentations, and hospitalizations. During the post-treatment period, for the BT group compared with the sham group, there was a 36% risk reduction in the proportion of subjects reporting worsening of asthma (PPS, 99.7%) and an 84% reduction in respiratory-related ED visits (PPS, 99.9%). The rate of severe exacerbations was also significantly reduced in the BT group (PPS, 95.5%).[54]

Although the validity of the sham control in AIR2 has been questioned, this study was the first placebo-controlled trial to demonstrate that BT improves asthma symptom activity and exacerbations.

Safety of Bronchial Thermoplasty

All of the pivotal BT studies were divided into a treatment period and a follow-up or study/post-treatment period. Most adverse events occurred during the treatment period, which was defined as the time a subject started the first BT procedure until after the third procedure was completed. This was 6 to 9 weeks in AIR, 6 weeks in RISA, and 12 weeks in AIR2. The post-treatment period, or study follow-up period, began at the end of the treatment period and lasted approximately 1 year for all the studies. The safety profile was monitored in each study through reporting of adverse events and was consistent across the three studies. Subjects who underwent BT experienced a significantly higher rate of adverse events during the treatment period compared with control groups. Most adverse events occurred within 1 day of the procedure, resolved within 7 days, and were reported as mild, such as wheezing, cough, dyspnea, and sputum production. There were also more serious events. The RISA study reported that 4/15 (27%) BT subjects had at least one hospitalization during the treatment period, compared with none in the control group. These hospitalizations were for asthma exacerbations or partial lobar collapse in lower lobes that occurred 1 to 2 days after BT. In AIR2, 8.4% of BT patients required hospitalization during the treatment period, mostly because of worsening asthma symptoms or segmental atelectasis, compared with 2% in the sham group. In contrast, during the post-treatment periods, the BT group did not experience an increase in the rate of adverse events and, as described previously, may have seen improvement in respiratory symptoms.[52–54]

Open Label Extension Studies

An open-label component of the AIR study continued to follow BT subjects up to 5 years post-procedure and control subjects up to 3 years post-procedure to monitor for safety (AIR Extension Trial). A total of 87% of BT subjects and 49% of control subjects enrolled in the extension trial. The year 1 data, which was the focus of the initial study, served as comparison data for matched pairs. Subjects were also asked about changes in maintenance medications, exacerbations necessitating emergent medication regimens, and any ED or hospital admissions related to asthma. These events were confirmed in the electronic medical record when possible (80% of subjects). Across years 2 to 5 of the extension study, for BT subjects, the rate of respiratory-related adverse events (adverse events/subject) remained stable. This rate could not be compared with the year 1 rate because during year 1, individual symptoms were recorded rather than events, prohibiting numerical comparison. There was no significant difference in the adverse event rate between the BT subjects and control subjects during years 2 to 3 (when control subjects were followed). There were no significant differences in ED or hospitalization rates in BT subjects in years 2 to 5 compared with year 1 or in years 2 to 3 compared with control subjects. There was no significant difference in OCS use or maintenance medication use or FEV_1 or forced vital capacity in the BT group in years 2 to 5 compared with year 1 or in years 2 to 3 compared with the control group in years 2 to 3. Overall these data suggest a stable safety profile in the years following the BT treatment. The BT group showed a significantly higher PC_{20} compared with control subjects at years 2 and 3 that was not present at year 1.[55]

An extension of the RISA trial enrolled 14 of the 15 patients that had been randomized to undergo BT for an additional 4 years. Control patients were not included in the extension. Over the course of years 2 to 5, there was no significant change in the subjects' rate of adverse events, hospitalizations, or ED use compared with year 1 following the procedure. There was no development of radiographic abnormalities and no change in pre-bronchodilator or post-bronchodilator FEV_1. The authors concluded that there was no deterioration in lung function or structural compromise in the 5 years following BT treatment.[56]

Two studies followed AIR2 subjects out beyond the initial 1-year study. The first enrolled 92% of the initial BT subjects to follow for a second year to evaluate for the persistence of treatment effect in a noninferiority study comparing the proportion of subjects who experienced a severe exacerbation during year 2 with year 1. The year 2 data showed no inferiority compared with year 1 in terms of proportions and rates of severe exacerbations, asthma symptoms, and respiratory-related ED visits.[57] Another study followed BT subjects out for a total of 5 years after the treatment period. During this extended period, patients were contacted by telephone every 3 months to assess for exacerbations, ED visits, hospitalizations, need for OCS, or change in maintenance medications. Patients who had had high-resolution computed tomography (CT) at baseline and after year 1 also had one at year 3 and year 5. The results showed no significant change in the proportion of subjects with a severe exacerbation over years 2 to 5 and preservation of the improvement in severe exacerbation rates in year 1 compared with the year before BT. The same pattern was found for the proportion of patients who experienced respiratory-related ED visits or hospitalizations. The prebronchodilator and post-bronchodilator spirometry remained stable through 5 years. Most patients who had high-resolution CT imaging throughout the study showed either no change or improvement in year 5 compared with baseline.[58]

Limitations and Conclusions

There are some important considerations that have limited the interpretation of the pivotal BT studies and therefore of BT itself. Perhaps the most commonly mentioned criticism is the lack of and difficulty in achieving a study with a true placebo control. In AIR and RISA, the control groups did not undergo procedures and were managed medically, which could bias the self-reported data from these trials compared with a nontreated control group. In addition, even though the control group did undergo a sham procedure in the AIR2 trial, some critics have questioned whether this study was truly blinded given that the BT procedure is often accompanied by increased dyspnea, cough, wheezing, and other respiratory symptoms that would likely clue a study participant in to his or her study group assignment. Another criticism regarding AIR2 questioned whether the statistical analysis reflected clinical significance[59] and whether it was appropriate to report comparisons of outcomes not matched at baseline.[60] Thus it is difficult to conclude with certainty whether BT improves asthma outcomes. This equipoise should be shared with patients in whom the procedure is considered.

To help clinicians assimilate the data from the three previously mentioned trials, a meta-analysis[61] examined the studies, which had largely overlapping patient characteristics and data collection points. A total of 429 participants were included. The authors found that BT results in a modest but not significant clinical benefit in quality of life, with a mean difference in AQLQ score of 0.28 (95% confidence interval, 0.07–0.5), and in asthma control, with a mean difference in ACQ score of −0.15 (95% confidence interval, −0.4 to 0.1). They also found a modest decrease in exacerbation rates, which came from comparisons of year 1 data with baseline in the AIR and RISA trials, and a comparison of the BT with sham group in the AIR2 trial. They noted that patients who underwent BT had a greater risk of hospitalization during the treatment period, with a risk ratio of 3.5, but that overall the procedure has a reasonable safety profile after the completion of the treatment period.[61] These data were not conclusive enough to encourage the routine use of BT in practice and instead demonstrated the need for further studies, particularly on the appropriate patient population and mechanism of the procedure.

The previously mentioned meta-analysis reflected that none of the studies showed a significant improvement in pulmonary function parameters, including prebronchodilator or post-bronchodilator FEV_1 or PC_{20}, following BT.[61] This was a puzzling result because the procedure was developed in response to the canine experiment by Danek and colleagues,[46] which showed a significant and sustained improvement in PC_{20} following the application of radiofrequency to the airways. This improvement is thought to reflect the decrease in bronchoconstrictive smooth muscle leading to a reduction in hyperresponsiveness and not an improvement in airflow (bronchodilation). In the human trials, however, there was no improvement in obstruction or hyperresponsiveness, making it difficult to explain the physiologic mechanism behind any observed clinical benefit.[62] In a meta-analysis comparing 5-year follow-up data from the open-label extension trials with 1-year data, the authors again found no significant change in prebronchodilator or post-bronchodilator FEV_1.[63] A limitation of the extension trials, however, was that with the exception of 2 years of the AIR Extension Trial, control subjects were not included.

MECHANISM OF ACTION

Given the lack of physiologic changes in AIR, RISA, and AIR2, there has been significant interest and debate about the mechanism of action of BT that could explain the improved clinical outcomes demonstrated in the pivotal trials.

Bronchial Wall Analyses

The first effort to study the histology of the airway wall before and after BT was conducted by Preto-lani and colleagues.[64] Endobronchial biopsies were obtained from 10 patients before and 3 months after BT. Histologic comparisons included ASM area, which was assessed by morphometry on alpha-actin-stained biopsy sections and expressed as ASM area over total biopsy area. The results showed a significant reduction in ASM after BT that ranged between 48.7% and 78.5% and was consistent across all lung areas (BT and non-BT treated areas). This finding was subsequently reproduced,[64] and, in another study, persisted on biopsies taken 27 to 48 months after the procedure.[65] That BT leads to a loss of ASM area is not surprising given prior observations.[46,51] Unexpectedly, however, the ASM reduction seen in the treated lobes was also seen in the right middle lobe, which was not treated, in 70% of the patients. The authors proposed that the mechanism was the diffusion of thermal energy generated by the procedure through incomplete interlobular fissures.

Another hypothesis for the mechanism of BT is that the application of radiofrequency energy has a generalized effect on the neuromuscular innervation to the smooth muscle compartment throughout the airway. In a study of 12 subjects, endobronchial biopsies showed a significant reduction of nerve fibers in the submucosa and ASM compared with baseline, suggesting that nerve ablation may contribute to the beneficial effects of BT.[66]

Any explanation for the effect of BT must consider that it is a procedure performed on the large airways but seems to affect asthma, which is a disease predominantly of small- and medium-sized airways. It has been proposed that pulmonary pacemakers that control ASM contractility reside in the proximal airways. Ablation of this pacemaker function, therefore, may explain downstream small airway effects.[67]

Inflammation

In addition to BT's effect on the contribution of ASM to abnormal bronchoconstriction in asthma,[68] the possibility that it's mechanism of action could also impact ASM's potent immunomodulatory role in airway inflammation remains an important consideration.[69] Attempts to characterize the changes in a variety of airway components following BT have hoped to explain the procedure's effects on inflammation. A small patient series demonstrated an increase in $CD4^+$ $CD25^+$ T-regulatory cells following BT, which could lead to decreased cytokines and eosino-philia.[70] Examination of bronchoalveolar lavage fluid and endobronchial biopsies of 11 subjects at 3 and 6 weeks after BT, compared with baseline, showed a significant decrease in transforming growth factor-β1 and RANTES and an increase in TRAIL.[71] More studies are needed to characterize the implications of these changes.

USE IN CLINICAL PRACTICE
Real World Data

The FDA approved BT in 2010.[72] It remains unclear whether real patient populations experience the same safety and efficacy of BT as those in the clinical trials. Results from small case series of nontrial patients have yielded variable results. One study found that fewer patient achieved clinical improvement after BT compared with patients from the AIR1, RISA, or AIR2 trials.[73,74] Another showed that a higher proportion of patients from a British registry experienced adverse events compared with the clinical trial patients.[75] The discrepancies were attributed to the treatment of an older and sicker population in real practice. In contrast, other series have shown significant improvement in control and quality-of-life scores, severe exacerbation rates, and controller medication use at 12 months compared with the year before BT.[64,73]

The Post-FDA Approval Clinical Trial Evaluating Bronchial Thermoplasty in Severe Persistent Asthma (PAS2) study is a prospective, open-label, multicenter observational clinical trial to assess the short- and long-term safety and efficacy of BT in clinical practice by following patients for 5 years.[76] The patients are contacted by telephone every 3 months to discuss asthma control and adverse events and seen annually for a physical examination and spirometry. An interim analysis comparing the PAS2 with AIR2 population showed the patients to be older, more obese, and taking more controller medications (ICS, OCS, and omalizumab) before BT. Following treatment, subjects followed in PAS2 showed significant decreases in ICS and OCS doses and decreases in severe exacerbations and hospitalizations in year 3 compared with the year before BT. Consistent with prior studies, there was no change in prebronchodilator or post-bronchodilator FEV_1 following BT. The adverse effect profile mimicked that seen in AIR2. The last patients are expected to exit the study in January 2020. Responder analyses hope to characterize those patients who particularly benefit from BT and may include stratification, such as by blood inflammatory markers.

Complications

As BT moves into clinical practice, expected and unexpected adverse events have been reported (**Fig. 2**). The adverse events during the treatment period seen in the clinical trials were mostly mild and self-limited and included dyspnea, wheezing, respiratory tract infection, and atelectasis.[52–54] A case report of a "real life" patient described a 43-year-old woman[77] who developed a lung abscess 3 days after BT. Another reported recurrent bronchial plugging with lobar collapse and respiratory failure shortly following both of two BT procedures in a 49-year-old man.[78] Interestingly, the bronchial plug was not composed of mucous but predominantly of fibrin mixed with inflammatory cells. A pulmonary cyst complicated by pneumothorax formed in a 47-year-old man in the setting of bilateral upper lobe atelectasis following BT; this resolved with chest tube insertion and reinflation of the upper lobes.[79] A ruptured bronchial artery pseudoaneurysm was reported in a 66-year-old woman 3 days after BT, following the initiation of unfractionated heparin for an acute pulmonary embolism. The pseudoaneurysm was successfully embolized. Bronchial artery pseudoaneurysm is a rare entity[80] but has been reported to occur following the use of radiofrequency energy for

ablation of a metastatic lung tumor,[80] suggesting a possible thermal mechanism. One reported adverse event in the AIR2 study was hemoptysis treated with bronchial artery embolization[54]; it is unclear whether this was related to a pseudoaneurysm.

Cost Considerations

In addition to possible adverse events, the financial cost of BT must be considered. The procedure requires endoscopy space, a multidisciplinary team, and procedural expertise, and as such is only cost effective in the proper patient population.[81] A cost analysis of a hypothetical cohort of patients with severe asthma in a third-party payer system in Italy calculated that the high cost of BT versus standard of care during the first year would be offset by reduced spending in the third and fourth years, resulting in net savings by the fifth year.[82] Multiple cost-effectiveness analyses using Markov modeling have shown a high probability that BT is cost effective compared with high-dose combination therapy among patients with severe asthma[81,83] or omalizumab among patients with severe allergic asthma.[84] The consistency of these results is unclear, however, given considerable variation in figures including the estimated procedural cost, which ranged from $6690 in the

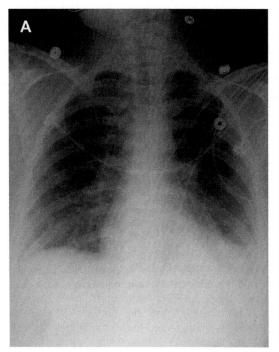
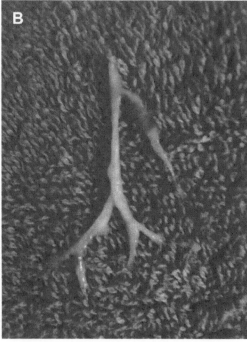

Fig. 2. Complications of bronchial thermoplasty. (*A*) Chest radiograph showing left lower lung collapse 1 day following bronchial thermoplasty procedure. (*B*) Bronchial cast expectorated 2 weeks post-bronchial thermoplasty.

study by Zein and colleagues[81] to $14,500 in Zafari and colleagues.[84]

Securing insurance coverage for BT requires proving that it is reasonable and necessary. Until a few years ago, the Current Procedural Terminology code for BT was in category III, which consists of temporary codes for emerging technology, services, or procedures.[85] It is now category I, which indicates consistency with current medical practice and performance with adequate frequency.[86] Boston Scientific reports that some payers are covering the procedure, whereas others may or may not cover it with preauthorization. Medicare includes BT as part of a covered benefit category and has approved the procedure for qualified patients nationwide, but does not have a formal coverage policy for the procedure.[87]

Role of Bronchial Thermoplasty in the Biologics Era

As more therapies develop for severe asthma, selecting the proper management strategy for a given patient depends on various characteristics. Severe asthma is clinically and phenotypically diverse[88,89]; this heterogeneity may not be adequately addressed in stepwise management plans, such as the GINA guidelines.[2] In an endorsement of phenotyping patients with asthma to help guide treatment, in 2017 a consensus panel published a recommendation for testing IgE level, blood eosinophils, and possibly sputum eosinophils or fractional exhaled nitric oxide at the time of asthma diagnosis, rather than when it becomes difficult to treat.[30] This testing is important because allergic or inflammatory asthma may respond to cytokine-targeted biologic therapies, whereas patients with nonphenotyped asthma are unlikely to benefit from biologics.[90]

In contrast to biologic therapies, the American Thoracic Society/European Respiratory Society guidelines recommended that BT be performed only in the context of an institutional review board–approved independent systematic registry or clinical study because evidence remains inadequate.[8] This approach has not been widely adopted in the United States or other countries and has contributed to a decline in preauthorization for the procedure in the United States. BT can be considered before regular OCS treatment of nonallergic or noninflammatory asthma, or in the case of biologic therapy failure in patients with allergic or eosinophilic asthma.[30] Patients may prefer BT to biologics because it is completed in three sessions in contrast to the burden of taking an injected therapy indefinitely.[91] As with other advanced asthma therapies, proper patient selection is

central to the success of BT,[92] but remains a challenge. There is currently no definitive clinical, imaging, or biologic marker to predict how patients will respond to BT.[93] Parameters of multidetector CT, such as air trapping, lung density, and airway wall thickness, may correlate with clinical improvement following BT[94,95] but require further studies.

In addition to BT, another nonpharmacologic technique under investigation for chronic lung disease is targeted lung denervation, a bronchoscopic technique whose goal is to ablate the pulmonary parasympathetic innervation that normally contributes to ASM tone, mucous secretion, and potentially inflammation.[96] The procedure involves delivery of radiofrequency energy through a cooled catheter (Nuvaira, Inc, Minneapolis, MN) during two bronchoscopies 30 days apart. The safety and efficacy of this procedure have been investigated in patients with chronic obstructive pulmonary disease[97,98] but it has not been reported in asthma; studies in Europe are ongoing.

SUMMARY

BT is a device-based advanced therapy for severe asthma that has been shown to significantly reduce ASM mass. Data from large randomized trials and smaller real-world patient series have shown promising short- and long-term clinical benefit and have consistently shown an acceptable short- and long-term safety profile. Although in the initial canine studies BT reduced airway hyperresponsiveness, the procedure in humans has not resulted in improvement in lung function parameters. Thus, a complete understanding of the physiologic mechanism of BT in asthma remains unclear. As the understanding of asthma changes and the role of ASM in asthma is further elucidated, a population of patients with severe asthma may emerge of particularly appropriate candidates for treatment with BT. Until then, BT remains a safe nonpharmacologic option for the properly selected patient with severe asthma.

REFERENCES

1. Panettierei RA, Kotlikoff MI, Gerthoffer WT, et al. Airway smooth muscle in bronchial tone, inflammation, and remodeling: basic knowledge to clinical relevance. Am J Respir Crit Care Med 2008; 177(3):248–52.
2. Global Initiative for Asthma. Global strategy for asthma management and prevention. 2017.
3. Lozano R, Naghavi M, Foreman K, et al. Global and regional mortality from 235 causes of death for 20 age groups in 1990 and 2010: a systematic analysis

for the Global Burden of Disease Study. Lancet 2010;380:2095–128.

4. Anandan C, Nurmatov U, van Schayck OC, et al. Is the prevalence of asthma declining? Systematic review of epidemiological studies. Allergy 2010; 65(2):152–67.

5. Sears MR. Trends in the prevalence of asthma. Chest 2014;145(2):219–25.

6. Nurmagambetov T, Kuwahara R, Garbe P. The economic burden of asthma in the United States, 2008-2013. Ann Am Thorac Soc 2018;15(3):348–56.

7. Cisternas MG, Blanc PD, Yen IH, et al. A comprehensive study of the direct and indirect costs of adult asthma. J Allergy Clin Immunol 2003;111(6):1212–8.

8. Chung KF, Wenzel SE, Brozek JL, et al. International ERS/ATS guidelines on definition, evaluation and treatment of severe asthma. Eur Respir J 2014; 43(2):343–73.

9. Bel EH, Sousa A, Fleming L, et al. Diagnosis and definition of severe refractory asthma: an international consensus statement from the Innovative Medicine Initiative (IMI). Thorax 2011;66:910–7.

10. Araujo AC, Ferraz E, Borges MC, et al. Investigation of factors associated with difficult-to-control asthma. J Bras Pneumol 2007;33(5):495–501.

11. Sheehan W, Phipatanakul W. Difficult to control asthma: epidemiology and its link with environmental factors. Curr Opin Allergy Clin Immunol 2015;15(5):397–401.

12. Haahtela T, Jarvenin M, Kava T, et al. Comparison of a beta 2-agonist, terbutaline, with an inhaled corticosteroid, budesonide, in newly detected asthma. N Engl J Med 1991;325(6):388–92.

13. Sin DD, Man J, Sharpe H, et al. Pharmacological management to reduce exacerbations in adults with asthma: a systematic review and meta-analysis. JAMA 2004;292(3):367–76.

14. Moore WC, Bleecker ER, Curran-Everett D, et al, National Heart, Lung, Blood Institute's Severe Asthma Research Program. Characterization of the severe asthma phenotype by the National Heart, Lung, and Blood Institute's Severe Asthma Research Program. J Allergy Clin Immunol 2007; 119(2):405–13.

15. Pain M, Bermudez O, Lacoste P, et al. Tissue remodelling in chronic bronchial diseases: from the epithelial to mesenchymal phenotype. Eur Respir Rev 2014;23(131):118–30.

16. Johnson SR, Knox AJ. Synthetic functions of airway smooth muscle cells in asthma. Trends Pharmacol Sci 1997;18(8):288–92.

17. Fehrenbach H, Wagner C, Wegmann M. Airway remodeling in asthma: what really matters. Cell Tissue Res 2017;367(3):551–69.

18. Prakash YS. Emerging concepts in smooth muscle contributions to airway structure and function: implications for health and disease. Am J Physiol Lung Cell Mol Physiol 2016;311(6):L1113–40.

19. Huber H, Koessler K. The pathology of bronchial asthma. Arch Intern Med (Chic) 1922;30(6): 689–760.

20. Bergeron C, Boulet LP. Structural changes in airway diseases: characteristics, mechanism, consequences, and pharmacologic modulation. Chest 2006;129:1068–87.

21. Kuwano K, Bosken CH, Pare PD, et al. Small airways dimensions in asthma and in chronic obstructive pulmonary disease. Am Rev Respir Dis 1993; 148(5):1220–5.

22. Roche WR, Beasley R, Williams JH, et al. Subepithelial fibrosis in the bronchi of asthmatics. Lancet 1989;1(8637):520–4.

23. Brewster CE, Howarth PH, Djukanovic R, et al. Myofibroblasts and subepithelial fibrosis in bronchial asthma. Am J Respir Cell Mol Biol 1990;3(5):507–11.

24. Benayoun L, Druilhe A, Dombret MC, et al. Airway structural alterations selectively associated with severe asthma. Am J Respir Crit Care Med 2003; 167(10):1360–8.

25. Elias JA, Zhu Z, Chupp G, et al. Airway remodeling in asthma. J Clin Invest 1999;104(8):1001–6.

26. Wenzel S. Asthma: defining of the persistent adult phenotypes. Lancet 2006;368(9537):804–13.

27. Barlow JL, McKenzie AN. Type-2 innate lymphoid cells in human allergic disease. Curr Opin Allergy Clin Immunol 2014;14(5):397–403.

28. Robinson D, Humbert M, Buhl R, et al. Revisiting type 2-high and type 2-ow airway inflammation in asthma: current knowledge and therapeutic implications. Clin Exp Allergy 2017;47(2):161–75.

29. King GG, James A, Harkness L, et al. Pathophysiology of severe asthma: we've only just started. Respirology 2018;23(3):262–71.

30. Blaiss MS, Castro M, Chipps BE, et al. Guiding principles for use of newer biologic and bronchial thermoplasty for patients with severe asthma. Ann Allergy Asthma Immunol 2017;119(6):533–40.

31. Normansell R, Walker S, Milan SJ, et al. Omalizumab for asthma in adults and children. Cochrane Database Syst Rev 2014;(1):CD003559.

32. Haldar P, Brightling CE, Hargadon B, et al. Mepolizumab and exacerbations of refractory eosinophilic asthma. N Engl J Med 2009;360(10):973.

33. Castro M, Zangrilli J, Wechsler ME, et al. Reslizumab for inadequately controlled asthma with elevated eosinophil counts: results from two multicentre, parallel, double-blind, randomised, placebo-controlled, phase 3 trials. Lancet Respir Med 2015;3(5):355–66.

34. Ferguson GT, FitzGerald JM, Bleecker ER, et al, BISE Study Investigators. BISE Study Investigators, Benralizumab for patients with mild to moderate, persistent asthma (BISE): a randomised,

double-blind, placebo-controlled, phase 3 trial. Lancet Respir Med 2017;5(7):568–76.

35. Ebina M, Takahashi T, Chiba T, et al. Cellular hypertrophy and hyperplasia of airway smooth muscles underlying bronchial asthma. A 3-D morphometric study. Am Rev Respir Dis 1993; 148(3):720–6.

36. Hirst SJ. Regulation of airway smooth muscle cell immunomodulatory function: role in asthma. Respir Physiol Neurobiol 2003;137(2–3):309–26.

37. James AL, Elliot JG, Jones RL, et al. Airway smooth muscle hypertrophy and hyperplasia in asthma. Am J Respir Crit Care Med 2012; 185(10):1058–64.

38. Tang DD. Critical role of actin-associated proteins in smooth muscle contraction, cell proliferation, airway hyperresponsiveness and airway remodeling. Respir Res 2015;16:134.

39. Dulin NO, Fernandes DJ, Dowell M, et al. What evidence implicates airway smooth muscle in the cause of BHR? Clin Rev Allergy Immunol 2003; 24(1):73–84.

40. Ma X, Cheng Z, Kong H, et al. Changes in biophysical and biochemical properties of single bronchial smooth muscle cells from asthmatic subjects. Am J Physiol Lung Cell Mol Physiol 2002;283(6): L1181–9.

41. Tliba O, Panettieri RA Jr. Noncontractile functions of airway smooth muscle cells in asthma. Annu Rev Physiol 2009;71:509–35.

42. Xia YC, Redhu NS, Moir LM, et al. Pro-inflammatory and immunomodulatory functions of airway smooth muscle: emerging concepts. Pulm Pharmacol Ther 2013;26(1):64–74.

43. Naveed SU, Clements D, Jackson DJ, et al. Metrix metalloproteinase-1 activation contributes to airway smooth muscle growth and asthma severity. Am J Respir Crit Care Med 2017; 195(8):1000–9.

44. Seow CY, Fredberg JJ. Historical perspective on airway smooth muscle: the saga of a frustrated cell. J Appl Physiol 2001;91:938–52.

45. Ni Y, Mulier S, Maio Y, et al. A review of the general aspects of radiofrequency ablation. Abdom Imaging 2005;30(4):381–400.

46. Danek CJ, Lombard CM, Dungworth DL, et al. Reduction in airway hyperresponsiveness to methacholine by the application of RF energy in dogs. J Appl Physiol 2004;97(5):1946–53.

47. Pedley TJ, Schroter RC, Sudlow MF. The prediction of pressure drop and variation of resistance within the human bronchial airways. Respir Physiol 1970; 9(3):387–405.

48. Cox PG, Miller J, Mitzner W, et al. Radiofrequency ablation of airway smooth muscle for sustained treatment of asthma: preliminary investigation. Eur Respir J 2004;24(4):659–63.

49. Kwon KY, Myers JL, Swensen SJ, et al. Middle lobe syndrome: a clinicopathological study of 21 patients. Hum Pathol 1995;26(3):302–7.

50. Cox G, Miller JD, McWilliams A, et al. Bronchial thermoplasty for asthma. Am J Respir Crit Care Med 2006;173(9):965–9.

51. Miller JD, Cox G, Vincic L, et al. A prospective feasibility study of bronchial thermoplasty in the human airway. Chest 2005;127(6):1999–2006.

52. Cox G, Thomson NC, Rubin AS, et al, AIR Trial Study Group. Asthma control during the year after bronchial thermoplasty. N Engl J Med 2007;356(13): 1327–37.

53. Pavord ID, Cox G, Thomson NC, et al, RISA Trial Study Group. Safety and efficacy of bronchial thermoplasty in symptomatic, severe asthma. Am J Respir Crit Care Med 2007;176(12):1185–91.

54. Castro M, Rubin AS, Laviolette M, et al, AIR2 Trial Study Group. Effectiveness and safety of bronchial thermoplasty in the treatment of severe asthma: a multicenter, randomized, double-blind, sham-controlled clinical trial. Am J Respir Crit Care Med 2010;181(2):116–24.

55. Thomson NC, Rubin AS, Niven RM, et al, AIR Trial Study Group. Long-term (5 year) safety of bronchial thermoplasty: asthma intervention research (AIR) trial. BMC Pulm Med 2011;11:8.

56. Pavord ID, Thomson NC, Niven RM, et al, RISA Trial Study Group. Safety of bronchial thermoplasty in patients with severe refractory asthma. Ann Allergy Asthma Immunol 2013;111(5):402–7.

57. Castro M, Rubin A, Laviolette M, et al, AIR2 Trial Study Group. Persistence of effectiveness of bronchial thermoplasty in patients with severe asthma. Ann Allergy Asthma Immunol 2011; 107(1):65–70.

58. Wechsler ME, Laviolette M, Rubin AS, et al, AIR2 Trial Study Group. Bronchial thermoplasty: long-term safety and effectiveness in patients with severe persistent asthma. J Allergy Clin Immunol 2013; 132(6):1295–302.

59. Bel EH, Zwinderman AH. Outcome reporting in asthma research. Am J Respir Crit Care Med 2011;183(1):132.

60. Ibrahim W. Bronchial thermoplasty: misleading differences in asthma exacerbation rates! Chest 2016;149(2):608–9.

61. Torrego A, Sola I, Munoz AM, et al. Bronchial thermoplasty for moderate to severe persistent asthma in adults. Cochrane Database Syst Rev 2014;(3): CD009910.

62. Bel EH. Bronchial thermoplasty: has the promise been met? Am J Respir Crit Care Med 2010; 181(2):101–2.

63. Zhou JP, Feng Y, Wang Q, et al. Long term efficacy and safety of bronchial thermoplasty in patients with moderate-to-severe persistent asthma: a systemic

review and meta-analysis. J Asthma 2016;53(1): 94–100.

64. Pretolani M, Bergqvist A, Thabut G, et al. Effectiveness of bronchial thermoplasty in patients with severe refractory asthma: clinical and histopathologic correlations. J Allergy Clin Immunol 2017;139(4): 1176–85.

65. Salem IH, Boulet LP, Biardel S, et al. Long-term effects of bronchial thermoplasty on airway smooth muscle and reticular basement membrane thickness in severe asthma. Ann Am Thorac Soc 2016;13(8): 1426–8.

66. Facciolongo N, DiStefano A, Pietrini V, et al. Nerve ablation after bronchial thermoplasty and sustained improvement in severe asthma. BMC Pulm Med 2018;18(1):29.

67. Jesudason EC. Airway smooth muscle: an architect of the lung? Thorax 2009;64(6):541–5.

68. d'Hooghe JNS, Ten Hacken NHT, Weersink EJM, et al. Emerging understanding of the mechanism of action of bronchial thermoplasty in asthma. Pharmacol Ther 2018;181:101–7.

69. Hirst SJ. Regulation of airway smooth muscle cell immunomodulatory function: role in asthma. Respir Physiol Neurobiol 2003;137(2–3):309–26.

70. Marc Malovrh M, Rozman A, Skrgat S, et al. Bronchial thermoplasty induces immunomodulation with a significant increase in pulmonary CD4+25+ regulatory T cells. Ann Allergy Asthma Immunol 2017; 119(3):289–90.

71. Denner DR, Doeing DC, Hogarth DK, et al. Airway inflammation after bronchial thermoplasty for severe asthma. Ann Am Thorac Soc 2015;12(9):1302–9.

72. Chrisy Foreman, Acting Director, Office of Device Evaluation, Food and Drug Administration, Silver Spring, MD. Letter to Debera Brown, Vice President, Regulatory Affairs, Asthmatx, Inc, Sunnyvale, CA. 2010.

73. Arrigo R, Failla G, Scichilone N, et al. How effective and safe is bronchial thermoplasty in "real life" asthmatics compared to those enrolled in randomized controlled trials? Biomed Res Int 2016;2016: 9132198.

74. Bicknell S, Chaudhuri R, Lee N, et al. Effectiveness of bronchial thermoplasty in severe asthma in "real life" patients compared to those recruited to clinical trials in the same centre. Ther Adv Respir Dis 2015; 9(6):267–71.

75. Burn J, Sims AJ, Keltie K, et al. Procedural and short-term safety of bronchial thermoplasty in clinical practice: evidence from a national registry and Hospital Episode Statistics. J Asthma 2017;54(8): 872–9.

76. Chupp G, Laviolette M, Cohn L, et al, Other Members of the PAS2 Study Group. Long-term outcomes of bronchial thermoplasty in subjects with severe asthma: a comparison of 3-year follow-up results

from two prospective multicentre studies. Eur Respir J 2017;50(2) [pii:1700017].

77. Balu A, Ryan D, Niven R. Lung abscess as a complication of bronchial thermoplasty. J Asthma 2015; 52(7):740–2.

78. Facciolongo N, Menzella F, Lusuardi M, et al. Recurrent lung atelectasis from fibrin plugs as a very early complication of bronchial thermoplasty: a case report. Multidiscip Respir Med 2015;10(1):9.

79. Funatsu A, Kobayashi K, Iikura M, et al. A case of pulmonary cyst and pneumothorax after bronchial thermoplasty. Respirol Case Rep 2017;6(2):e00286.

80. Restrepo CS, Carswell AP. Aneurysms and pseudoaneurysms of the pulmonary vasculature. Semin Ultrasound CT MR 2012;33(6):552–66.

81. Zein JG, Menegay MC, Singer ME, et al. Cost effectiveness of bronchial thermoplasty in patients with severe uncontrolled asthma. J Asthma 2016;53(2):194–200.

82. Menzella F, Zucchi L, Piro R, et al. A budget impact analysis of bronchial thermoplasty for severe asthma in clinical practice. Adv Ther 2014;31(7):751–61.

83. Cangelosi MJ, Ortendahl JD, Meckley LM, et al. Cost-effectiveness of bronchial thermoplasty in commercially-insured patients with poorly controlled, severe, persistent asthma. Expert Rev Pharmacoecon Outcomes Res 2015;15(2):357–64.

84. Zafari Z, Sadatsafavi M, Marra C, et al. Cost-effectiveness of bronchial thermoplasty, omalizumab, and standard therapy for moderate-to-severe allergic asthma. PLoS One 2016;11(1):e0146003.

85. Mahajan AK, Hogarth DK. Payer coverage for bronchial thermoplasty: shifting the traditional paradigm for refractory asthma therapy. Chest 2013;14(3):1051–4.

86. American Medical Association. Criteria for CPT Category I and Category III Codes. 2018. Available at: https://www.ama-assn.org/practice-management/criteria-cpt-category-i-and-category-iii-codes. Accessed February 1, 2018.

87. Boston Scientific. 2017 coding & payment quick reference: bronchial thermoplasty. 2017.

88. Moore WC, Meyers DA, Wenzel SE, et al, National Heart, Lung, and Blood Institute's Severe Asthma Research Program. Identification of asthma phenotypes using cluster analysis in the severe asthma research program. Am J Respir Crit Care Med 2010;181(4):315–23.

89. Chung KF. Asthma phenotyping: a necessity for improved therapeutic precision and new targeted therapies. J Intern Med 2016;279(2):192–204.

90. Fajt ML, Wenzel SE. Biologic therapy in asthma: entering the new age of personalized medicine. J Asthma 2014;51(7):669–76.

91. Trivedi A, Pavord ID, Castro M. Bronchial thermoplasty and biological therapy as targeted treatments for severe uncontrolled asthma. Lancet 2016;4(7):585–92.

92. Menzella F, Galeone C, Bertolini F, et al. Innovative treatments for severe refractory asthma: how to

choose the right option for the right patient? J Asthma Allergy 2017;10:237–47.

93. Beghe B, Fabbri LM, Controll M, et al. Update in asthma 2016. Am J Respir Crit Care Med 2017;196(5):548–57.

94. Sarikonda K, Sheshadri A, Koch T, et al. Predictors of bronchial thermoplasty response in patients with severe refractory asthma. Minisymposium B13. Mechanisms and Treatment Considerations for Severe Asthma, 2014.

95. Zanon M, Strieder DL, Rubin AS, et al. Use of MDCT to assess the results of bronchial thermoplasty. Am J Roentgenol 2017;209(4):752–6.

96. Kistemaker LE, Slebos DJ, Meurs H, et al. Anti-inflammatory effects of targeted lung denervation in patients with COPD. Eur Respir J 2015;46(5): 1489–92.

97. Koegelenberg CF, Theron J, Slebos DJ, et al. Antimuscarinic bronchodilator response retained after bronchoscopic vagal denervation in chronic obstructive pulmonary disease patients. Respiration 2016;92(1):58–60.

98. Slebos DJ, Klooster K, Koegelenberg CF, et al. Targeted lung denervation for moderate to severe COPD: a pilot study. Thorax 2015;70(5):411–9.

The Use of Geographic Data to Improve Asthma Care Delivery and Population Health

Margaret E. Samuels-Kalow, MD, MPhil, MSHP[a],*,
Carlos A. Camargo Jr, MD, DrPH[b]

KEYWORDS

- Asthma • Geographic information system • Spatial epidemiology • Care delivery
- Population health

KEY POINTS

- Geographic data are increasingly used to examine asthma risk factors and care delivery and to develop and test interventions.
- There are significant methodological challenges to using geographic data that need to be carefully addressed.
- The advent of smaller geographic positioning system units and novel data linkage strategies holds promise for improving asthma care delivery and population health.

INTRODUCTION

Geographic, or place-based, analyses can be used for epidemiologic analyses of asthma risk factors (exposures) and disease clustering,[1,2] for better understanding care delivery and health system factors, and to develop and test interventions to improve care. Geographic information systems (GIS) are computer programs that enable the manipulation of geographic and place-based information. Nongeographic data (such as income level or disease rate) can be described by geographic boundaries (such as zip code or census tract). Spatial data (such as the location of a home or hospital) can be assigned to a specific geographic location through geocoding.[3] GIS maps can describe relationships in several different ways, such as within a geographic boundary or at a particular distance from a feature (such as a hospital).[4] Maps can be layered to show relationships between different types of data (such as residential housing quality, asthma prevalence, emergency medical services response time) and can be used to understand how disease trends have changed over time, or to model areas at higher risk of exposure or disease.[5] Identification of geographic disease trends can prompt research questions about exposure risk or disease management strategies.[6] Multilevel modeling approaches allow researchers to examine asthma clustering by neighborhood, explore clustering of risk factors, and examine the relative importance of individual and neighborhood risk factors.[7,8]

A systematic review of GIS studies found that asthma was the second most common noninfectious disease analyzed (after cancer).[5] The goal of the current review was to assess the uses of

Disclosure Statement: The authors have no commercial relationships to disclose.
[a] Department of Emergency Medicine, Massachusetts General Hospital, Harvard Medical School, Zero Emerson Place Suite 104, Boston, MA 02114, USA; [b] Department of Emergency Medicine, Massachusetts General Hospital, Harvard Medical School, 125 Nashua Street, Suite 920, Boston MA 02114, USA
* Corresponding author.
E-mail address: msamuels-kalow@partners.org

Clin Chest Med 40 (2019) 209–225
https://doi.org/10.1016/j.ccm.2018.10.012

geographic data on asthma care delivery and population health, with a focus on methodology and technique, and to describe areas for future research.

Methods

The authors conducted a scoping review, which describes key concepts and sources of evidence and identifies areas for future research. Scoping reviews are often conducted when the literature of interest crosses multiple disciplines,[9] and they do not include a formal quality assessment or quantitative synthesis.[10] Instead, a scoping review provides a narrative synthesis to guide subsequent work.[10] The authors searched PubMed, Embase, Cochrane, and Web of Science for articles involving geographic analysis of asthma or asthma care delivery, geographic-based interventions for asthma, and proposed practice changes and research based on geographic data. **Table 1** shows the search strategy. One additional article was obtained by manual review of the table of contents for core journals following the initial search.

The authors aimed to capture studies focused on geomarkers, or "geographic measures that influence or predict the incidence of outcome or disease."[11] Articles were eligible for inclusion if they were available in English and involved asthma and geographic data or small area geographic analysis. Articles were excluded if they provided only summary data on "respiratory diseases" without separating out results for asthma or examined neighborhood effects without geographic analysis. For example, studies discussing neighborhood factors that were obtained without geographic analysis (ie, surveys asking people about neighborhood crime or exposure to violence) were not included.

The authors identified 5523 records, after duplicates were removed. All abstracts were reviewed for eligibility by the first author (M.S.K.), and 369 were determined to be potentially eligible for inclusion based on the abstract and were reviewed in full; 162 were included in the final article (**Fig. 1**). Papers were separated into those describing risk factors, care delivery/health system management, and potential interventions.

SUMMARY
Geographic Distribution of Asthma Risk Factors

Studies have reported variance in asthma prevalence by neighborhood that was not fully explained by standard risk factors (such as age, sex, race/ethnicity, household members with asthma, and income).[12,13] These findings suggest the importance of neighborhood-level risk factors, such as those shown in **Table 2**.

Environmental exposures

The influence of environmental risk factors on asthma prevalence and severity has been widely described.[13–15] For example, GIS modeling has been used for assessing exposure to traffic-related air pollution[16] and for improved estimates of air pollution in areas that do not have sampling stations.[17] Although some studies have not found an association between air pollution and asthma,[18–21] most have found that air pollution is linked to asthma outcomes.[22–29] Multiple studies have specifically examined the associations of traffic-related air pollution and roadway proximity with asthma.[30–45]

One study suggests that the distance from and type of traffic that infants are exposed to may be of particular importance in the development of wheeze[46] as compared with overall traffic volume. Urban land-use was associated with increased wheeze severity, but was no longer significant after adjustment for nitrogen dioxide levels, suggesting a strong role for traffic in the association between urban land-use and wheeze.[47] In addition, the relationship between traffic exposure and asthma may vary by race,[46] although it is unclear if that represents underlying differences in susceptibilities or unmeasured confounders.

GIS has also been used to investigate the association between tree canopy coverage and asthma, with some studies finding no effects[48] or associations with worse asthma[49] and others finding that trees[50] and green space was associated with less asthma or wheezing.[51,52]

Overall, geographic data provide the opportunity to link the spatial distribution of risk factors with asthma outcomes.

Socioeconomic status

Most, but not all,[53–55] studies with small area or neighborhood analysis have shown associations between asthma and socioeconomic factors, including poverty, race,[56–59] and violence.[11] Asthma hospitalization has been positively correlated with poverty rate and the proportion of nonwhite residents and inversely with income and education.[60,61] Even after controlling for socioeconomic status (SES) and urbanicity, the strong associations between black race and asthma persist.[62]

The associations between neighborhood factors and asthma in patients of Hispanic ethnicity are complex. One report suggested that neighborhood deprivation was associated with reduced odds of wheezing in urban children of Mexican

Table 1
Search strategy

Provider/Interface	NLM	Elsevier	Ovid	Clarivate Analytics
Database	PubMed	Embase	Cochrane library (EBM Reso)	Web of Science Core Collection
Items found	1986	3956	326	2715
Internal duplicates (within	9	N/A	0	N/A
External duplicates (between	0	1650	107	1694
Unique items found	1977	2316	219	1022
Search strategy	(asthma[tiab] OR asthma [MeSH]) AND (mapping [tiab] OR map[tiab] OR maps [tiab] OR mapped[tiab] OR geograph*[tiab] OR geospatial[tiab] OR GIS [tiab] OR mapping[OT] OR map[OT] OR maps[OT] OR mapped[OT] OR geograph* [OT] OR geospatial[OT] OR GIS[OT] OR "geographic mapping"[MeSH] OR "geographic information systems"[MeSH] OR "small area analysis"[MeSH] OR neighborhood*[tiab] OR neighborhood*[tiab] OR neighborhood*[OT] OR neighborhood*[OT]) NOT ("gene mapping"[tiab] OR "genetic mapping"[tiab])	asthma'/exp OR asthma:ab,ti geographic mapping'/de OR 'geographic distribution'/de OR 'geographic information system'/exp OR 'neighborhood'/exp OR mapping:ab,ti OR map:ab,ti OR maps:ab,ti OR	asthma.ti,ab. or exp asthma/ (mapping or map or maps or mapped or geograph* or geospatial or GIS or neighborhood* or neighborhood*).ti,ab. or geographic mapping/or geographic information	TOPIC: (asthma) TOPIC: (mapping or map or maps or mapped or geograph* or geospatial or GIS or neighborhood* or neighborhood*)

(continued on next page)

Table 1
(continued)

Provider/Interface	NLM	Elsevier	Ovid	Clarivate Analytics
		mapped:ab,ti OR geograph*:ab,ti OR geospatial:ab,ti OR gis:ab,ti OR neighborhood*:ab,ti OR neighborhood*:ab,ti gene mapping/exp OR 'gene mapping':ab,ti OR 'genetic mapping':ab,ti	systems/or small area analysis/ ("gene mapping" or "genetic mapping").ti,ab.	TOPIC: ("gene mapping" or "genetic mapping")
		#1 AND #2 #4 NOT #3	1 AND 2 NOT 3 remove duplicates from 4	(#1 AND #2) NOT #3

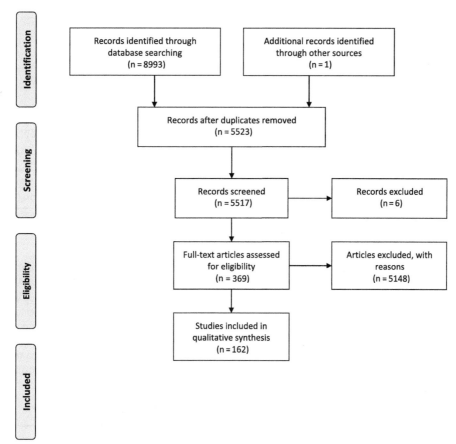

Fig. 1. PRISMA diagram.

descent.[63] In another study, geocoded addresses were used to examine the relations of acculturation and neighborhood ethnic density to asthma among Hispanic children. The study found that acculturation was a risk factor, but ethnic density was not.[64] Geocoded addresses have also been used to look at the relationship between immigration density and individual risk factors as predictors of wheezing, finding that higher neighborhood immigrant density was associated with reduced odds of wheezing.[65]

Beck and colleagues[66] developed a geographic risk index incorporating census tract poverty, home value, and education. Children with higher geographic risk had a higher likelihood of readmission for asthma[66] after adjustment for age, sex, insurance, and clustering.[66] Another multidimensional measure of child opportunity has also been associated with acute health care use for asthma.[67]

The density of asthma-relevant housing code violations (such as mold) was associated with asthma, even after adjustment for poverty, and explained 22% of the variation in asthma emergency department (ED) visits and hospitalizations.[68]

A combined score, including number of bedrooms, number of bathrooms, housing unit square footage, and taxable property value, was associated with uncontrolled asthma in a small (n = 58) study.[69]

There have been a few random or quasi-random assignments of families to neighborhoods that allow for an improved understanding of neighborhood effects with reduced risk of confounding. In the Moving to Opportunity randomized housing voucher experiment, being in the experimental (vouchers given) group did not improve asthma outcomes.[70,71] A natural experiment of quasi-random assignment of households to neighborhoods in the Denver Housing Authority investigated the direct effect of residential segregation (% of Latino and African American residents in housing tract) and indirect effects (SES, safety, housing stock, environmental conditions) on asthma.[72] Low-income African American children in a neighborhood with a higher percentage of African American residents had greater odds of an asthma diagnosis in their initial model, but lower odds when the remainder of the neighborhood context variables was included in the model. In

Table 2
Neighborhood level factors

Neighborhood Factors	Examples
Structural characteristics of buildings	State of repair, density
Infrastructure characteristics	Roads, sidewalks
Demographic characteristics of residents	Race/ethnicity
Class status characteristics of residents	Income, occupation, education
Public services	Schools, parks
Environmental characteristics	Environmental hazards
Proximity characteristics	Employment, grocery stores
Social interactive characteristics	Neighborhood cohesion, diversity

Data from DePriest K, Butz A. Neighborhood-level factors related to asthma in children living in urban areas. J Sch Nurs 2017;33(1):8–17.

particular, higher property crime rate and lower occupational prestige among residents were associated with higher odds of asthma diagnosis. The authors conclude that the "adverse developmental consequences of ethnic segregation appeared to be generated primarily by concentrating minority children in neighborhoods with higher rates of property crime and lower occupational prestige, not by higher minority concentrations per se."[72]

Environmental exposures and socioeconomic status

GIS research has often been used at the intersection of SES and environmental exposure, exploring questions of environmental injustice or the increased exposure of vulnerable communities to pollution and resulting effects on health.[73] Individuals living near sources of pollution have been found to have higher rates of asthma hospitalizations and are more likely to be poor or minority,[73] so it can be difficult to determine if asthma clusters are due to environmental pollution or SES factors or both.[74] For example, the association between urban land-use and wheeze was stronger for infants in low SES families, potentially relating to decreased access to air conditioning or decreased access to health care.[47] There may be also unmeasured aspects of the environmental and social context or diagnostic differences at the clinic level.[75]

Physiologic alterations from life stressors may underlie part of the causal pathway linking SES, environmental exposures, and disparities in asthma. For example, one study found an association between traffic-related air pollution and asthma only in children exposed to violence.[76] Other studies have reported that social factors modify the influence of environmental factors in predicting asthma.[77,78]

The intersection of environmental and SES factors is not limited to race or poverty. Recent work has demonstrated that after adjusting for racial/ethnic and SES, population density, urban location, and geographic clustering, living in census tracts with high proportions of same-sex partners is associated with significantly greater respiratory risks from hazardous air pollutants.[79]

Care Delivery and Health System Measurement

Geographic data have also been used for health system planning to optimize system capacity, public health, and prevention efforts.[5] One example is a Web-based application that enables the geographic monitoring of asthma symptoms, smoking rates, and pollution levels.[80] GIS data can also be used to improve epidemiologic surveillance of disease and identify potential disparities.[6] For example, prescription data from Medicaid and commercial pharmacies have been used to examine disparities in asthma in Chicago.[81] Particularly with prescription data, it is important to separate out regional variations in need for care from regional variations in care delivery.[82] For example, one study of children with Medicaid insurance found wide variation in inhaled corticosteroid use by area that was not explained by the measured demographic and clinical characteristics of the children in the area.[83]

Geographic data have been used to facilitate discussion among stakeholders to address asthma disparities in communities.[84] Appropriate selection of regions can improve data utility for policy making. For example, small area estimation has been used to create asthma symptom prevalence estimates for legislative districts,[85] and **Fig. 2** shows pediatric asthma prevalence per 100 students.

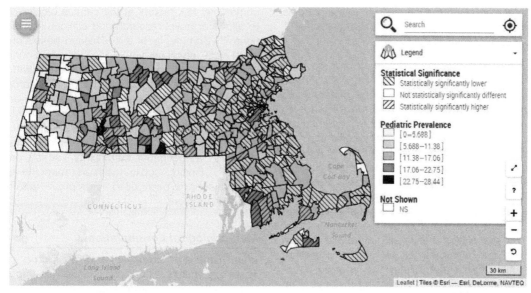

Fig. 2. Pediatric asthma prevalence per 100 students for school year 2014 to 2015. NS indicates number/prevalence not shown due to small numbers. These data are suppressed for confidentiality reasons. Statistical significance indicates that prevalence is different from the state prevalence and the difference is unlikely due to chance. Community prevalence is based on the residential address of the student. Data source: Bureau of Environmental Health Massachusetts Department of Public Health. (*From* the Massachusetts Environmental Public Health Tracking system, Bureau of Environmental Health, Massachusetts Department of Public Health. Available at: https://matracking.ehs.state.ma.us/Health-Data/Asthma/pediatric.html. Accessed May 9, 2018.)

Data sources and regions

Geocoding of electronic health record (EHR) data has been used to identify spatial patterns of asthma exacerbation that were independent of known risk factors.[86] In this study, however, the records were obtained only from one health system, so they may represent patterns of health system use instead of different patterns of risk. In addition, the system only captures one address and so is susceptible to bias if patients move frequently. A study in Australia used an automated system to abstract data from primary care visits for similar surveillance purposes. Interestingly, they found a lower than national average age-adjusted prevalence of asthma[87] and suggest they may not have identified appropriately representative sites for data collection. A study using data from an HMO in Israel was able to identify children with inadequate pharmaceutical treatment of asthma and generate maps of clinics with high prevalence of non–guideline compliant treatment.[88] A study examining areas with high risk of potentially preventable hospitalizations for adult asthma in Spain used a Shared Component Model to examine several kinds of potentially preventable hospitalization and examine the spatial pattern shared by all conditions as compared with the spatial pattern specific to a single condition,[89] potentially allowing for the examination of asthma care quality

separate from overall quality. GeoMedStat is an example of a surveillance system that can use satellite and ground monitor data from the US National Aeronautics and Space Administration and the US Environmental Protection Agency (EPA), as well as hospital systems for chief complaint and disease classification codes for asthma.[90] The health data are geographically coded and linked with census data and the air quality observations.[90]

Geographic analysis of ED visits for asthma has been used to identify at-risk patient populations for subsequent public health intervention,[91,92] with some investigators proposing using geographic analyses of ED visits for public health surveillance.[93] To generate accurate estimates, however, hospitals need geographically dispersed patient populations, a racial/ethnic distribution matching the Census, and high-quality data coding.[94] ED-based methods may be less biased by health care accessibility than claims data[93] and so could improve the understanding of the health status of minority patients as well as provide data at smaller geographic scale.[95] One study used emergency medical services data to identify high-risk areas for ambulance-treated asthma[96] and analyzed ambulance-treated asthma attacks by school zone, arguing that these data could provide guidance for school districts on targeting asthma plans and resources to high-risk schools and improving school-community partnerships.[97]

Geographic access to care

Models examining geographic access to care have used several different measures. These measures include county-average distances to care, variation between counties in distance to care,[98] straight line distance to the nearest hospital (not necessarily in the same district),[99] or various definitions of neighborhood.[100] Another approach uses street reference databases to measure distance and travel time.[5] However, GIS-calculated travel time may not accurately predict travel time to clinic for patients with lung disease.[101]

The association between geographic access and asthma outcomes has been reported to differ by state.[98] Several studies have reported an increase in mortality with increasing distance from the hospital,[99,102] and lower levels of health care utilization has been reported for asthmatics living further from primary care or hospital providers.[103] In other settings, living at a greater distance from the ED was associated with increased ED visits,[104] and asthma deaths were concentrated in the poorest neighborhoods, with the largest number of public primary health facilities.[105] The challenges in measuring geographic access to care may, in part, explain the differences in association that have been reported.

Interventions, Advocacy, and Policy

GIS-enabled projects have been used for advocacy and policy change. In Minnesota, local air pollution and public health data were combined to examine air-pollution attributable respiratory hospitalizations. The results were described in 3 key messages, and a Web site was provided for community information and to promote actions to reduce pollution.[106] Another air-pollution monitoring project that grew out of neighborhood advocacy around air pollution and asthma created multiple avenues for information dissemination, including a Web site, telephone and flag notification system, youth training, and community outreach.[107]

Several papers reported on projects using geographic data to improve clinical care or community programs. Geographic data can assist with identification of place-based risks and improved tailored recommendations and can help reduce disparities.[108] In addition, smaller global positioning system (GPS) units are enabling new research protocols that can track movement over time.[5] A project in Wisconsin describes the linkage of EHR data to a database listing community risk factors at the census block level to allow for novel research and clinical interventions.[109] CommunityRx is a Chicago-based program that employs youth to map community assets and generate personalized referrals within the electronic medical record. The top 3 resources for asthma were pharmacies, mold removal, and smoking cessation classes, but only 3% of asthmatics had access to all 3 resources within their home zip code.[110] GIS analysis has also been used for evaluation of community asthma programs.[111] Finally, mobile health and mapping applications have been used to improve asthma self-management.[112]

Methodological Considerations

Identification of exposures and risk factors

There are multiple challenges in the geographic identification of environmental hazards. Often, studies have used the Toxic Release Inventory from the EPA, but many relevant facilities may not be included because their volume is below the regulatory reporting requirements.[73] In addition, the time of sampling frames for measuring air pollution may not match the time of collection for health outcomes data. For example, one study linked a 2-week sampling of air pollutants to annual health outcomes.[113]

Descriptions of environmental exposure can be derived in several ways.[114] Self-reported exposure to air pollution is subject to potential bias as patients with chronic diseases report more pollution problems, despite adjustment for modeled level of pollution and other potential confounders.[115] Similarly, self-reported traffic exposure is only weakly associated with modeled exposure to traffic-related air pollution.[16] Air dispersion modeling uses "emission quantities, meteorological and topographical factors"[116] over time and space to describe air-pollution exposure. In the spatial coincidence method, populations are defined by a geographic unit (such as census tract or zip code). Populations within a unit containing an environmental hazard are presumed to be exposed. However, this has a significant limitation that the borders of the geographic units may not represent the boundary of an exposure. Proximity analysis includes the population within a prespecified buffer distance from the polluting source.[73] Studies have used GIS to calculate distance to roadways and length and density of roadways,[117] with different cutoff values to define traffic exposures.[118] However, using a buffer distance to define exposure from a single address (ie, defining children who lived >200 m from traffic flow as unexposed) may inadequately capture overall exposure.[43] One study of traffic-related air pollution used multiple "buffer" zones around each study subject to examine how the association changes with increased ascertainment of road segment exposure.[42] For the smallest buffer zones, no association was found between traffic and asthma, but there was an association in the larger buffer areas.[42] In some studies, traffic counts have been obtained from the local government, but may only be available for major roads,[43] which could lead to bias from unmeasured exposures from smaller roads. Other approaches include boundary analysis, which describes "naturally occurring shifts of magnitude in socio-environmental and health outcomes across the wider urban area,"[119] or conducting sensitivity analyses with varied buffer sizes.[47] In addition, air pollutants from traffic have varied spatial patterns within urban areas, suggesting the importance of modeling several pollutants and accounting for site-specific modification of the traffic-disease relationship.[120]

SES measurements can be obtained directly from the individual or by using values collated at a geographic level (such as a census tract). Information at the census tract level can serve as a proxy for the individual characteristic, but also potentially describes contextual factors that arise from the neighborhood.[66] Some countries have standardized deprivation indices that can be applied to small areas.[58]

Studies have also used inconsistent definitions of neighborhood, often described as "spatially based attributes associated with clusters of residences."[121] For example, studies looking at violence have used police beat,[122] census tract,[123] or different walking distances around a child's house.[124] Some investigators have proposed the creation of new synthetic areas rather than existing administrative units.[125]

Geocoding and geographic units
The modifiable areal unit problem is when geographic analyses provide different results depending on the geographic unit of analysis chosen.[6,126] Although the extent of the study (scale) and the spatial resolution (unit of analysis) are often limited by the availability of data,[73] the smallest possible unit of analysis is usually recommended.[73]

Geocoded data can have several sources of error. Positional accuracy is the relationship between the database description of an object and the object's real-world position. Error can occur at the initial measurement, at the coding between measurement and a GIS database,[73] or in the non-repeatability of geocoding.[127] Studies report a geocoding error range from 5%[128] to 30%.[129]

The strength of the odds ratios between exposures and disease declined with decreased geocoding accuracy.[130] In addition, geocoding errors have been found to be nonrandom in nature and can overestimate the number of exposed.[131] Differential failure to geocode could also bias risk estimation if the cases have a different rate of failure to code than the controls. Zimmerman and Fang[132] provide nonparametric estimation methods for incompletely geocoded data.

Different geocoding strategies can substantially alter the observed association. For example, a French study examining air pollution and markers of asthma found changes in the magnitude of association depending on the method of geocoding (manual vs software).[133] In this study, the residential outdoor exposures were higher in the software-geocoded addresses where the software assigned locations that were closer to the street and traffic as compared with the manual coding, which assigned address coordinates at the center of the building. The software-assigned addresses were also based on averages of the street numbers (50 would be assigned halfway between 1 and 100), whereas the manual coding assigned the actual location of the building.[133] Other studies have incorporated sensitivity analyses for geocoding exposure misclassifications to examine these effects.[134]

Movement and measurement
Although many studies only code one address to assess environmental exposures, it is probably better to examine a combination of residential and school[25,43] or occupational exposures. For example, a Swedish study found that asthma prevalence was associated with traffic exposure at residential address, but not with workplace address or time spent in traffic.[135] Personal GPS units can be used to more specifically quantify environmental exposures and may provide more accurate information on location compared with a diary.[136]

A study in France found that SES had no influence on the association between air pollution and emergency calls made for asthma exacerbations.[137] However, this may not include patients who self-presented to the hospital or doctor's office without calling. In addition, the exposure measurement assigned to each subject was derived from the location where the emergency was called, which may not accurately represent their exposure.[137] The questions about how the impact of environmental effects on health varies across space can be addressed by geographically weighted regression models.[138]

Creating databases for GIS analysis may be more complicated in countries with fragmented health care systems[6] because it often requires the collection of health data from more than one source. Using only data from an individual health system creates the potential for error in that the areas of high utilization/high risk identified in such work may reflect geographic patterns of health system use rather than of underlying disease. High disease rates in a community that uses a different health care system would be invisible to a single-system EHR-based analysis.

Study design, confounding, and bias

An early study in Harlem described the importance of collecting and analyzing multiple levels of geographic data: housing violations, sources of pollution, bus route proximity, construction permits, vacancy, and distance from local health clinics to each street segment.[8] Another study emphasized the importance of controlling for migration and travel in studying pollution and asthma. In particular, the investigators examined the potential of "selective migration" into and out of the affected area, and the likelihood that factory workers were more likely to live there and perhaps had occupational exposure rather than residential exposure (see earlier text for more discussion of migration error).[139]

Case-crossover designs have been widely used in air-pollution analysis, in which each case can serve as its own control before and after the pollution event or increase in the measured level of pollutant. In addition to controlling for case characteristics (such as sex, race/ethnicity) and seasonal variation (if the referent days are close to the event days), this also has the advantage of controlling for case-level spatial exposure variation.[134] Others have proposed using a propensity score approach to improve balance of confounders between exposed and unexposed groups.[140]

Another approach to assess the relationship between asthma and air pollution is to examine the spatial pattern of the disease of interest (asthma) as compared with a more common control disease that would not be expected to be related to environmental air pollution (such as gastroenteritis).[141] Similar approaches use existing asthma morbidity patterns to rank potential environmental hazards based on wind-direction weighted proximity[142] or air pollution and other characteristics of those areas.[143]

Similar to studying other environmental exposures, research examining neighborhood effects of SES also needs to account for geographic selection bias in which unmeasured behaviors, values, traits, or skills related to the outcome of interest may cause selective movement to and from particular types of neighborhoods.[144] Methodological responses to this bias are summarized in **Table 3**.

Table 3
Methodological responses to geographic selection bias

Technique Name	Comment
Propensity score matching	Outcomes within neighborhood compared with sample of nonneighborhood on basis of probability model of similar likelihood of being in neighborhood
Sibling model	Measurement of differences between 2 siblings eliminates biases from unobserved, time-invariant, parental characteristics
Difference model based on longitudinal data	Measure differences between 2 periods eliminates unobserved, time-invariant, individual characteristics
Fixed-effects models	Use individual dummy variables to measure unobserved, tie-invariant, characteristics of individuals that may lead to neighborhood selection and outcomes
Instrumental variables for neighborhood characteristics	Proxy variables for neighborhood characteristics that vary only due to exogenous attributes
Residents of same block	Very localized neighbors may have less geographic selection bias
Natural quasi-experiments	Exogenous variation in neighborhood for selected individuals (such as public housing construction, refugee resettlement); important to assess randomness of individual assignment and bias from subsequent mobility
Random assignment experiments	Households randomly assigned to different neighborhoods

Data from Galster GC, Santiago AM. Evaluating the potential of a natural experiment to provide unbiased evidence of neighborhood effects on health. Health Serv Outcomes Res Methodol 2015;15(2):99–135.

Another challenge is making sure that the reported constructs actually capture the characteristics of interest. For example, neighborhood interaction has been shown to be significantly higher in neighborhoods with high asthma prevalence.[145] However, interaction was "measured by the percent of households not linguistically isolated or comprised of a single person living alone," which may represent crowding from poverty, potentially associated increased exposure to environmental triggers for asthma. Another study examined associations of neighborhood with asthma after adjustment for individual characteristics and found weak associations, with the exception of neighborhood education, with lower levels of neighborhood education associated with higher rates of asthma.[146] However, in this study the researchers included a housing variable as an individual characteristic, and that variable included direct observation of the child's housing and immediate block. In other studies, the direct observation factors have been coded as neighborhood rather than individual factors, which may limit the ability to compare findings across studies.

As with all observational studies, GIS analyses remain vulnerable to other sources of unmeasured confounding. For example, one study examined spatial correlations between fast food outlets and asthma without adjusting for SES or obesity.[147] Of particular importance to geographic data is the challenge of accounting for confounding or bias from underlying population differences, a particular concern in areas with high residential segregation. "Structural confounding" describes the absence of a complete set of distributions to enable a multivariable model to be reliable. For example, if there are too few low-income people living in high-income neighborhoods and too few high-income people living in low-income neighborhoods, it will be difficult to disentangle the contributions of individual and neighborhood income.[148]

Modeling challenges

In most studies, only one location is geocoded. As discussed earlier, geocoding based purely on residence ignores other potential areas of exposure, such as work or school.[5] In addition, single address assessments of environmental exposures also have the potential to be biased by moving to a new residence. One study found that 54% of a pediatric cohort in Cincinnati, Ohio moved once before age 7 and the move was associated with a median decrease of 4.4% in traffic-related air pollution (ie, moving away from air pollution).[149] Furthermore, models often have very straightforward assumptions about space and exposure,

and it is important to remember that exposure is not necessarily related to geographic nearness. There could be undescribed barriers in the way (such as all buildings on the side of a roadway), and the analysis does not account for how individuals actually move through the world or the "time geography"[148] of exposure.

Accounting for spatial and temporal variation[134] is of key importance.[126] A study in New York examined the sensitivity of the association between air-pollution asthma based on the geographic and temporal resolution of the health data. The association between air pollution and asthma did not change when different geographic regions were used (country vs neighborhood), but the association of ozone did change with temporal resolution, appearing 15% lower when seasonal, instead of annual, morbidity was used.[150] Models combining spatial and temporal data have been proposed and studied in relation to asthma.[151,152] Asthma has also been used as the case study for the development of several complex temporal modeling techniques,[153–157] whose description is outside the scope of this review.

Next Steps: Practice Changes and Research Agenda

Improved health information exchanges will enable more rigorous analyses of neighborhood factors and asthma and will improve public health programs.[109,158] For example, geographic-based social-risk targeting can improve identification of asthmatic children at risk for ED utilization,[11,67] or readmission, to improve outcomes and reduce disparities.[66] On an individual clinical level, a geographic medical history could collect information on spatial and temporal environmental exposures to assist physicians with better understanding of disease risk factors.[159]

From a research perspective, additional work is needed to identify how geographic data can best be used to improve health and the efficiency of the health system, to define the optimal technological solutions for data linkage and analysis across health systems, and to identify the most useful geomarkers and geographic units of analyses.[108] Additional qualitative research may help identify the importance of particular neighborhood factors to patient populations[160] With increasing research and clinical use of geographic data, continued work is needed to develop best practices in data display.[161] The authors encourage future studies to investigate the integration of geographic data into clinical and population health decision making to improve outcomes and reduce disparities.

ACKNOWLEDGMENTS

The authors thank Lisa Phillpotts (Treadwell Library, Massachusetts General Hospital, Boston, MA) for her assistance with the literature search.

REFERENCES

1. Variations in the prevalence of respiratory symptoms, self-reported asthma attacks, and use of asthma medication in the European Community Respiratory Health Survey (ECRHS). Eur Respir J 1996;9(4):687–95.

2. Crighton EJ, Feng J, Gershon A, et al. A spatial analysis of asthma prevalence in Ontario. Can J Public Health 2012;103(5):e384–9.

3. Choi M, Afzal B, Sattler B. Geographic information systems: a new tool for environmental health assessments. Public Health Nurs 2006;23(5):381–91.

4. Boothby J, Dummer TJB. Facilitating mobility? The role of GIS. Geography 2003;88:300–11.

5. Lyseen AK, Nøhr C, Sorensen EM, et al. A review and framework for categorizing current research and development in health related geographical information systems (GIS) studies. Yearb Med Inform 2014;9:110–24.

6. Yiannakoulias N, Svenson LW, Schopflocher DP. An integrated framework for the geographic surveillance of chronic disease. Int J Health Geogr 2009;8:15.

7. Wright RJ, Subramanian SV. Advancing a multilevel framework for epidemiologic research on asthma disparities. Chest 2007;132(5 Suppl):757s–69s.

8. Allacci MS. Identifying environmental risk factors for asthma emergency care" a multilevel approach for ecological study. J Ambul Care Manage 2005; 28(1):2–15.

9. Wilson MG, Lavis JN, Guta A. Community-based organizations in the health sector: a scoping review. Health Res Policy Syst 2012;10:36.

10. Grant MJ, Booth A. A typology of reviews: an analysis of 14 review types and associated methodologies. Health Info Libr J 2009;26(2):91–108.

11. Beck AF, Huang B, Ryan PH, et al. Areas with high rates of police-reported violent crime have higher rates of childhood asthma morbidity. J Pediatr 2016;173:175–82.e1.

12. Gupta RS, Zhang X, Sharp LK, et al. Geographic variability in childhood asthma prevalence in Chicago. J Allergy Clin Immunol 2008;121(3):639–45.e1.

13. Farah C, Hosgood HD 3rd, Hock JM. Spatial prevalence and associations among respiratory diseases in Maine. Spat Spatiotemporal Epidemiol 2014;11:11–22.

14. Cabieses B, Uphoff E, Pinart M, et al. A systematic review on the development of asthma and allergic diseases in relation to international immigration: the leading role of the environment confirmed. PLoS one 2014;9(8):e105347.

15. Goldstein IF, Arthur SP. "Asthma Alley": a space clustering study of asthma in Brooklyn, New York City. J Asthma Res 1978;15(2):81–93.

16. Heinrich J, Gehring U, Cyrys J, et al. Exposure to traffic related air pollutants: self reported traffic intensity versus GIS modelled exposure. Occup Environ Med 2005;62(8):517–23.

17. Alizadeh MG, Ghasemi Hashtroodi L, Chavoshzadeh Z, et al. Effect of air pollution in frequency of hospitalizations in asthmatic children. Acta Med Iran 2016;54(8):542–6.

18. Seo S, Kim D, Min S, et al. GIS-based association between PM10 and allergic diseases in seoul: implications for health and environmental policy. Allergy Asthma Immunol Res 2016;8(1):32–40.

19. Wilkinson PE, Elliott P, Grundy C, et al. Case-control study of hospital admission with asthma in children aged 5-14 years: relation with road traffic in north west London. Thorax 1999;54(12):1070–4.

20. Lewis SA, Antoniak M, Venn AJ, et al. Secondhand smoke, dietary fruit intake, road traffic exposures, and the prevalence of asthma: a cross-sectional study in young children. Am J Epidemiol 2005; 161(5):406–11.

21. Pujades-Rodriguez M, Lewis S, McKeever T, et al. Effect of living close to a main road on asthma, allergy, lung function and chronic obstructive pulmonary disease. Occup Environ Med 2009;66(10): 679–84.

22. Akinbami LJ, Lynch CD, Parker JD, et al. The association between childhood asthma prevalence and monitored air pollutants in metropolitan areas, United States, 2001-2004. Environ Res 2010; 110(3):294–301.

23. Gorai AK, Tuluri F, Tchounwou PB. A GIS based approach for assessing the association between air pollution and asthma in New York State, USA. Int J Environ Res Public Health 2014;11(5): 4845–69.

24. Hruba F, Fabiánová E, Koppova K, et al. Childhood respiratory symptoms, hospital admissions, and long-term exposure to airborne particulate matter. J Expo Anal Environ Epidemiol 2001;11(1):33–40.

25. Pikhart H, Bobak M, Gorynski P, et al. Outdoor sulphur dioxide and respiratory symptoms in Czech and Polish school children: a small-area study (SAVIAH). Small-Area Variation in Air Pollution and Health. Int Arch Occup Environ Health 2001;74(8):574–8.

26. Skarkova P, Kadlubiec R, Fischer M, et al. Refining of asthma prevalence spatial distribution and visualization of outdoor environment factors using GIS and its application for identification of mutual associations. Cent Eur J Public Health 2015;23(3): 258–66.

27. Girardi P, Marcon A, Rava M, et al. Spatial analysis of binary health indicators with local smoothing techniques the Viadana study. Sci Total Environ 2012;414:380–6.

28. Patel MM, Quinn JW, Jung KH, et al. Traffic density and stationary sources of air pollution associated with wheeze, asthma, and immunoglobulin E from birth to age 5 years among New York City children. Environ Res 2011;111(8):1222–9.

29. Oyana TJ, Rogerson P, Lwebuga-Mukasa JS. Geographic clustering of adult asthma hospitalization and residential exposure to pollution at a United States-Canada border crossing. Am J Public Health 2004;94(7):1250–7.

30. Brauer M, Hoek G, van Vliet P, et al. Estimating long-term average particulate air pollution concentrations: application of traffic indicators and geographic information systems. Epidemiology 2003;14(2):228–39.

31. Gordian ME, Hoek S, Wakefield J. An investigation of the association between traffic exposure and the diagnosis of asthma in children. J Expo Sci Environ Epidemiol 2006;16(1):49–55.

32. Kim JJ, Huen K, Adams S, et al. Residential traffic and children's respiratory health. Environ Health Perspect 2008;116(9):1274–9.

33. Lindgren A, Stroh E, Montnemery P, et al. Traffic-related air pollution associated with prevalence of asthma and COPD/chronic bronchitis. A cross-sectional study in Southern Sweden. Int J Health Geogr 2009;8:2.

34. Nuvolone D, Della Maggiore R, Maio S, et al. Geographical information system and environmental epidemiology: a cross-sectional spatial analysis of the effects of traffic-related air pollution on population respiratory health. Environ Health 2011;10:12.

35. Skrzypek M, Zejda JE, Kowalska M, et al. Effect of residential proximity to traffic on respiratory disorders in school children in upper Silesian Industrial Zone, Poland. Int J Occup Med Environ Health 2013;26(1):83–91.

36. Svendsen ER, Gonzales M, Mukerjee S, et al. GIS-modeled indicators of traffic-related air pollutants and adverse pulmonary health among children in El Paso, Texas. Am J Epidemiol 2012;176(Suppl 7):S131–41.

37. Miyake Y, Tanaka K, Fujiwara H, et al. Residential proximity to main roads during pregnancy and the risk of allergic disorders in Japanese infants: the Osaka Maternal and Child Health Study. Pediatr Allergy Immunol 2010;21(1 Pt 1):22–8.

38. Cakmak S, Mahmud M, Grgicak-Mannion A, et al. The influence of neighborhood traffic density on the respiratory health of elementary schoolchildren. Environ Int 2012;39(1):128–32.

39. Dales R, Wheeler A, Mahmud M, et al. The influence of living near roadways on spirometry and exhaled nitric oxide in elementary schoolchildren. Environ Health Perspect 2008;116(10):1423–7.

40. Sapkota A, Eftim S, Nachman K, et al. Traffic exposure and asthma exacerbation among a nationally representative sample of the us population. Epidemiology 2011;22:S64.

41. Brown MS, Sarnat SE, DeMuth KA, et al. Residential proximity to a major roadway is associated with features of asthma control in children. PLoS One 2012;7(5):e37044.

42. Cook AG, deVos AJ, Pereira G, et al. Use of a total traffic count metric to investigate the impact of roadways on asthma severity: a case-control study. Environ Health 2011;10:52.

43. Andersson M, Modig L, Hedman L, et al. Heavy vehicle traffic is related to wheeze among schoolchildren: a population-based study in an area with low traffic flows. Environ Health 2011; 10:91.

44. Shankardass K, Jerrett M, Dell SD, et al. Spatial analysis of exposure to traffic-related air pollution at birth and childhood atopic asthma in Toronto, Ontario. Health Place 2015;34:287–95.

45. Delfino RJ, Wu J, Tjoa T, et al. Asthma morbidity and ambient air pollution: effect modification by residential traffic-related air pollution. Epidemiology 2014;25(1):48–57.

46. Ryan PH, LeMasters G, Biagini J, et al. Is it traffic type, volume, or distance? Wheezing in infants living near truck and bus traffic. J Allergy Clin Immunol 2005;116(2):279–84.

47. Ebisu K, Holford TR, Belanger KD, et al. Urban land-use and respiratory symptoms in infants. Environ Res 2011;111(5):677–84.

48. Lovasi GS, O'Neil-Dunne JP, Lu JW, et al. Urban tree canopy and asthma, wheeze, rhinitis, and allergic sensitization to tree pollen in a New York City birth cohort. Environ Health Perspect 2013; 121(4):494–500.

49. Khan IA, Arsalan MH, Siddiqui MF, et al. Spatial association of asthma and vegetation in karachi: a GIS perspective. Pak J Bot 2010;42(5):3547–54.

50. Ulmer JM, Wolf KL, Backman DR, et al. Multiple health benefits of urban tree canopy: the mounting evidence for a green prescription. Health Place 2016;42:54–62.

51. Eldeirawi KM, Kunzweiler C, Rosenberg N, et al. Associations of residential greenness with asthma and asthma symptoms among a sample of Mexican American children in Chicago. Am J Respir Crit Care Med 2017;195.

52. Feng X, Astell-Burt T. Is neighborhood green space protective against associations between child asthma, neighborhood traffic volume and perceived lack of area safety? Multilevel analysis of 4447 Australian Children. Int J Environ Res Public Health 2017;14(5) [pii:E543].

53. Coogan PF, Castro-Webb N, Yu J, et al. Neighborhood and individual socioeconomic status and asthma incidence in African American Women. Ethn Dis 2016;26(1):113–22.

54. Chen Y, Stewart P, Dales R, et al. Ecological measures of socioeconomic status and hospital readmissions for asthma among Canadian adults. Respir Med 2004;98(5):446–53.

55. Saha C, Riner ME, Liu G. Individual and neighborhood-level factors in predicting asthma. Arch Pediatr Adolesc Med 2005;159(8):759–63.

56. Claudio L, Tulton L, Doucette J, et al. Socioeconomic factors and asthma hospitalization rates in New York City. J Asthma 1999;36(4):343–50.

57. Beck AF, Moncrief T, Huang B, et al. Inequalities in neighborhood child asthma admission rates and underlying community characteristics in one US county. J Pediatr 2013;163(2):574–80.

58. Salmond C, Crampton P, Hales S, et al. Asthma prevalence and deprivation: a small area analysis. J Epidemiol Community Health 1999;53(8):476–80.

59. Carr W, Zeitel L, Weiss K. Variations in asthma hospitalizations and deaths in New York City. Am J Public Health 1992;82(1):59–65.

60. Gottlieb DJ, Beiser AS, O'Connor GT. Poverty, race, and medication use are correlates of asthma hospitalization rates. A small area analysis in Boston. Chest 1995;108(1):28–35.

61. Castro M, Schechtman KB, Halstead J, et al. Risk factors for asthma morbidity and mortality in a large metropolitan city. J Asthma 2001;38(8):625–35.

62. Ray NF, Thamer M, Fadillioglu B, et al. Race, income, urbanicity, and asthma hospitalization in California: a small area analysis. Chest 1998; 113(5):1277–84.

63. Eldeirawi K, Riley B, Kunzweiler C. Effect of neighborhood deprivation on respiratory health of inner-city children of mexican origin. Study of asthma in children of mexican descent. Am J Respir Crit Care Med 2015;191.

64. Grineski SE, Collins TW, Kim YA. Contributions of individual acculturation and neighborhood ethnic density to variations in Hispanic children's respiratory health in a US-Mexican border metropolis. J Public Health (Oxf) 2016;38(3):441–9.

65. Kim YA, Collins TW, Grineski SE. Neighborhood context and the Hispanic health paradox: differential effects of immigrant density on childrens wheezing by poverty, nativity and medical history. Health Place 2014;27:1–8.

66. Beck AF, Simmons JM, Huang B, et al. Geomedicine: area-based socioeconomic measures for assessing risk of hospital reutilization among children admitted for asthma. Am J Public Health 2012;102(12):2308–14.

67. Kersten EE, Adler NE, Gottlieb L, et al. Neighborhood child opportunity and individual-level pediatric acute care use and diagnoses. Pediatrics 2018;141(5) [pii:e20172309].

68. Beck AF, Huang B, Chundur R, et al. Housing code violation density associated with emergency department and hospital use by children with asthma. Health Aff (Millwood) 2014;33(11):1993–2002.

69. Harris MN, Lundien MC, Finnie DM, et al. Application of a novel socioeconomic measure using individual housing data in asthma research: an exploratory study. NPJ Prim Care Respir Med 2014;24:14018.

70. Fortson JG, Sanbonmatsu L. Child health and neighborhood conditions results from a randomized housing voucher experiment. J Hum Resour 2010;45(4):840–64.

71. Schmidt NM, Lincoln AK, Nguyen QC, et al. Examining mediators of housing mobility on adolescent asthma: results from a housing voucher experiment. Soc Sci Med 2014;107:136–44.

72. Galster G, Santiago AM. Neighbourhood ethnic composition and outcomes for low-income Latino and African American children. Urban Stud 2017; 54(2):482–500.

73. Maantay J. Asthma and air pollution in the Bronx: methodological and data considerations in using GIS for environmental justice and health research. Health Place 2007;13(1):32–56.

74. Meliker JR, Nriagu JO, Hammad AS, et al. Spatial clustering of emergency department visits by asthmatic children in an urban area: South-western Detroit, Michigan. Ambul Child Health 2001;7(3–4): 297–312.

75. Brewer M, Kimbro RT, Denney JT, et al. Does neighborhood social and environmental context impact race/ethnic disparities in childhood asthma? Health Place 2017;44:86–93.

76. Clougherty JE, Levy JI, Kubzansky LD, et al. Synergistic effects of traffic-related air pollution and exposure to violence on urban asthma etiology. Environ Health Perspect 2007;115(8):1140–6.

77. Magzamen S, Gale SA, Richards M, et al. Social and environmental determinants of childhood asthma: a GIS approach. Am J Epidemiol 2011; 173:S144.

78. Shmool JL, Kubzansky LD, Newman OD, et al. Social stressors and air pollution across New York City communities: a spatial approach for assessing correlations among multiple exposures. Environ Health 2014;13:91.

79. Collins TW, Grineski SE, Morales DX. Environmental injustice and sexual minority health disparities: a national study of inequitable health risks from air pollution among same-sex partners. Soc Sci Med 2017;191:38–47.

80. Maclachlan JC, Jerrett M, Abernathy T, et al. Mapping health on the internet: a new tool for environmental justice and public health research. Health Place 2007;13(1):72–86.

81. Naureckas ET, Thomas S. Are we closing the disparities gap? Small-area analysis of asthma in Chicago. Chest 2007;132(5 Suppl):858s–65s.

82. Goodman DC, Fisher ES, Gittelsohn A, et al. Why are children hospitalized? The role of non-clinical factors in pediatric hospitalizations. Pediatrics 1994;93(6 Pt 1):896–902.

83. Goedken AM, Brooks JM, Milavetz G, et al. Geographic variation in inhaled corticosteroid use for children with persistent asthma in Medicaid. J Asthma 2018;55(8):851–8.

84. Roberts EM, English PB, Wong M, et al. Progress in pediatric asthma surveillance II: geospatial patterns of asthma in Alameda County, California. Prev Chronic Dis 2006;3(3):A92.

85. Mendez-Luck CA, Yu H, Meng YY, et al. Estimating health conditions for small areas: asthma symptom prevalence for state legislative districts. Health Serv Res 2007;42(6 Pt 2):2389–409.

86. Xie S, Greenblatt R, Levy M, et al. Assessing the geospatial distribution of asthma exacerbations using electronic health record (EHR)-derived data. Am J Respir Crit Care Med 2017;195.

87. Ghosh A, Charlton KE, Girdo L, et al. Using data from patient interactions in primary care for population level chronic disease surveillance: the Sentinel Practices Data Sourcing (SPDS) project. BMC Public Health 2014;14:557.

88. Peled R, Reuveni H, Pliskin JS, et al. Defining localities of inadequate treatment for childhood asthma: a GIS approach. Int J Health Geogr 2006;5:3.

89. Ibanez-Beroiz B, Librero J, Bernal-Delgado E, et al. Joint spatial modeling to identify shared patterns among chronic related potentially preventable hospitalizations. BMC Med Res Methodol 2014;14:74.

90. Faruque FS, Li H, Williams WB, et al. GeoMedStat: an integrated spatial surveillance system to track air pollution and associated healthcare events. Geospat Health 2014;8(3):S631–46.

91. Lajoie P, Laberge A, Lebel G, et al. Cartography of emergency department visits for asthma - targeting high-morbidity populations. Can Respir J 2004;11(6):427–33.

92. Lee DC, Yi SS, Fong HF, et al. Identifying local hot spots of pediatric chronic diseases using emergency department surveillance. Acad Pediatr 2017;17(3):267–74.

93. Lee DC, Long JA, Wall SP, et al. Determining chronic disease prevalence in local populations using emergency department surveillance. Am J Public Health 2015;105(9):e67–74.

94. Lee DC, Swartz JL, Koziatek CA, et al. Assessing the reliability of performing citywide chronic disease surveillance using emergency department data from sentinel hospitals. Popul Health Manag 2017;20(6):427–34.

95. Lee DC, Yi SS, Athens JK, et al. Using geospatial analysis and emergency claims data to improve minority health surveillance. J Racial Ethn Health Disparities 2018;5(4):712–20.

96. Raun LH, Ensor KB, Campos LA, et al. Factors affecting ambulance utilization for asthma attack treatment: understanding where to target interventions. Public Health 2015;129(5):501–8.

97. Raun LH, Campos LA, Stevenson E, et al. Analyzing who, when, and where: data for better targeting of resources for school-based asthma interventions. J Sch Health 2017;87(4):253–61.

98. Garcia E, Serban N, Swann J, et al. The effect of geographic access on severe health outcomes for pediatric asthma. J Allergy Clin Immunol 2015;136(3):610–8.

99. Jones AP, Bentham G. Health service accessibility and deaths from asthma in 401 local authority districts in England and Wales, 1988-92. Thorax 1997;52(3):218–22.

100. Spernak SM, Mintz M, Paulson J, et al. Neighborhood racial composition and availability of asthma drugs in retail pharmacies. J Asthma 2005;42(9):731–5.

101. Thakur N, Jalluri C, Burchard EG, et al. Average travel time to clinic in patients with and without lung disease utilizing a safety-net clinic. Am J Respir Crit Care Med 2012;185.

102. Jones AP, Bentham G, Horwell C. Health service accessibility and deaths from asthma. Int J Epidemiol 1999;28(1):101–5.

103. Jones AP, Bentham G, Harrison BD, et al. Accessibility and health service utilization for asthma in Norfolk, England. J Public Health Med 1998;20(3):312–7.

104. Lewis-Land C, Bellin M, Bollinger M, et al. Accessiblity to healthcare for inner city children with poorly controlled asthma. Am J Respir Crit Care Med 2013;187.

105. Souza-Machado C, Souza-Machado A, Da Natividade MS, et al. Geographical distribution of deaths from asthma in Salvador, Brazil (2000-2009). World Allergy Organ J 2012;5:S195.

106. Johnson JE, Bael DL, Sample JM, et al. Estimating the public health impact of air pollution for informing policy in the twin cities: a Minnesota tracking collaboration. J Public Health Manag Pract 2017;23(Suppl 5 Supplement, Environmental Public Health Tracking):S45–52.

107. Loh P, Sugerman-Brozan J, Wiggins S, et al. From asthma to AirBeat: community-driven monitoring of fine particles and black carbon in Roxbury, Massachusetts. Environ Health Perspect 2002;110(Suppl 2):297–301.

108. Beck AF, Sandel MT, Ryan PH, et al. Mapping neighborhood health geomarkers to clinical care decisions to promote equity in child health. Health Aff (Millwood) 2017;36(6):999–1005.

109. Guilbert TW, Arndt B, Temte J, et al. The theory and application of UW ehealth-PHINEX, a clinical electronic health record-public health information exchange. WMJ 2012;111(3):124–33.

110. Beiser DG, Makelarski JA, Escamilla V, et al. Communityrx: connecting health care to self care in an academic emergency department on Chicago's south side. Acad Emerg Med 2016;23:S150.

111. Woods ER, Fleegler E, Chan E, et al. Evaluation of the community asthma initiative: adolescent vs. child outcomes and GIS mapping. J Adolesc Health 2012;50(2):S83–4.

112. Van Sickle D, Barrett M, Humblet O, et al. Impact of a mobile health and sensor-driven asthma management pilot study on symptoms, control, and self-management. J Allergy Clin Immunol 2016; 137(2):AB9.

113. Lemke LD, Lamerato LE, Xu X, et al. Geospatial relationships of air pollution and acute asthma events across the Detroit-Windsor international border: study design and preliminary results. J Expo Sci Environ Epidemiol 2014;24(4):346–57.

114. Sahsuvaroglu T, Jerrett M, Sears MR, et al. Spatial analysis of air pollution and childhood asthma in Hamilton, Canada: comparing exposure methods in sensitive subgroups. Environ Health 2009;8(1):14.

115. Piro FN, Madsen C, Naess O, et al. A comparison of self reported air pollution problems and GIS-modeled levels of air pollution in people with and without chronic diseases. Environ Health 2008;7:10.

116. Maantay JA, Tu J, Maroko AR. Loose-coupling an air dispersion model and a geographic information system (GIS) for studying air pollution and asthma in the Bronx, New York City. Int J Environ Health Res 2009;19(1):59–79.

117. Patel MM, Quinn JW, Jung K, et al. Residential density of roadways associated with cough and asthma in Urban children through age 5 years. J Allergy Clin Immunol 2010;125(2):AB232.

118. English P, Neutra R, Scalf R, et al. Examining associations between childhood asthma and traffic flow using a geographic information system. Environ Health Perspect 1999;107(9):761–7.

119. Jephcote C, Chen H. Geospatial analysis of naturally occurring boundaries in road-transport emissions and children's respiratory health across a demographically diverse cityscape. Soc Sci Med 2013;82:87–99.

120. Clougherty JE, Wright RJ, Baxter LK, et al. Land use regression modeling of intra-urban residential variability in multiple traffic-related air pollutants. Environ Health 2008;7:17.

121. DePriest K, Butz A. Neighborhood-level factors related to asthma in children living in urban areas. J Sch Nurs 2017;33(1):8–17.

122. Gupta RS, Zhang X, Springston EE, et al. The association between community crime and childhood asthma prevalence in Chicago. Ann Allergy Asthma Immunol 2010;104(4):299–306.

123. Eldeirawi K, Kunzweiler C, Rosenberg N, et al. Association of neighborhood crime with asthma and asthma morbidity among Mexican American children in Chicago, Illinois. Ann Allergy Asthma Immunol 2016;117(5):502–7.e1.

124. Gale SL, Magzamen SL, Radke JD, et al. Crime, neighborhood deprivation, and asthma: a GIS approach to define and assess neighborhoods. Spat Spatiotemporal Epidemiol 2011;2(2):59–67.

125. Sabel CE, Kihal W, Bard D, et al. Creation of synthetic homogeneous neighbourhoods using zone design algorithms to explore relationships between asthma and deprivation in Strasbourg, France. Soc Sci Med 2013;91:110–21.

126. Yang TC, Shoff C, Noah AJ. Spatialising health research: what we know and where we are heading. Geospatial health 2013;7(2):161–8.

127. Zandbergen PA, Green JW. Error and bias in determining exposure potential of children at school locations using proximity-based GIS techniques. Environ Health Perspect 2007;115(9):1363–70.

128. Ganguly R, Batterman S, Isakov V, et al. Effect of geocoding errors on traffic-related air pollutant exposure and concentration estimates. J Expo Sci Environ Epidemiol 2015;25(5):490–8.

129. Schootman M, Sterling DA, Struthers J, et al. Positional accuracy and geographic bias of four methods of geocoding in epidemiologic research. Ann Epidemiol 2007;17(6):464–70.

130. Mazumdar S, Rushton G, Smith BJ, et al. Geocoding accuracy and the recovery of relationships between environmental exposures and health. Int J Health Geogr 2008;7:18.

131. Zandbergen PA. Influence of geocoding quality on environmental exposure assessment of children living near high traffic roads. BMC Public Health 2007;7:13.

132. Zimmerman DL, Fang X. Estimating spatial variation in disease risk from locations coarsened by incomplete geocoding. Stat Methodol 2012;9(1–2):239–50.

133. Jacquemin B, Lepeule J, Boudier A, et al. Impact of geocoding methods on associations between long-term exposure to urban air pollution and lung function. Environ Health Perspect 2013;121(9):1054–60.

134. Shmool JL, Kinnee E, Sheffield PE, et al. Spatiotemporal ozone variation in a case-crossover analysis of childhood asthma hospital visits in New York City. Environ Res 2016;147:108–14.

135. Lindgren A, Björk J, Stroh E, et al. Adult asthma and traffic exposure at residential address, workplace address, and self-reported daily time

outdoor in traffic: a two-stage case-control study. BMC Public Health 2010;10:716.

136. Nethery E, Mallach G, Rainham D, et al. Using Global Positioning Systems (GPS) and temperature data to generate time-activity classifications for estimating personal exposure in air monitoring studies: an automated method. Environ Health 2014;13(1):33.

137. Laurent O, Pedrono G, Segala C, et al. Air pollution, asthma attacks, and socioeconomic deprivation: a small-area case-crossover study. Am J Epidemiol 2008;168(1):58–65.

138. Grineski SE, Collins TW, Olvera HA. Local variability in the impacts of residential particulate matter and pest exposure on children's wheezing severity: a geographically weighted regression analysis of environmental health justice. Popul Environ 2015;37(1):22–43.

139. Dunn CE, Woodhouse J, Bhopal RS, et al. Asthma and factory emissions in northern England: addressing public concern by combining geographical and epidemiological methods. J Epidemiol Community Health 1995;49(4):395–400.

140. Juhn YJ, Qin R, Urm S, et al. The influence of neighborhood environment on the incidence of childhood asthma: a propensity score approach. J Allergy Clin Immunol 2010;125(4):838–43.e2.

141. Oyana TJ, Rivers PA. Geographic variations of childhood asthma hospitalization and outpatient visits and proximity to ambient pollution sources at a U.S.-Canada border crossing. Int J Health Geogr 2005;4:14.

142. Svechkina A, Portnov BA. A new approach to spatial identification of potential health hazards associated with childhood asthma. Sci Total Environ 2017;595:413–24.

143. Corburn J, Osleeb J, Porter M. Urban asthma and the neighbourhood environment in New York City. Health Place 2006;12(2):167–79.

144. Galster GC, Santiago AM. Evaluating the potential of a natural experiment to provide unbiased evidence of neighborhood effects on health. Health Serv Outcomes Res Methodol 2015;15(2):99–135.

145. Gupta RS, Zhang X, Sharp LK, et al. The protective effect of community factors on childhood asthma. J Allergy Clin Immunol 2009;123(6):1297–304.e2.

146. Holt EW, Theall KP, Rabito FA. Individual, housing, and neighborhood correlates of asthma among young urban children. J Urban Health 2013;90(1):116–29.

147. Sheth A, Asher MI, Ellwood P, et al. Can geodata be used to determine the distribution of fast food outlets in relation to the prevalence and severity of asthma? A novel methodology. Allergol Immunopathol (Madr) 2016;44(4):307–13.

148. Shankardass K, Dunn JR. How goes the neighbourhood? Rethinking neighbourhoods and health research in social epidemiology. Dordrecht (Netherlands): Springer; 2012.

149. Brokamp C, LeMasters GK, Ryan PH. Residential mobility impacts exposure assessment and community socioeconomic characteristics in longitudinal epidemiology studies. J Expo Sci Environ Epidemiol 2016;26(4):428–34.

150. Kheirbek I, Wheeler K, Walters S, et al. PM2.5 and ozone health impacts and disparities in New York City: sensitivity to spatial and temporal resolution. Air Qual Atmos Health 2013;6(2):473–86.

151. Torabi M, Rosychuk RJ. Spatio-temporal modelling of disease mapping of rates. Can J Stat 2010; 38(4):698–715.

152. Zhu L, C BP, English P, et al. Hierarchical modeling of spatio-temporally misaligned data: relating traffic density to pediatric asthma hospitalizations. Environmetrics 2000;11(1):43–61.

153. Torabi M. Zero-inflated spatio-temporal models for disease mapping. Biom J 2017;59(3):430–44.

154. Quick H, Banerjee S, Carlin BP. Modeling temporal gradients in regionally aggregated California asthma hospitalization data. Ann Appl Stat 2013; 7(1):154–76.

155. Torabi M. Spatio-temporal modeling for disease mapping using CAR and B-spline smoothing. Environmetrics 2013;24(3):180–8.

156. Cook AJ, Gold DR, Li Y. Spatial cluster detection for repeatedly measured outcomes while accounting for residential history. Biom J 2009;51(5):801–18.

157. Cook AJ, Gold DR, Li Y. Spatial cluster detection for longitudinal outcomes using administrative regions. Commun Stat Theory Methods 2013; 42(12):2105–17.

158. Chute CG, Hart LA, Alexander AK, et al. The Southeastern Minnesota beacon project for community-driven health information technology: origins, achievements, and legacy. EGEMS (Wash DC) 2014;2(3):1101.

159. Faruque FS, Finley RW. Geographic medical history: advances in geospatial technology present new potentials in medical practice. In: Halounova L, Safar V, Raju PLN, et al, editors. Xxiii ISPRS Congress, Commission Viii, vol. 41. Gottingen (Germany): Copernicus Gesellschaft Mbh; 2016. p. 191–5.

160. Keddem S, Barg FK, Glanz K, et al. Mapping the urban asthma experience: using qualitative GIS to understand contextual factors affecting asthma control. Soc Sci Med 2015;140:9–17.

161. Pereira G, De Vos AJ, Cook A, et al. Vector fields of risk: a new approach to the geographical representation of childhood asthma. Health Place 2010;16(1):140–6.

The Future of Asthma Care
Personalized Asthma Treatment

Stephen T. Holgate, MD, FMedSci[a],*, Samantha Walker, PhD[b], Brigitte West, BSc[b], Kay Boycott, BA[b]

KEYWORDS

- Asthma • Personalized health care • Biologics • Companion diagnostics • mHealth
- Digital self-management

KEY POINTS

- Asthma is a complex disease with different causal pathways (endotypes).
- With appropriate diagnostic tests that identify engagement of a specific causal mechanism (eg, involvement of a specific type 2 cytokine), use of appropriate targeted therapy can be disease transforming.
- Improved diagnostic precision beyond type 2 inflammatory responses are required and multi-omics are being used to uncover such biomarkers.
- Real-time monitoring is creating the basis for mHealth in asthma management.
- To realize the impact of digital asthma technologies, interdisciplinary working across many sectors is required to create self-management tools that are simple, attractive, and of value to those who would benefit from them.

INTRODUCTION

The introduction of international and national guidelines for the day-to-day management of asthma has undoubtedly achieved considerable benefits for patients with this common disease, especially through the focus on reducing airway inflammation and frequency of exacerbation toward improved disease control.[1] However, countries vary greatly in their capacity to implement management guidelines in "real-world" settings.[2] This trend is beginning to reflect in a plateauing in asthma health gains and in some countries even a reduction.[3,4] Guided self-management is strongly advocated, but a recent Cochrane analysis has raised questions about its effectiveness in achieving asthma control especially at the severe end of the disease spectrum.[5,6] Indeed, it seems counterintuitive that approximately 60% of asthma deaths in the developed economies occur in patients not classified as conforming to the widely accepted definition of having severe asthma.[7]

PERSONALIZED HEALTH CARE VERSUS PERSONALIZED MEDICINE

A need to confront defects in current asthma management is leading to a revaluation of approach of personalized health care, which is strongly incentivized by the availability of new biologic treatments and methods for monitoring disease

Disclosure Statement: The authors declare that they have no commercial or financial interests that relate to the research described in this article. Asthma UK is a UK medical charity that receives donations from a wide variety of sources including industry. Neither S. Walker, B. West, nor K. Boycott has any personal conflicts of interest to declare; S. Holgate is a Non-executive Director of Synairgen and shareholder. He also undertakes occasional Scientific Advisory Boards and Speaker engagements speaking engagements activities for Dyson, Novartis, Teva, and Sanofi.
[a] Clinical and Experimental Sciences, Faculty of Medicine, University of Southampton, The Sir Henry Wellcome Research Laboratories, Southampton General Hospital, Mail Point 810, Level, Southampton SO166YD, UK;
[b] Asthma UK, 18 Mansell Street, London E1 8AA, UK
* Corresponding author.
E-mail address: sth@soton.ac.uk

Clin Chest Med 40 (2019) 227–241
https://doi.org/10.1016/j.ccm.2018.10.013
0272-5231/19/© 2018 Elsevier Inc. All rights reserved.

activity.[8] Personalized health and care means empowering people to have greater choice and control over the way their health and care is delivered. The result is better health and well-being for individuals with asthma, better quality and experience of care that is integrated and tailored around what really matters to them, and more sustainable health services. This change requires positioning patients and carers at the center of asthma management and redesigning care pathways accordingly, especially because the new biologics are costly. The potential for using mobile health care approaches will also help patient empowerment.

A component of personalized health care is personalized medicine: the design of therapeutic interventions that target underlying disease mechanisms more precisely. Although sometimes referred to as stratified, precision medicine, or P4 medicine, personalized medicine aims to treat the right patients with the right interventions at the right time. Cancer has led the way by using genetic sequencing to identify embryonic and somatic mutations within a tumor to enable selected targeted treatments that act on the functional consequences of the mutations. In cancer, this approach is rapidly extending to whole genome sequencing,[9] liquid biopsy,[10] and identification of immunotherapy targets.[11] However, even within the field of cancer, intratumor heterogeneity may hinder precision medicine strategies.[12]

PERSONALIZED TREATMENTS FOR ASTHMA

Although airway inflammation and remodeling underpin pathophysiology, in the case of asthma, it is becoming increasingly clear that the disease is a heterogeneous disorder comprising several different phenotypes each driven by a combination of separate causative pathways (**Fig. 1**). Unlike cancer, there are no clear genetic markers that can be used to identify disease subtypes; so far, associations between asthma and changes in more than 400 genes have been identified.[13] Studying asthma susceptibility genetics has been valuable in identifying novel underlying mechanisms, but no single cluster of mutations identify with particular asthma subtypes. There occur rare genetic variants linked to adverse asthma outcomes, but these have not helped in identifying those at most risk of adverse outcomes.[14]

That is not to say that stratification of asthma is not possible. Indeed, one may consider more conventional methods, such as lung function, symptoms, and quality-of-life assessments, as tools successfully used to stratify the disease by severity that underpins current therapeutic

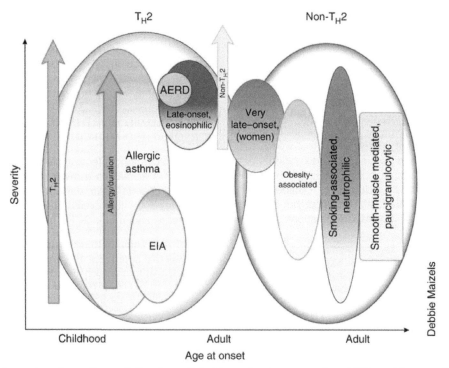

Fig. 1. Asthma phenotypes: the evolution from clinical to molecular approaches. AERD, aspirin-exacerbated respiratory disease; EIA, exercise-induced asthma; T_H2, T helper 2 lymphocyte. (*From* Wenzel SE. Asthma phenotypes: the evolution from clinical to molecular approaches. Nat Med 2012;18(5):720; with permission.)

approaches to "severity phenotypes" (any observable characteristic or trait of a disease, without any implication of a mechanism).[15] Such an approach, focusing on reducing disease severity and preventing exacerbations in large part using a combination of inhaled corticosteroids with or without long-acting bronchodilators in relation to 4 to 5 bands of disease severity, has been the accepted norm for asthma treatment over the last 2 decades.

However, it is the very heterogeneity of asthma, which is stimulating a new, more personalized approach to its management, especially at the severe end of the disease spectrum. This change has been made possible by the uncovering of specific cellular and molecular drivers of the disease leading to different phenotypic endotypes (phenotypes defined by biological mechanisms[16]); biomarkers are able to help identify particular patients suitable for specific targeted therapies, especially the use of biologics. To be clinically useful, biomarkers need to be linked to point-of-care diagnostics, which can be readily measured in exhaled breath or biological fluids.[17] Although in the past, subtypes of asthma have been described, such as allergic asthma, late-onset asthma, aspirin-intolerant asthma, and occupational asthma, these have largely been descriptive. With a few exceptions, such asthma subtypes have not been associated with the identification of specific causal pathways amenable to focused therapies. One exception to this view might be aspirin- and nonsteroidal anti-inflammatory drug (NSAID)-intolerant asthma with enhanced cysteinyl leukotriene production and benefit from leukotriene receptor antagonists.[18]

IDENTIFICATION OF IMMUNOLOGIC/INFLAMMATORY ENDOTYPES IN SEVERE ASTHMA

Most asthma begins in early childhood and is associated with atopy, especially sensitization to indoor allergens (dust mite, fungal, and pet allergens). Although allergic asthma may fluctuate across the year influenced by environmental exposures, its persistence and severity track across the life course.[19] However, reduced lung function seen in adults with this type of asthma is established in childhood and does not appear to decline more rapidly in adult years despite continuing symptoms. Severity of this type of asthma is predicated on sensitization in infancy[20] and the coexistence of atopic dermatitis and food allergy,[21] although after adolescence, atopic dermatitis generally diminishes over time.[22] It is established that this type of asthma, in which allergy plays a significant role, involves allergen sensitization of the airways, recruitment and activation of Th2-type lymphocytes, isotype switching of B cells from immunoglobulin M (IgM) to IgE with subsequent sensitization, and activation of airway mast cells and basophils culminating in the recruitment of effector leukocytes, especially eosinophils.[23] It is also clear that after the teenage years, new-onset or late-onset asthma may occur. Adults with early-onset current asthma are more likely to be atopic and have a higher frequency of asthma attacks, whereas adults with late-onset disease were more likely to be women and smokers and had greater levels of fixed airflow obstruction.[24]

Although allergic pathways involving type 2 (T2) cytokines, such as interleukin-3 (IL-3), -4, -5 and granulocyte-macrophage colony-stimulating factor (GM-CSF), are amenable to suppression by allergen-specific (subcutaneous or sublingual) immunotherapy through the induction of allergen-specific tolerance linked to regulatory T cells, multiple allergen sensitization and risks of side effects have limited this approach.[25] Nevertheless, so far, immunotherapy is the only known mechanism of influencing the natural history of allergic asthma especially if given early in the course of the disease and when the number of causative driver allergens is low.[26]

Although allergen-associated asthma became normalized as the classical "asthma paradigm" and was used to develop animal models to screen for new antiasthma drugs, such a "simple pathophysiological concept" flew in the face of clinical experiences showing asthma to be a heterogeneous disorder. This view was particularly the case when considering asthma that had a poor or no response to corticosteroids. Indeed, identification of a prominent allergic Th2 signature and accompanying eosinophil infiltration of the airways was considered paramount to identifying corticosteroid responsiveness. However, it has been known for many years that eosinophilic asthma occurred in the absence of atopy and allergic sensitization. Of particular note was late-onset severe asthma first identified by Rackemann[27] in 1947 and given the label of intrinsic asthma. Brown[28] noticed as far back as 1958 that the presence of eosinophils in the sputum was a biomarker of responsiveness to oral prednisolone. In 1960, Samter[29] identified circulating eosinophilia to be a marker of asthma irrespective of whether atopy was present or not, including his pioneer work on aspirin-exacerbated respiratory disease (Samter's Triad: asthma, nasal polyps, and a sensitivity to aspirin). Since then, there have been numerable descriptions of eosinophils being a prominent feature of nonallergic asthma,[30] but so far, environmental or infectious mechanisms accounting for this have eluded identification.

Beyond these early descriptions, it is only relatively recently that a serious attempt has been made to apply current knowledge to the classification of asthma subtypes. Wenzel and colleagues[31] were the first to describe a specific phenotype of severe asthma characterized by persistent eosinophils in bronchial biopsies in the presence of high-dose inhaled and/or oral corticosteroid treatment, which they called eosinophil-positive severe asthma (or severe eosinophilic asthma). Subsequently, Wenzel has gone on to classify asthma according to a range of clinical, physiologic, and laboratory characteristics[32] (see **Fig. 1**). These disease subtypes were predicated on pioneer observations by Woodruff and colleagues,[33] who, using messenger RNA microarray applied to airway epithelial brushings from patients with mild to moderate asthma and healthy control subjects, were able to classify subjects based on high or low epithelial expression of IL-13-inducible genes. Gene expression analyses identified 2 evenly sized and distinct subgroups, "Th2-high" and "Th2-low" asthma, the latter being indistinguishable from control subjects. These subgroups differed in expression of IL-5 and IL-13 in bronchial biopsies and in airway hyperresponsiveness, serum levels of total IgE, blood and airway eosinophilia, subepithelial fibrosis, and airway mucin gene expression as well as noted that lung function improvements with inhaled corticosteroid treatment only occurred in the Th2-high asthmatics. Thus, the era of molecular asthma phenotyping was born.

SUB-PHENOTYPING ASTHMA

The greater understanding of asthma being made up of separate phenotypes with their own mechanisms has great implications for the future management of the disease. Although currently focusing on the more severe end of the disease spectrum, the "one-size-fits-all" view of asthma and its management is being challenged. A wide range of hierarchical and nonhierarchical statistical methods have been used to identify different asthma clusters.[34–37] Statistical machine-learning methods are facilitating greater levels of efficiency in exploring data to identify and analyze disease patterns. As recently pointed out, these new digital approaches interrogate vast arrays of data generated from birth and patient cohorts in order to cluster, classify, regress, and make predictions based on inherent patterns within large and complex data sets.[38] What all of these approaches have in common is the identification of clusters

that do not clearly map well onto the 4 to 5 severity bands currently used to guide asthma management. Moreover, clusters may not always be stable with features extracted at any one specific time point not always being seen at different time points, with longitudinal analyses being needed to visualize how the clusters vary over time.[39,40]

Although dividing asthma into subtypes is helping differentiate patients with respect to initiating and exacerbating factors, treatment responses, and prognosis, the strength of these comes into their own when biological and biomarker data are incorporated.[41,42] A biomarker is a biologic feature that is used to measure the presence or progress of disease or the effects of treatment. From the foregoing discussion, measurement of lung function or a measure of bronchial responsiveness to a nonspecific challenge could be considered a biomarker of asthma severity because it directly relates to some clinical manifestations of the disease. However, although useful to make an initial diagnosis or monitor disease progress, it does not inform on underlying biological mechanisms.[43,44] On the other hand, eosinophils present in the sputum or blood identify a clear T2 inflammatory pathway with enhanced production of cytokines of the IL-4 gene cluster encoded on chromosome $5q_{31-33}$, IL-3, -4, -5, -9 ,and GM-CSF.

TYPE 2 BIOMARKERS IN DEFINING TREATMENT RESPONSES

Thus, although T2 pathways are implicated in the pathobiology of allergic asthma, they are equally important in nonallergic disease, especially in late-onset eosinophilic asthma, which is usually more severe than its allergic counterpart. Eosinophils are found in high levels in mucosal tissue, sputum, and blood, and the levels are associated with poor control and fatal/near-fatal attacks.[45] Late-onset eosinophilic asthma is characterized by lower forced expiratory volume in 1 second (FEV_1), incomplete bronchodilator reversibility, and small airway involvement accompanied by air trapping. Another characteristic feature of late-onset eosinophilic asthma is comorbid chronic rhinosinusitis with nasal polyposis,[46] a feature known for many years and in some cases linked with aspirin and other NSAID hypersensitivity.

Interest in nonallergic severe eosinophilic asthma and its associated comorbidities has increased with the recognition that in this subtype, high levels of the pro-eosinophilic cytokine IL-5 are produced by a unique population of T2 innate lymphoid cells.[47] These cells produce large amounts of IL-5 and IL-13 in response to epithelial-derived cytokines[48] and are increased in numbers in the airways of severe asthma patients.[49]

The importance of eosinophils as a biomarker of asthma severity and response to corticosteroid treatment has been known for many years as emphasized by the pioneer studies of Green and colleagues[50] and Yancey and colleagues.[51] What is difficult to explain is why, until relatively recently, the use of this relatively simple T2 inflammatory biomarker has not gained traction in asthma management. The emergence of the biologics targeting IL-5 and their close therapeutic efficacy link to eosinophils is creating an imperative for its use when choosing which patients with severe corticosteroid refractory asthma to try with one of the 3 available anti-IL-5/IL5 receptor-directed biologics (mepolizumab, reslizumab, and benralizumab) as discussed in Mauli Desai and colleagues' article, "Immunomodulators and Biologics: Beyond Stepped-Care Therapy," in this issue. The consensus currently lies at a peripheral blood eosinophil count on several occasions of greater than 300 cells per microliter. However, a recent analysis of several mepolizumab trials indicates a baseline blood eosinophil threshold of 150 cells per microliter or greater or a historical blood eosinophil threshold of 300 cells per microliter or greater, will allow selection of patients with severe eosinophilic asthma who are most likely to achieve clinically significant reductions in the rate of exacerbations with treatment.[51] IL-5 blockade can produce dramatic improvements in asthma symptoms as well as beneficial effects on comorbidities, such as rhinosinusitis and nasal polyposis,[52] as well as enabling reductions and withdrawal of oral corticosteroids,[53] with their attendant side effects. The antibody-dependent cell cytotoxic monoclonal antibody (mAb) benralizumab directed against the IL-5 receptor alpha chain, resulting in the killing of eosinophils by cytotoxic T cells, has also revealed efficacy in a phase 2 trial in T2 asthma.[54] Whether this will prove more effective than IL-5 blockade alone is not yet known.

Another key T2 target is signaling through the IL-4/IL-13 pathways. Although initial results with IL-13 blocking monoclonal antibodies such as lebrikizumab looked promising when patients were selected on the basis of elevated circulating periostin levels, a peptide secreted by airway epithelial cells in the presence of IL-13,[55] subsequent phase 2 trials selecting T2 high-type asthmatics proved disappointing.[56,57] By contrast, blockade of the IL4rα with dupilumab has proven efficacious in a corticosteroid reduction trial in moderate to severe T2 asthma, possibly because the receptor subunit is involved in both IL-4 and IL-13 signaling.[58] The importance of the combined IL-4/-13 pathway in atopic dermatitis has also been shown in positive clinical trials with dupilumab.[59,60]

Thus, with multiple biologics now becoming available to treat severe allergic and nonallergic T2 asthma, the paradigm of therapy is changing from ever-increasing doses of inhaled/oral corticosteroids with their attendant problems over adherence and side effects to a pathway specific targeted approach. This pathway-specific research is still in the early days, but as more becomes known about why one biologic targeting a T2 pathway is preferable to another, the personalized precision approach to treatment will begin to be the norm. This approach will be made easier with the availability of further biomarkers that will delineate subtypes of T2 response and enable selection of the most appropriate therapy. As biologics give way to biosimilars, especially if they are of small molecular weight that can be taken by inhalation or orally, this approach of using a companion diagnostic to select a specific therapy will become cheaper and more widely available.

BEYOND THE T2 ASTHMA SUBTYPE

Recognizing how effective mAb targeting of T2-type asthma is, there has been a concerted effort to uncover other asthma endotypes because only ~50% of severe asthma is eosinophilic. Although other types of asthma have been described such as neutrophilic,[61] just as there are different endotypes of eosinophilic asthma, the same is true of asthma in which neutrophils are present in the relative absent of eosinophils. Known causative factors include high-dose corticosteroid therapy,[62] tobacco smoking,[63] bacterial infection (especially with *Haemophilus influenzae*),[64–66] obesity,[67] and epithelial injury itself.[68] Although there have been several attempts to treat neutrophilic asthma, most have failed with the exception of macrolides, such as azithromycin.[69,70] Another asthma subtype that has been identified is paucigranulocytic (ie, normal levels of both eosinophils and neutrophils in sputum),[71] although it has been suggested that this asthma subtype represents simply a lower level of inflammation.[72]

MULTI-OMIC TECHNOLOGIES ARE UNCOVERING NEW ASTHMA DISEASE MECHANISMS

Application of 'omic technologies to asthma in an agnostic way is identifying novel clusters linked to biomarkers. Among the first of these was that of Baines and colleagues,[73] who examined gene expression profiles from induced sputum of 47 asthmatic patients. They identified 6 gene biomarkers (Charcot-Leydon crystal protein, carboxypeptidase A3, deoxyribonuclease I-like 3, IL-1β, alkaline phosphatase, tissue-nonspecific isozyme and chemokine [C-X-C motif] receptor 2), which could significantly discriminate eosinophilic asthma from other phenotypes, including patients with noneosinophilic, paucigranulocytic, neutrophilic asthma, and healthy control subjects, as well as discriminating patients with neutrophilic asthma from those with paucigranulocytic asthma and healthy control subjects. The NIH Severe Asthma Research Program (SARP) has also provided a window on asthma subtypes in severe disease, including airway epithelial cell gene expression profiles indicative of heterogeneous mechanisms of severe disease.[74] SARP was also able to identify refractory airway T2 inflammation in a large subgroup of asthmatic patients treated with inhaled corticosteroids,[75] and a lipoxin A receptor biochemical endotype for severe asthma[76] and asthma subgroups associated with circulating YKL-40 levels.[77] However, although such studies have helped expose different molecular and cellular subtypes of asthma, at this time, it is difficult to determine how one subtype and its endotype might relate to another.

There is general agreement that standardized definitions and concepts of asthma severity, risk, and level of control are critical if targeted interventions and pathways to deliver them are to transform asthma care.[78] A systematic approach has been made in several EU projects starting with the cross-sectional European Network for Understanding the Mechanisms of severe asthma study,[79] evolving into a biomarker 1-year prospective longitudinal study of severe asthma (BIOAIR).[80] Most recently, the EU-supported Innovative Medicine's Initiative Unbiased BIOmarkers in PREDiction of respiratory disease outcomes (UBIOPRED) study has used common datasets to build a cohort of severe and less severe asthma compared with normal controls suitable for multiomic analyses.[81,82]

UBIOPRED, as described in some detail in R. Stokes Peebles Jr and Mark A. Aronica's article, Proinflammatory Pathways in the Pathogenesis of Asthma," in this issue, is providing valuable insights into possible new causal pathways comprising this complex phenotype. Although full integration of the different 'omic technologies applied to sputum, blood, and exhaled breath is ongoing, some new pathways have been uncovered. Sputum, epithelial, and biopsy transcriptomics have proven especially valuable in defining 3 transcriptome-associated clusters (TACs)[83,84]:

TAC1 (characterized by immune receptors IL33R, CCR3, and TSLP receptor), TAC2 (characterized by interferon-, tumor necrosis factor-α-, and inflammasome-associated genes), and TAC3 (characterized by genes of metabolic pathways, ubiquitination, and mitochondrial function). TAC1 showed the highest enrichment of gene signatures for IL-13/T-helper cell Th2 and innate lymphoid cell T2 and most closely resembles the T2 eosinophil-driven asthma with the highest sputum eosinophilia and exhaled nitric oxide fraction and was restricted to severe asthma with oral corticosteroid dependency, frequent exacerbations, and severe airflow obstruction. TAC2 revealed the highest sputum neutrophilia, serum C-reactive protein levels, and prevalence of eczema. TAC3 had normal to moderately high sputum eosinophils and better-preserved lung function (FEV_1). Gene-protein coexpression networks extended the molecular classification of TAC2 and TAC3, characterized by inflammasome-associated and metabolic/mitochondrial pathways, respectively. The former neutrophilic-type has a high proportion of bacterial infected features, whereas the latter paucigranulocytic-type most closely links to smooth muscle mitochondrial oxidant stress and pollutant exposure. TAC2 inflammasome-linked endotype is a particularly interesting subtype because involvement of the nucleotide-binding domain and leucine-rich repeat-containing 3 (NLRP3) inflammasome in some severe asthma patients has been documented in other cohorts, including asthmatic children.[85,86] The function of the NLRP3 inflammasome is to activate caspase-1, which leads to the processing of IL-1β and IL-18 into active forms, and the induction of pyroptosis, a highly inflammatory form of programmed cell death occurring most frequently upon infection with intracellular pathogens.

THE START OF A NEW JOURNEY: EMBEDDING PRECISION MEDICINE OF ASTHMA INTO PRACTICE

Although the relentless identification of asthma subtypes continues, it is highly likely that asthma treatment, especially of the more severe disease, will become increasingly dependent on the use of companion diagnostics linked to specific use of pathway-selective targeted treatments. This is to be welcomed if it increases efficacy and reduces side effects, but we are some way off this approach becoming routine practice. There have been early attempts to generate biomarker decision algorithms to choose whether to use a biologic or advise a particular biologic over another.[87,88] For the present, these and other algorithms require testing in practice. Moreover, greater granularity in the matching of biomarker/ diagnostic to treatment decision making will be required, but this exciting new journey has begun and is likely to open the door for an entirely new approach to asthma treatment (and prevention) based on detailed knowledge of causal pathways. Such an approach is long overdue. Apart from improved and simple point-of-care diagnostics, more needs to be understood about whether interfering with sentinel asthma pathways will influence the natural history of the disease and even be able to prevent asthma from evolving in the first place. As confidence in biologics increases and biosimilars become available,[89] the future may well see the introduction of biologics earlier in the course of the disease, combinations with other potential disease modifying agents, such as low-dose methotrexate, and even combinations of biologics,[90] as are now being adopted in the standard treatment of autoimmune diseases.

It is still not known whether targeted treatments with biologics are capable of reversing remodeling of the airways. Mucus plugging of the airways in chronic severe asthma may persist in the same lung segment for years[91]; smooth muscle increases and associated hyperresponsiveness seem only partly reversible with anti-inflammatory and thermoplasty treatments,[92] and airway wall fibrosis[93] and pruning of the microvasculature[94] are all components of severe persistent asthma that deserve much more attention. At the time of writing, very few, if any, interventions influence the natural history of chronic asthma.

THE FUTURE OF ASTHMA CARE: PERSONALIZED ASTHMA MANAGEMENT

As already discussed, asthma is a complex, episodic condition with multiple triggers, which can vary in severity across the life course.[95] For example, in the United Kingdom, an estimated 5.4 million people have asthma, the annual cost of which is estimated at £1.1 billion, presenting a considerable and increasing burden to the National Health Service.[96] In many countries, most people with asthma are looked after in primary care (general practice),[97] and although asthma accounts for a small minority of primary care appointments, many of these are routine annual checkups that are not personalized to an individual; given the dynamic nature of asthma symptoms over time, it could be questioned how much value this brings to either the clinician or the patient. Despite there being effective medication for a large proportion of people with asthma and an extensive evidence base demonstrating that supported self-management improves asthma control, reduces exacerbations and admissions, and improves quality of life,[98,99] asthma remains poorly controlled in a substantial proportion of people.[100] In most health care systems, most of the asthma management takes place outside the health care setting and relies on people independently managing their symptoms effectively. Although there are relatively few hospital admissions for asthma compared with its prevalence,[96] the National Review of Asthma Deaths in the United Kingdom found that 45% of people who died of an asthma attack did so without seeking medical assistance or before emergency medical care could be provided.[101] The situation is likely to be similar in other countries and illustrates that, despite good intentions, self-management is not always effective. To improve asthma outcomes and prevent avoidable asthma deaths, asthma management needs to be highly personalized and delivered to people in their everyday lives. The emergence of mobile and electronic health (mHealth) internet-linked applications (apps) and improved data sharing and analysis capabilities offer a great opportunity to deliver personalized asthma care,[102–104] especially for those who are at higher than average risk of an asthma attack but who are highly digitally literate.[105]

Increasingly, advanced mHealth apps and electronic dashboards will collect multiple streams of external information, such as adherence to inhaled treatments, weather, pollen count, pollution levels as well as activity and geographic locations, analyze this information, and then present it in a user-friendly way to help people adjust their treatments, manage their asthma triggers, and manage their interactions with health care professionals more effectively.[106–108] These data would provide a more complete picture of an individual's asthma, which could then be used to predict asthma attacks, aid clinical decision making, and drive better targeting of health care resources. It is important that these data are collected passively (ie, data are collected during routine use) because it is unlikely that they, like most other populations who sign up to use disease-management apps, would continue to actively enter data for the extended periods of time necessary to get a detailed picture of their asthma.

DIGITAL SELF-MANAGEMENT INTERVENTIONS FOR PEOPLE WITH ASTHMA

"Smart" inhalers, inhalers that contain sensors and trackers that can connect via Bluetooth to smart phones and tablet devices, are a particularly promising technology to drive technology-enabled asthma management.[109–112] Smart inhalers can passively monitor inhaler usage and offer the most accurate solution for recording adherence to inhaled medication; however, their real-world impact is not yet clear.[110,113]

At the time of this writing, many mHealth studies have been of moderate quality and show significant heterogeneity in both designs and study end points.[114,115] A dose counter and a remote monitoring adherence device that recorded a participant's inhaler use have shown a trend toward positive impact on adherence, but the investigators concluded that although remotely monitored adherence holds important clinical information, future research should focus on refining adherence and exacerbation measures.[107] An exploration of the utility of telemonitoring data for building machine learning algorithms that predict asthma exacerbations before they occur has revealed that machine learning techniques have significant potential in developing personalized decision support for chronic disease telemonitoring systems.[116] A digital asthma management intervention has demonstrated significant reductions in the use of inhaled short-acting bronchodilator (SABA) use, increased number of symptom-free days, and improvements in asthma control.[109] In a further study that has investigated whether a self-care system would achieve better asthma control through a mobile telephone-based interactive program, the group using the mobile telephone program had better quality of life after 3 months (determined using the Short Form-12 physical component score) and fewer episodes of exacerbation and unscheduled visits than the control group.[117] A randomized clinical trial of electronic adherence monitoring with reminder alarms and feedback use in children found that electronic monitoring with feedback-improved adherence decreased hospital admissions and courses of oral corticosteroids required.[106]

Finally, a systematic review of the beneficial effects of mobile health applications on asthma outcomes has concluded that multifunctional mHealth apps have potential to improve asthma control and improve quality of life compared with traditional interventions, but that further studies are needed to identify the effectiveness of these interventions on outcomes related to medication adherence and costs.[118]

DIGITAL ASTHMA DIAGNOSIS AND BETTER DISEASE UNDERSTANDING

As referred to in relation to the use of targeted biologics, personalized medicine in asthma requires better diagnostics. As highlighted in this and other articles in this issue, asthma is increasingly being recognized as a heterogeneous condition that is characterized by mechanistically distinct symptoms. Diagnostic tests have not kept pace with these advances in scientific understanding, and there are still no widely used tests that can accurately differentiate between different types of asthma. This lack of diagnostic tests results in underdiagnosis and overdiagnosis, and people potentially receiving the wrong treatment. A diagnostic process that combined objective tests with the use of real-time data from connected technologies, such as smart inhalers, could significantly advance the both the diagnosis and the management of asthma in the future.[119]

Although it appears that technology could play a significant role in the real-time identification of those at risk of an asthma attack using data gathered through mobile platforms, it is important that such technologies improve asthma outcomes and are acceptable and useful to people with asthma. Accurate and timely assessment of asthma control, identification of future risk, and the subsequent targeting of an appropriate intervention form the basis of digital health approaches[104,108] (**Fig. 2**). However, although there is increasing evidence that these are promising approaches with potentially beneficial effects on asthma control and adherence to medication, there is currently a lack of standardized and validated risk tools for asthma available in primary care.[120] Desktop alerts such as prescribing alerts and personal action plans offer promise but so far have been poorly adopted.

Current clinical decision support systems that offer advice to health care professionals on how to manage their patients based on risk are rarely used and the advice is rarely followed.[121] Big data and artificial intelligence offer the opportunity to develop more advanced and user-focused risk and population management tools that use new streams of data (eg, remote adherence data) to predict asthma attacks in real time and develop personalized decision support.[107,116]

WHAT IS NEEDED IN THE FUTURE?

To prepare the world for an exciting future using digital innovation in asthma management, it is crucial to develop, agree, and adopt quality standards for conducting trials of e-health interventions.[122] Research on specific needs and barriers in target populations and development of appropriate strategies for use of new digital technology for adherence monitoring are also required.[123] For successful applications to be developed, and most importantly used, it is vital that people with asthma and their health care professionals are

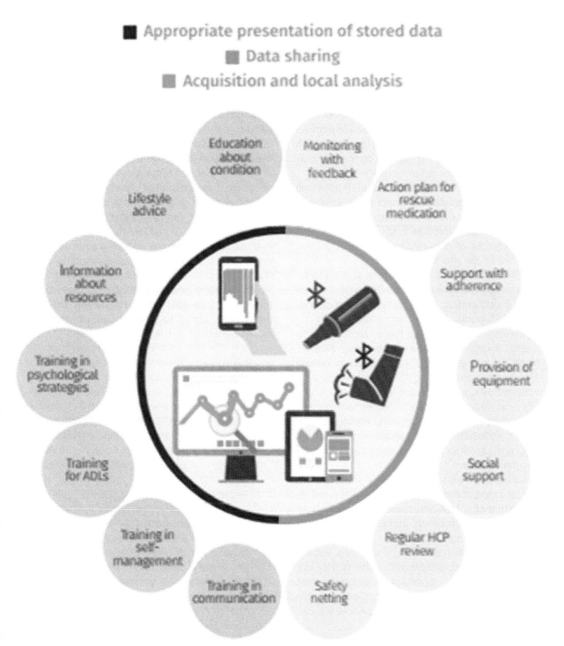

Fig. 2. Connected asthma: the potential for technology to transform care. ADLs, activities of daily living. HCP, heath care professional. (*Reproduced* with permission of the © ERS 2018: European Respiratory Journal Dec 2017; 50(6). pii: 1701782. DOI: 10.1183/13993003.01782-2017.)

involved in the development of mHealth asthma tools because there are often discrepancies between the needs and expectations of different groups.[124] Significant barriers to implementation of asthma digital health technology exist, including the lack of a patient-professional partnership and a lack of perceived benefit in improving asthma symptoms.[125] Barriers identified among primary care physicians include a low sense of urgency toward asthma care and current work routines. Practice nurses identified a low level of structured asthma care and a lack of support by colleagues as barriers. The cost of adopting the innovation needs to be lower than the benefit, understanding the health economics of introducing new technologies is key; otherwise, the technology will not be adopted by the health care system,[126] and more research is needed to evaluate the impact of health technologies on health outcomes and health economics.

Developers of digital technologies also need to recognize that people with asthma are a heterogeneous group and that in the same way that the "one-size-fits-all" approach to routine use of inhaled corticosteroids does not work for everyone, a "one-size-fits-all" approach to asthma technology will not work either. Most important will be the ability to be able to personalize the technology easily for multiple different users.

Digital asthma applications and platforms will need effective regulation to ensure that interventions are evidence based and that they add value to the population expected to use them. One recent example of a public/private collaboration that successfully reduced the burden of asthma was AIR Louisville, one of the largest studies looking at an integrated solution for asthma conducted in a real-world setting. AIR Louisville was a collaboration of 25 public, private, and philanthropic organizations that used digital health technology to try and improve asthma outcomes. Results showed an impressive 78% reduction in rescue SABA inhaler use and a 48% improvement in symptom-free days. Data also informed municipal policy recommendations, including enhancing tree canopy, tree removal mitigation, zoning for air pollution emission buffers, recommended truck routes, and development of a community asthma notification system.[127]

In summary, mHealth/technology solutions are currently being developed, but how they will fit into self-management and routine care is not yet clear. Some key problems include that apps for asthma self-management often contain limited and inaccurate information[128,129] and that, even if the content is good, people with asthma may not use them.[121,130] It is important to recognize that proving efficacy is different, both methodologically and scientifically, from proving that people will use it in everyday practice.

Although asthma digital health is a promising area, existing supporting evidence is only of moderate quality, and there is significant heterogeneity in study end points and trial designs.[114,115,131] A systematic review of the effects of mobile health applications on asthma outcomes concluded that multifunctional mHealth apps show good potential, but further studies are needed to identify the effectiveness of these interventions on outcomes related to medication adherence and costs.[118] Current asthma applications are often poor quality,[128,129] and more research is needed to validate digital health solutions to ensure they drive improved asthma outcomes and efficiencies.[108,131]

Considering the current rate of technological development alongside new targeted therapeutic interventions and partner diagnostics, in the future there will be a plethora of software and information providers to choose from with greater or lesser degrees of assurance about the quality and safety of their products. However, even if well-validated, easy-to-use asthma tools are developed, mobile devices and computers will simultaneously be delivery platforms for a significant proportion of an individual's financial and utility management tasks, shopping, entertainment, socializing, and many other more necessary and interesting distractions from managing the life-long episodic condition that is asthma. To realize the impact of digital asthma technologies on reducing asthma attacks, preventing hospitalizations, and reducing asthma deaths, technology companies, clinicians, researchers, and people with asthma need to work together to create self-management tools that are simple, attractive, and of value to those that would benefit from them.

REFERENCES

1. Reddel HK, Bateman ED, Becker A, et al. A summary of the new GINA strategy: a roadmap to asthma control. Eur Respir J 2015;46:622–39.
2. Becker AB, Abrams EM. Asthma guidelines: the global initiative for asthma in relation to national guidelines. Curr Opin Allergy Clin Immunol 2017; 17:99–103.
3. Papaioannou AI, Kostikas K, Zervas E, et al. Control of asthma in real life: still a valuable goal? Eur Respir Rev 2015;24:361–9.
4. Bell MC, William WW. Busse severe asthma: an expanding and mounting clinical challenge. J Allergy Clin Immunol Pract 2013;1:110–22.
5. Pinnock H, Thomas M. Does self-management prevent severe exacerbations? Curr Opin Pulm Med 2015;21:95–102.
6. Lenferink A, Brusse-Keizer M, van der Valk PD, et al. Self-management interventions including action plans for exacerbations versus usual care in patients with chronic obstructive pulmonary disease. Cochrane Database Syst Rev 2017;(8): CD011682.
7. Levy ML, Winter R. Asthma deaths: what now? Thorax 2015;70:209–10.
8. Thomas M. Why aren't we doing better in asthma: time for personalised medicine? NPJ Prim Care Respir Med 2015;25:15004.
9. Nakagawa H, Fujita M. Whole genome sequencing analysis for cancer genomics and precision medicine. Cancer Sci 2018;109:513–22.
10. Maciejko L, Smalley M, Goldman A. Cancer immunotherapy and personalized medicine: emerging

technologies and biomarker-based approaches. J Mol Biomark Diagn 2017;8 [pii:350].

11. Raspollini MR, Montagnani I, Montironi R, et al. Intratumoural heterogeneity may hinder precision medicine strategies in patients with clear cell renal cell carcinoma. J Clin Pathol 2018;71:467–71.

12. Dive C, Shishido SN, Kuhn P. Cancer Moonshot connecting liternational liquid biopsy efforts through academic partnership. Clin Pharmacol Ther 2017;101:622–4.

13. Demenais F, Margaritte-Jeannin P, Barnes KC, et al. Multiancestry association study identifies new asthma risk loci that colocalize with immune-cell enhancer marks. Nat Genet 2018;50:42–53.

14. Ortega VE, Hawkins GA, Moore WC, et al. Effect of rare variants in ADRB2 on risk of severe exacerbations and symptom control during longacting β agonist treatment in a multiethnic asthma population: a genetic study. Lancet Respir Med 2014;2: 204–13.

15. Nathan RA, Sorkness CA, Kosinski M, et al. Development of the asthma control test: a survey for assessing asthma control. J Allergy Clin Immunol 2004;113:59–65.

16. Anderson GP. Endotyping asthma: new insights into key pathogenic mechanisms in a complex, heterogeneous disease. Lancet 2008;372:1107–19.

17. Medical Research Council. The MRC framework for the development, design and analysis of stratified medicine research. Swindon (UK): Medical Research Council. Available at: https://mrc.ukri.org/research/initiatives/stratified-medicine/stratified-medicine-methodology-framework/.

18. Dahlén SE, Malmström K, Nizankowska E, et al. Improvement of aspirin-intolerant asthma by montelukast, a leukotriene antagonist: a randomized, double-blind, placebo-controlled trial. Am J Respir Crit Care Med 2002;165:9–14.

19. Tai A, Tran H, Roberts M, et al. Outcomes of childhood asthma to the age of 50 years. J Allergy Clin Immunol 2014;133:1572–8.

20. Simpson A, Tan VY, Winn J, et al. Beyond atopy: multiple patterns of sensitization in relation to asthma in a birth cohort study. Am J Respir Crit Care Med 2010;181:1200–6.

21. Bantz SK, Zhu Z, Zheng T. The atopic march: progression from atopic dermatitis to allergic rhinitis and asthma. J Clin Cell Immunol 2014;5 [pii:202].

22. Tai A, Tran H, Roberts M, et al. Trends in eczema, rhinitis, and rye grass sensitization in a longitudinal asthma cohort. Ann Allergy Asthma Immunol 2014; 112:437–40.

23. Holgate ST, Wenzel S, Postma DS, et al. Asthma. Nat Rev Dis Primers 2015;1:15025.

24. Tan DJ, Walters EH, Perret JL, et al. Age-of-asthma onset as a determinant of different asthma phenotypes in adults: a systematic review and meta-

analysis of the literature. Expert Rev Respir Med 2015;9:109–23.

25. Dominguez-Ortega J, Delgado J, Blanco C, et al. Specific allergen immunotherapy for the treatment of allergic asthma: a review of current evidence. J Investig Allergol Clin Immunol 2017;27(Suppl. 1):1–35.

26. Incorvaia C. Preventive capacity of allergen immunotherapy on the natural history of allergy. J Prev Med Hyg 2013;54:71–4.

27. Rackemann FM. Intrinsic asthma. Bull N Y Acad Med 1947;23:302–6.

28. Brown HM. Treatment of chronic asthma with prednisolone: significance of eosinophils in the sputum. Lancet 1958;ii:1245.

29. Samter M. On eosinophils. Allerg Asthma (Leipz) 1960;6:195–9.

30. Ulrik CS. Peripheral eosinophil counts as a marker of disease activity in intrinsic and extrinsic asthma. Clin Exp Allergy 1995;25:820–7.

31. Wenzel SE, Schwartz LB, Langmack EL, et al. Evidence that severe asthma can be divided pathologically into two inflammatory subtypes with distinct physiologic and clinical characteristics. Am J Respir Crit Care Med 1999;160: 1001–8.

32. Wenzel SE. Asthma phenotypes: the evolution from clinical to molecular approaches. Nat Med 2012; 18:716–25.

33. Woodruff PG, Modrek B, Choy DF, et al. T-helper type 2-driven inflammation defines major subphenotypes of asthma. Am J Respir Crit Care Med 2009;180:388–95.

34. Amelink M, de Nijs SB, de Groot JC, et al. Three phenotypes of adult-onset asthma. Allergy 2013; 68:674–80.

35. Haldar P, Pavord ID, Shaw DE, et al. Cluster analysis and clinical asthma phenotypes. Am J Respir Crit Care Med 2008;178:218–24.

36. Moore WC, Meyers DA, Wenzel SE, et al. Identification of asthma phenotypes using cluster analysis in the Severe Asthma Research Program. Am J Respir Crit Care Med 2010;181:315–23.

37. Siroux V, Basagana X, Boudier A, et al. Identifying adult asthma phenotypes using a clustering approach. Eur Respir J 2011;38:310–7.

38. Deliu M, Sperrin M, Belgrave D, et al. Identification of asthma subtypes using clustering methodologies. Pulm Ther 2016;2:19–41.

39. Newby C, Heaney LG, Menzies-Gow A, et al. Statistical cluster analysis of the British Thoracic Society Severe refractory Asthma Registry: clinical outcomes and phenotype stability. PLoS One 2014;9:e102987.

40. Zaihra T, Walsh CJ, Ahmed S, et al. Phenotyping of difficult asthma using longitudinal physiological and biomarker measurements reveals significant

differences in stability between clusters. BMC Pulm Med 2016;16:74.

41. Ray A, Oriss TB, Wenzel SE. Emerging molecular phenotypes of asthma. Am J Physiol Lung Cell Mol Physiol 2015;308:L130–40.

42. Chung KF. Personalised medicine in asthma: time for action: number 1 in the Series "personalised medicine in respiratory diseases" Edited by Renaud Louis and Nicolas Roche. Eur Respir Rev 2017;26(145) [pii:170064].

43. Moeller A, Carlsen KH, Sly PD, et al. Monitoring asthma in childhood: lung function, bronchial responsiveness and inflammation. Eur Respir Rev 2015;24:204–15.

44. Giovannini M, Valli M, Ribuffo V, et al. Relationship between Methacholine Challenge Testing and exhaled nitric oxide in adult patients with suspected bronchial asthma. Eur Ann Allergy Clin Immunol 2014;46:109–13.

45. de Groot JC, Storm H, Amelink M, et al. Clinical profile of patients with adult-onset eosinophilic asthma. ERJ Open Res 2016;2 [pii:00100-2015].

46. Licari A, Brambilla I, De Filippo M, et al. The role of upper airway pathology as a co-morbidity in severe asthma. Expert Rev Respir Med 2017;11:855–65.

47. Morita H, Moro K, Koyasu S. Innate lymphoid cells in allergic and non-allergic inflammation. J Allergy Clin Immunol 2016;138:1253–64.

48. van Rijt L, von Richthofen H, van Ree R. Type 2 innate lymphoid cells: at the cross-roads in allergic asthma. Semin Immunopathol 2016;38:483–96.

49. Kortekaas Krohn I, Shikhagaie MM, Golebski K, et al. Emerging roles of innate lymphoid cells in inflammatory diseases: clinical implications. Allergy 2018;73:837–50.

50. Green RH, Brightling CE, McKenna S, et al. Asthma exacerbations and sputum eosinophil counts: a randomised controlled trial. Lancet 2002;360: 1715–21.

51. Yancey SW, Keene ON, Albers FC, et al. Biomarkers for severe eosinophilic asthma. J Allergy Clin Immunol 2017;140:1509–18.

52. Bachert C, Sousa AR, Lund VJ, et al. Reduced need for surgery in severe nasal polyposis with mepolizumab: randomized trial. J Allergy Clin Immunol 2017;140:1024–31.

53. Bel EH, Wenzel SE, Thompson PJ, et al. Oral glucocorticoid-sparing effect of mepolizumab in eosinophilic asthma. N Engl J Med 2014;371: 1189–97.

54. Tian BP, Zhang GS, Lou J, et al. Efficacy and safety of benralizumab for eosinophilic asthma: a systematic review and meta-analysis of randomized controlled trials. J Asthma 2017;6:1–10.

55. Corren J, Lemanske RF, Hanania NA, et al. Lebrikizumab treatment in adults with asthma. N Engl J Med 2011;365:1088–98.

56. Noonan M, Korenblat P, Mosesova S, et al. Dose-ranging study of lebrikizumab in asthmatic patients not receiving inhaled steroids. J Allergy Clin Immunol 2013;132:567–74.

57. Scheerens H, Arron JR, Zheng Y, et al. The effects of lebrikizumab in patients with mild asthma following whole lung allergen challenge. Clin Exp Allergy 2014;44:38–46.

58. Wenzel S, Ford L, Pearlman D, et al. Dupilumab in persistent asthma with elevated eosinophil levels. N Engl J Med 2013;368:2455–66.

59. Simpson EL, Bieber T, Guttman-Yassky E, et al. Two phase 3 trials of dupilumab versus placebo in atopic dermatitis. N Engl J Med 2016;375: 2335–48.

60. Gooderham MJ, Hong HC, Eshtiaghi P, et al. Dupilumab: a review of its use in the treatment of atopic dermatitis. J Am Acad Dermatol 2018;78: S28–36.

61. Chung KF. Neutrophilic asthma: a distinct target for treatment? Lancet Respir Med 2016;4:765–7.

62. Nguyen LT, Lim S, Oates T, et al. Increase in airway neutrophils after oral but not inhaled corticosteroid therapy in mild asthma. Respir Med 2005;99: 200–7.

63. Siew LQC, Wu SY, Ying S, et al. Cigarette smoking increases bronchial mucosal IL-17A expression in asthmatics, which acts in concert with environmental aeroallergens to engender neutrophilic inflammation. Clin Exp Allergy 2017;47:740–50.

64. Green BJ, Wiriyachaiporn S, Grainge C, et al. Potentially pathogenic airway bacteria and neutrophilic inflammation in treatment resistant severe asthma. PLoS One 2014;9:e100645.

65. Brusselle GG. Are the antimicrobial properties of macrolides required for their therapeutic efficacy in chronic neutrophilic airway diseases? Thorax 2015;70:401–3.

66. Alnahas S, Hagner S, Raifer H, et al. IL-17 and TNF-α are key mediators of Moraxella catarrhalis triggered exacerbation of allergic airway inflammation. Front Immunol 2017;8:1562.

67. Telenga ED, Tideman SW, Kerstjens HA, et al. Obesity in asthma: more neutrophilic inflammation as a possible explanation for a reduced treatment response. Allergy 2012;67:1060–8.

68. Uddin M, Lau LC, Seumois G, et al. EGF-induced bronchial epithelial cells drive neutrophil chemotactic and anti-apoptotic activity in asthma. PLoS One 2013;8:e72502.

69. Johnston SL, Szigeti M, Cross M, et al. Azithromycin for acute exacerbations of asthma: the AZALEA randomized clinical trial. JAMA Intern Med 2016; 176:1630–7.

70. Brusselle GG, Vanderstichele C, Jordens P, et al. Azithromycin for prevention of exacerbations in severe asthma (AZISAST): a multicentre randomised

double-blind placebo-controlled trial. Thorax 2013; 68:322–9.

71. Ntontsi P, Loukides S, Bakakos P, et al. Clinical, functional and inflammatory characteristics in patients with paucigranulocytic stable asthma: comparison with different sputum phenotypes. Allergy 2017;72:1761–7.

72. Demarche S, Schleich F, Henket M, et al. Detailed analysis of sputum and systemic inflammation in asthma phenotypes: are paucigranulocytic asthmatics really non-inflammatory? BMC Pulm Med 2016;16:46.

73. Baines KJ, Simpson JL, Wood LG, et al. Sputum gene expression signature of 6 biomarkers discriminates asthma inflammatory phenotypes. J Allergy Clin Immunol 2014;133:997–1007.

74. Li X, Hawkins GA, Moore WC, et al. Expression of asthma susceptibility genes in bronchial epithelial cells and bronchial alveolar lavage in the Severe Asthma Research Program (SARP) cohort. J Asthma 2016;53:775–82.

75. Peters MC, Kerr S, Dunican EM, et al. Refractory airway type 2 inflammation in a large subgroup of asthmatic patients treated with inhaled corticosteroids. J Allergy Clin Immunol 2018. [Epub ahead of print].

76. Ricklefs I, Barkas I, Duvall MG, et al. ALX receptor ligands define a biochemical endotype for severe asthma. JCI Insight 2018;3 [pii:120932].

77. Gomez JL, Yan X, Holm CT, et al. Characterisation of asthma subgroups associated with circulating YKL-40 levels. Eur Respir J 2017;50 [pii: 1700800].

78. Kupczyk M, Wenzel S. U.S. and European severe asthma cohorts: what can they teach us about severe asthma? J Intern Med 2012;272:121–32.

79. The ENFUMOSA cross-sectional European multi-centre study of the clinical phenotype of chronic severe asthma. European Network for Understanding Mechanisms of Severe Asthma. Eur Respir J 2003;22:470–7.

80. Kupczyk M, Dahlén B, Sterk PJ, et al. Stability of phenotypes defined by physiological variables and biomarkers in adults with asthma. Allergy 2014;69:1198–204.

81. Bel EH, Sousa A, Fleming L, et al. Diagnosis and definition of severe refractory asthma: an international consensus statement from the Innovative Medicine Initiative (IMI). Thorax 2011;66:910–7.

82. Wheelock CE, Goss VM, Balgoma D, et al. Application of 'omics technologies to biomarker discovery in inflammatory lung diseases. Eur Respir J 2013; 42:802–25.

83. Kuo CS, Pavlidis S, Loza M, et al. T-helper cell type 2 (Th2) and non-Th2 molecular phenotypes of asthma using sputum transcriptomics in U-BIO-PRED. Eur Respir J 2017;49 pii:1602135.

84. Kuo CS, Pavlidis S, Loza M, et al. A transcriptome-driven analysis of epithelial brushings and bronchial biopsies to define asthma phenotypes in U-BIOPRED. Am J Respir Crit Care Med 2017; 195:43–455.

85. Kim RY, Pinkerton JW, Gibson PG, et al. Inflammasomes in COPD and neutrophilic asthma. Thorax 2015;70:1199–201.

86. Herberth G, Offenberg K, Rolle-Kampczyk U, et al. Endogenous metabolites and inflammasome activity in early childhood and links to respiratory diseases. J Allergy Clin Immunol 2015;136:495–7.

87. Bousquet J, Brusselle G, Buhl R, et al. Care pathways for the selection of a biologic in severe asthma. Eur Respir J 2017;50 [pii:1701782].

88. Zervas E, Samitas K, Papaioannou AI, et al. An algorithmic approach for the treatment of severe uncontrolled asthma. ERJ Open Res 2018;4: 00125–2017.

89. Ferrando M, Bagnasco D, Braido F, et al. Biosimilars in allergic diseases. Curr Opin Allergy Clin Immunol 2016;16:68–73.

90. Dedaj R, Unsel L. Case study: a combination of mepolizumab and omaluzimab injections for severe asthma. J Asthma 2018;7:1–2.

91. Dunican EM, Elicker BM, Gierada DS, et al. Mucus plugs in patients with asthma linked to eosinophilia and airflow obstruction. J Clin Invest 2018;128: 997–1009.

92. Chernyavsky IL, Russell RJ, Saunders RM, et al. In vitro/, in silico/and in vivo/study challenges the impact of bronchial thermoplasty on acute airway smooth muscle mass loss. Eur Respir J 2018;51 [pii:1701680].

93. Gu BH, Madison MC, Corry D, et al. Matrix remodeling in chronic lung diseases. Matrix Biol 2018;73: 52–63.

94. Ash SY, Rahaghi FN, Come CE, et al. Pruning of the pulmonary vasculature in asthma: the SARP Cohort. Am J Respir Crit Care Med 2018. https://doi.org/10.1164/rccm.201712-2426OC.

95. Pavord ID, Beasley R, Agusti A, et al. After asthma: redefining airways diseases. Lancet 2018;391: 350–400.

96. Mukherjee M, Stoddart A, Gupta RP, et al. The epidemiology, healthcare and societal burden and costs of asthma in the UK and its member nations: analyses of standalone and linked national databases. BMC Med 2016;14:113.

97. Campbell S, Reeves D, Kontopantelis E, et al. Quality of primary care in England with the introduction of pay for performance. N Engl J Med 2007;357:181–90.

98. Pinnock H. Supported self-management for asthma. Breathe (Sheff) 2015;11:98–109.

99. Pinnock H, Parke HL, Panagioti M, et al. Systematic meta-review of supported self-management for

asthma: a healthcare perspective. BMC Med 2017; 15:64.

100. Cumella A. Annual asthma care survey. Asthma UK. 2018. Available at: https://www.asthma.org.uk/get-involved/campaigns/publications/survey/. Accessed June 15, 2018.

101. Royal College of Physicians. Why asthma still kills: the National Review of Asthma Deaths (NRAD) Confidential Enquiry report. London: RCP; 2014. Available at: file:///C:/Users/sth/Downloads/Why%20asthma%20still%20kills%20brief%20summary%20for%20patients%20and%20the%20public%20(1).pdf/.

102. Xiao Q, Wang J, Chiang V, et al. Effectiveness of mHealth Interventions for asthma self-management: a systematic review and meta-analysis. Stud Health Technol Inform 2018;250:144–5.

103. Garcia-Marcos L, Edwards JL, Kennington EJ, et al. What asthma self-management tools and systems should have higher priority in future research: a delphi exercise from the EU. In: A102 Highlights in patient-centred research: methods and outcomes. American Thoracic Society. 2016. p. A2669. (American Thoracic Society International Conference Abstracts). Available at: https://doi.org/10.1164/ajrccm-conference.2016.193.1_Meeting Abstracts.A2669/. Accessed June 15, 2018.

104. West B, and Cumella A. Data sharing and technology: exploring the attitudes of people with asthma. Asthma UK. 2018. Available at: https://www.asthma.org.uk/datareport/. Accessed June 14, 2018.

105. Lewis C, Bradley E, Chesterton J, et al. Identifying asthma sub-populations to improve self-management. Eur Respir J 2016;48(suppl 60): PA2889.

106. Morton RW, Elphick HE, Rigby AS, et al. STAAR: a randomised controlled trial of electronic adherence monitoring with reminder alarms and feedback to improve clinical outcomes for children with asthma. Thorax 2017;72:347–54.

107. Killane I, Sulaiman I, MacHale E, et al. Predicting asthma exacerbations employing remotely monitored adherence. Healthc Technol Lett 2016;3:51–5.

108. Clift J. Connected asthma report. Asthma UK. 2016. Available at: https://www.asthma.org.uk/connectedasthma/. Accessed June 15, 2018.

109. Barrett MA, Humblet O, Marcus JE, et al. Effect of a mobile health, sensor-driven asthma management platform on asthma control. Ann Allergy Asthma Immunol 2017;119:415–21.

110. Blakey J, and Clift J. Smart asthma report. Asthma UK. 2017. Available at: https://www.asthma.org.uk/smartasthma/. Accessed June 15, 2018.

111. Jochmann A, Artusio L, Jamalzadeh A, et al. Electronic monitoring of adherence to inhaled corticosteroids: an essential tool in identifying severe asthma in children. Eur Respir J 2017;50 [pii: 1700910].

112. Cushing A, Manice MP, Ting A, et al. Feasibility of a novel mHealth management system to capture and improve medication adherence among adolescents with asthma. Patient Prefer Adherence 2016;10:2271–5.

113. Patel M, Pilcher J, Travers J, et al. Use of metered-dose inhaler electronic monitoring in a real-world asthma randomized controlled trial. J Allergy Clin Immunol Pract 2013;1:83–91.

114. Bousquet J, Chavannes NH, Guldemond N, et al. Realising the potential of mHealth to improve asthma and allergy care: how to shape the future. Eur Respir J 2017;49 [pii:1700447].

115. Rudin RS, Fanta CH, Predmore Z, et al. Core components for a clinically integrated mHealth app for asthma symptom monitoring. Appl Clin Inform 2017;08:1031–43.

116. Finkelstein J, Jeong IC. Machine learning approaches to personalize early prediction of asthma exacerbations. Ann N Y Acad Sci 2017;1387:153–65.

117. Liu W-T, Huang C-D, Wang C-H, et al. A mobile telephone-based interactive self-care system improves asthma control. Eur Respir J 2011;37:310–7.

118. Farzandipour M, Nabovati E, Sharif R, et al. Patient self-management of asthma using mobile health applications: a systematic review of the functionalities and effects. Appl Clin Inform 2017;8:1068–81.

119. Poinasamy K, Ellis D, and Walker S. Diagnosing asthma: a 21st century challenge. Asthma UK. 2018. Available at: https://www.asthma.org.uk/diagnostics-report/Accessed June 15, 2018.

120. Baxter N. Service development: tools to help you stratify people with asthma who should be offered a priority review. 2016. Available at: https://www.pcrs-uk.org/sites/pcrs-uk.org/files/ServiceDevel AsthmaPyramidEMIS_FINAL.pdf/. Accessed June 15, 2018.

121. Matui P, Wyatt JC, Pinnock H, et al. Computer decision support systems for asthma: a systematic review. NPJ Prim Care Respir Med 2014;24:14005.

122. Bonini M. Electronic health (e-Health): emerging role in asthma. Curr Opin Pulm Med 2017;23:21–6.

123. Blake KV. Improving adherence to asthma medications: current knowledge and future perspectives. Curr Opin Pulm Med 2017;23:62–70.

124. Simpson AJ, Honkoop PJ, Kennington E, et al. Perspectives of patients and healthcare professionals on mHealth for asthma self-management. Eur Respir J 2017;49 [pii:1601966].

125. Van Gaalen JL, van Bodegom-Vos L, Bakker MJ, et al. Internet-based self-management support for adults with asthma: a qualitative study among patients, general practitioners and practice nurses on barriers to implementation. BMJ Open 2016;6: e010809.

126. McNamee P, Murray E, Kelly MP, et al. Designing and undertaking a health economics study of digital health interventions. Am J Prev Med 2016;51:852–60.

127. Barrett M, Combs V, Su JG, et al. AIR Louisville: addressing asthma with technology, crowdsourcing, cross-sector collaboration, and policy. Health Aff (Millwood) 2018;37:525–34.

128. Huckvale K, Car M, Morrison C, ot al. Apps for asthma self-management: a systematic assessment of content and tools. BMC Med 2012;10:144.

129. Tinschert P, Jakob R, Barata F, et al. The potential of mobile apps for improving asthma self-management: a review of publicly available and well-adopted asthma apps. Eysenbach G, editor. JMIR MHealth UHealth 2017;5:e113.

130. Hui CY, Walton R, McKinstry B, et al. The use of mobile applications to support self-management for people with asthma: a systematic review of controlled studies to identify features associated with clinical effectiveness and adherence. J Am Med Inform Assoc 2017;24:619–32.

131. Huckvale K, Morrison C, Ouyang J, et al. The evolution of mobile apps for asthma: an updated systematic assessment of content and tools. BMC Med 2015;13:58.

Printed and bound by CPI Group (UK) Ltd, Croydon, CR0 4YY

08/05/2025

01864741-0005